Nurse Practitioner Acute Care Protocols

For Emergency Departments, Urgent Care Centers, and Family Practices

FIFTH EDITION

Nurse Practitioner Acute Care Protocols

For Emergency Departments, Urgent Care Centers, and Family Practices

FIFTH EDITION

Donald C. Correll, M.D., FACEP

Acute Care Horizons

Jackson, TN

Nurse Practitioner Acute Care Protocols - FIFTH EDITION: For Emergency Departments, Urgent Care Centers, and Family Practices

Acute Care Horizons, LLC
Jackson, Tennessee
acutecarehorizons.com

Printed in the United States of America.
Library of Congress Control Number: 2012933980
ISBN: 978-1-7331575-0-6 (Paperback)

Publisher's Cataloging-in-Publication Data
Correll, Donald Charles.
Nurse practitioner acute care protocols - fifth edition : for emergency departments, urgent care centers, and family practices / Donald C. Correll.
p. cm.
Includes index.
ISBN 978-1-7331575-0-6 (Paperback)
1. Nurse Practitioners—Handbooks, manuals, etc. 2. Medical emergencies—Handbooks, manuals, etc. 3. Emergencies—handbooks. 4. Emergency Medicine—methods—handbooks. 5. Medical protocols. I. Title.

RC86.8 .C67 2010
616.02/5—dc22 2012933980

Version
COV - 2019-06-15 (1)
TXT - 2019-06-15 (4)

DEDICATION

To the reviewers of this work.

To my brother John for his creativity and work to make this book possible.

To my mother Glenna who worked two jobs to put me through college.

To my father-in-law Joe Keller for his wisdom over the past 35 years.

To my wife Christina for her steadfast love and devotion.

To my children Joanna, Donny and Diana for bringing more meaning into my life.

CONTENTS

REVIEWERS

(Since beginning)

Stephanie Young, NP-C
Emergency Department
Jackson-Madison County General Hospital
Jackson, TN

Twonia Goyer, MSN, FNP, BC
Emergency Department
Jackson-Madison County General Hospital
Jackson, TN

Katie Cepparulo, NP-C
Emergency Department
Jackson-Madison County General Hospital
Jackson, TN

LeAnne Wilhite, ACNP-BC
Assistant Professor of Nursing
Chair of Undergraduate Nursing
Union University; Jackson, Tennessee

Robert E. Turner III, M.D., FACEP
Emergency Physician
Jackson-Madison County General Hospital
Volunteer Clinical Instructor, University of Tennessee Family Medicine; Jackson, Tennessee

Sharai C Amaya, M.D.
Obstetrics and Gynecology
Women's Advanced Care of Self Regional Healthcare
Greenwood, SC

Neil Wangstrom, M.D.
Otolaryngology
La Porte, Indiana

Austin Bancroft, D.O.
Otolaryngology
La Porte, Indiana

Karl E. Misulis, M.D., PhD
West Tennessee Neurosciences
Jackson-Madison County General Hospital
Jackson, Tennessee
Associate Clinical Professor of Neurology, Vanderbilt University School of Medicine; Nashville, Tennessee

Frederick (Rick) E. Barr, M.D., MSCI
Professor of Pediatrics and Anesthesiology

Timothy F. Linder, M.D., FAAFP
Family Physician Selmer, Tennessee
Volunteer Clinical Instructor, University of Tennessee Family Medicine; Jackson, Tennessee
Past President – Tennessee Academy of Family Physicians

David Roberts, M.D., FAAFP
Medical Director Jackson-Madison County General Hospital
Family and Geriatric Medicine
Past Director of University of Tennessee Family Medicine

E. Scott Yarbro, M.D.
Jackson Urological Associates PC
Volunteer Clinical Instructor, University of Tennessee Family Medicine; Jackson, Tennessee

Gregg Mitchell, M.D.
Program Director – University of Tennessee Family Medicine
Jackson, Tennessee

Thomas Ellis, M.D., FCCP
The Jackson Clinic
Pulmonary and Critical Care

Robert Gilroy, M.D., FCCP
The Jackson Clinic
Pulmonary and Critical Care

E. Lee Murray, M.D.
Clinical Assistant Professor of Neurology
University of Tennessee Health Science Center
Memphis, TN
Attending Neurologist
West Tennessee Neuroscience
Jackson, TN

John Baker, M.D., FACC
The Jackson Clinic
Cardiology
Jackson, Tennessee

Robert Daggett, M.D.
Rheumatology
Brentwood, Tennessee

Jacob A Aelion, M.D., FACR, CCD
Arthritis Clinic, Jackson, TN
Clinical Professor of Medicine
The University of Tennessee Health Science Center
Memphis, Tennessee

John Guidi, M.D.
Past District Health Officer, State of Tennessee Dept of Health
Medical Director of the CDC Clinics for the West TN Region

Lucius Wright, M.D.
The Jackson Clinic
Nephrology
Jackson, TN

Christin Gray, NP-C
Emergency Department
Jackson-Madison County General Hospital
Jackson, TN

Steven Williams, D.O., MBA
Staff Hospitalist
Jackson-Madison County General Hospital
Jackson, Tennessee

PURPOSE

This book of protocols has been created to assist Nurse Practitioners and the physicians they work with. It focuses on acute care medicine as practiced in emergency departments, urgent care centers, and family practices.

These protocols are intended to be concise and yet reasonably comprehensive, and to have parameters that determine physician interaction with the Nurse Practitioner, where applicable, while permitting flexibility in patient care by the Nurse Practitioner.

~ Read This! ~

NOTICE

The protocols presented in this book are *model guidelines.* Accordingly, they should be used — and, when necessary, modified — per any agreement that may exist between the supervising physician and Nurse Practitioner. In states, regions, or institutions where a supervisory model is in place, this agreement should be established *prior to use* of these protocols.

In writing these protocols the author has checked with sources believed to be reliable. However, medicine is an ever-changing science and art. As new research and clinical experience expand the knowledge base, changes in treatment and protocols are required.

Further, there is a possibility of human error or of changes in medical science. Neither the author nor any party involved in the preparation or publication of this work warrants that the information contained herein is in every respect accurate or complete, and they disclaim all responsibility for any errors or omissions, or for results obtained from use of the information contained in these protocols or this publication.

Users are recommended and encouraged to confirm the information contained herein with other sources and by their own experience and knowledge. This recommendation is of particular importance with new or infrequently used drugs and therapies.

GUIDELINES OF PROPER USE

It is recommended that the protocols and other information provided in this book are to be used in accordance with the following understandings, concepts, and guidelines:

1. The protocols presented herein are *model guidelines.* Accordingly, they only should be used per written agreement between any supervising physician and Nurse Practitioner where applicable. Any agreement should be established *prior to use* of any of the protocols by the Nurse Practitioner.

2. When deemed appropriate, any protocol should be modified to reflect any authorized policies, procedures, or practices at a particular medical facility.

3. Not all patient presentations can be covered in these protocols. Those presentations not covered in protocols should be evaluated and managed according to the Nurse Practitioner's training and experience, and according to the usual scope of practice of any supervising physician where applicable.

4. The Nurse Practitioner should perform only those tasks that are within the Nurse Practitioner's skills and competence, and that are within the usual scope of practice of any supervising physician, if applicable, and that are consistent with the protection and safety of the health and well-being of the patient.

5. Any perceived potential conflict between patient safety and the Protocols book should be resolved by consultation with a physician, if applicable, and in favor of patient safely.

6. Specific protocols override the General Patient Criteria Protocol if there is a disparity between the specific protocol and the General Patient Criteria Protocol.

7. Sanford Guide to Antimicrobial Therapy can be used for infections in lieu of protocol-specified antimicrobial treatments.

8. "Consult criteria" means to initially discuss the patient with a physician.

9. Life-saving care should not be withheld because of protocol instructions.

10. The Nurse Practitioner should discuss with a physician any patient care and safety concerns regardless of protocols.

11. Deviations from protocols should be reviewed by a supervising physician where applicable, feasible and appropriate.

12. Inclusion criteria of each protocol should be modified to reflect the accepted Nurse Practitioner practice at a specific institution

13. **Read the Notice (page 17) before applying the protocols contained herein. If you do not accept the limitations and disclaimers contained in the Notice you should refrain from using this book and the information and protocols contained herein.**

PROTOCOL GUIDELINE AGREEMENT

(Where needed for State regulations or institutional policies only)

By signing this Protocol Guideline Agreement each party acknowledges that he or she has read both the Notice section and the Guidelines of Proper Use section.

Provider's signature	Date
Provider's signature	Date
Provider's signature	Date
Provider's signature	Date
Provider's signature	Date
Provider's signature	Date
Provider's signature	Date
Provider's signature	Date
Provider's signature	Date
Provider's signature	Date
Provider's signature	Date
Provider's signature	Date
Provider's signature	Date

General

Section Contents — one protocol

When using any protocol, always follow the Guidelines of Proper Use (page 18).

GENERAL PATIENT CRITERIA PROTOCOL

When using any protocol, always follow the Guidelines of Proper Use (page 18).

Notify physician promptly during or after Nurse Practitioner initial assessment

- Acute myocardial infarction (AMI) or symptoms consistent with AMI — notify physician when AMI identified
- Acute central nervous system deficits
- Severe CHF
- Severe respiratory distress
- O_2 Saturation < 90% on room air, if acute
- Hypotension
- Acute altered mental status unless intoxicated
- Adult heart rate ≥ 140
- Emergency hypertension
- Age ≤ 28 days

Consult physician when:

- Age ≤ 28 days
- Age > 28 days and < 3 months (unless experienced with this age group)
- Moderate CHF
- SBP ≥ 240 or DBP ≥ 140 at presentation (that is asymptomatic) with preexisting hypertension history
- Adult heart rate ≥ 110 at time of disposition
- Patients sent to the ED or clinic from an outlying hospital, clinic, or from home by a medical provider
- Age ≥ 70 with systemic symptoms
- Patient receives more than one pain injection
- Patient returns ≤ 14 days for same acute complaint (Does not apply to chronic recurrent complaints unless a change in the complaint.)
- Elevated BP or heart rate in pregnancy or ≤ 6 weeks postpartum

- Pregnancy complications
- Chest pain (potentially consistent with angina or anginal equivalent symptoms)
- Nonspecific chest pain age ≥ 30 with history of
  - Hypertension
  - Diabetes
  - Smoking
  - Coronary artery disease history
  - Hyperlipidemia
  - Family history of coronary artery disease by age of 60

    OR
  - Age ≥ 50 without risk factors
- Abdominal pain
  - Requiring narcotics
  - Age ≥ 70
  - Diabetic
  - Uncertain diagnosis

Lab consult criteria

- Adult WBC ≥ 15,000 or < 1,000 neutrophils
- Pediatric WBC ≥ 15,000 or < 1,000 neutrophils
- Bandemia ≥ 15%
- Acute thrombocytopenia
- Hemoglobin 8–10 gms (unless chronic and stable)
- Hemoglobin < 8 gms even if chronic
- O_2 Sat ≤ 94% on room air if acute (or moderate dyspnea)
- O_2 Sat 2% less than chronic levels

Vital sign and age consult criteria

Fever

- Adult ≥ 104°F or 40°C
- Pediatric ≥ 104.5°F or 40.3°C

Hypothermia

- Temperature ≤ 95°F or 35°C

Heart rate/minute

- Adult heart rate ≥ 115
- Pediatric heart rate:
  - 0–4 months ≥ 180

- 5–7 months ≥ 175
- 8–12 months ≥ 170
- 1–3 years ≥ 160
- 4–5 years ≥ 145
- 6–8 years ≥ 130
- 9–11 years ≥ 125
- 12–15 years ≥ 120
- 16 years or older ≥ 115

Inappropriate sinus tachycardia (no clinical explanation)

Hypertension

- Adult asymptomatic hypertension of SBP > 220 or DBP > 120 at time of disposition with history of hypertension
- Adult asymptomatic SBP > 195 or DBP > 115 at discharge without history of hypertension
- Pediatric hypertension — age < 14 years

NOTE: Specific protocols override this General Patient Criteria Protocol

Shared decision making (SDM)

- Information transfer is two-way, with clinician providing medical information needed for decision-making, the patient providing information about preferences, and clinician and patient deciding together on the best evaluation and treatment to implement

Criteria that must be met for an interaction between a clinician and a patient to be classified as SDM:

- It must involve at least two participants, the clinician and the patient (or the patient's designated representative)
- Both parties must share information
- Both parties must take steps to build consensus on the preferred treatment
- Agreement on which treatment to implement must be reached
- Highly desirable model in certain circumstances
- Not appropriate for all clinical situations

Notes

References:

Hess EP, Grudzen CR, Thomson R, Raja AS, Carpenter CR. Shared decision-making in the emergency department: respecting patient autonomy when seconds count. Acad Emerg Med 2015 Jul;22(7):856-64

Cardiovascular

Section Contents

When using any protocol, always follow the Guidelines of Proper Use (page 18).

CHEST PAIN PROTOCOL

When using any protocol, always follow the Guidelines of Proper Use (page 18).

Definition

- Patient perception of discomfort in anterior chest or upper half of back

Differential Diagnosis

Pneumonia

- Cough
- Fever
- Chills
- Dyspnea
- Sweats
- Tachycardia

Pulmonary embolism

- Dyspnea
- Tachycardia
- Biphasic ST–T wave changes in V1–3 mimicking acute coronary syndrome
- Hypoxia
- Pleuritic chest pain
- Well's criteria moderate-to-high probability
- Troponin may be elevated in moderate to massive pulmonary embolism

Chest wall pain

- Chest tenderness
- Pleuritic chest pain
- Pain with movement

Angina/AMI

- Anterior chest pressure or tightness
- **EKG changes**
    - Acute ST elevation in 2 or more contiguous leads or acute ST elevation in AVR even if isolated— ≥ 2mm in men and ≥ 1.5 mm in women
        - **AVR acute ST elevation** may indicate left main disease, proximal LAD or left

main equivalent blockage—**treat as a STEMI**

- ST depression in V1–4 may indicate a posterior MI
- Hyperacute T waves with reciprocal changes
- **Sgarbossa AMI criteria for LBBB and pacemaker (repolarization of ST segment normally is opposite direction of QRS complex)**
    - Concordant repolarization, same direction as QRS, ≥ 1 mm
    - ST disconcordant elevation or depression (opposite direction as QRS) ≥ 25%height of QRS
    - ST disconcordant changes ≥ 5 mm
- New T wave inversion or ST depression may indicate NSTEMI

- Left or right arm pain
- Jaw pain
- Right arm pain only with chest pain highly specific for cardiac ischemia
- Approximately 50% of patients with angina pectoris have normal findings on a resting EKG
- Dyspnea (may be only presenting complaint in very elderly: age ≥ 80)
- Nausea and/or vomiting
- Diaphoresis
- Indigestion
- Angina may be exertional only
- Levine sign (characterized by the patient's fist clenched over the sternum when describing the discomfort) is suggestive of angina pectoris
- Angina decubitus is a variant of angina pectoris that occurs at night while the patient is recumbent
    - May be from an increase in myocardial oxygen demand caused by expansion of the blood volume from increased venous return during recumbency

Considerations

- All NSAIDs increase the risk of MI and death from CV disease, even with short-term use (7–10 days)
    - Celecoxib (Celebrex) causes the least amount of CV side effects, and is the

preferred NSAID for patients taking prophylactic low-dose aspirin

- Medium-size coronary plaques (30%–40% stenosis) may be vulnerable to cause occlusion because they are less mature, with a large lipid core and a thin cap prone to rupture or erode, exposing the thrombogenic subendothelial components
- Cocaine metabolites which persist in circulation up to 24 hours can cause delayed or recurrent coronary vasospasm

Pleurisy

- Pain occurs or worsens with breathing
- No other comorbid symptoms or signs

Pericarditis

- Pleuritic pain
- Fever
- Worse lying down
- Better sitting and leaning forward
- Diffuse ST segment elevation
- Diffuse PR segment depression
- Pericardial effusion
- Elevated C-reactive protein
- Echocardiogram for pericardial effusion

Pericarditis treatment

- Pericarditis: NSAID's and/or colchicine (if uncomplicated)
    - Colchicine 1–1.2 mg qday for 3 months
    - Dexamethasone 6 mg qday for 2–4 weeks then slow taper if failure of NSAID's and/or colchicine

Myopericarditis

- Elevated troponin
- Similar symptoms and findings as Pericarditis

Herpes zoster

- Vesicular dermatomal rash
- May have pain 4 days prior to rash

Aortic dissection

- Tearing pain
- Located or radiates to back

- Signs and symptoms above and below diaphragm frequently
- Ascending aorta most common location of thoracic dissection
- The mediastinum is considered widened on an AP radiograph if its width is > 8 cm at the level of aortic knob
    - This is not an absolute number and in general the more the width, the higher the probability of underlying aortic dissection

Chest Pain with Respiratory (Pleuritic) or Movement Exacerbation

- May need no further testing if vital signs and O_2 Sat are normal and clinical suspicion is low for cardiac or serious pulmonary disease
- Consider chest x-ray and D-dimer
- Consider EKG and troponin if diagnosis is uncertain for a non-cardiac etiology
- Consider CTA chest to evaluate for pulmonary embolism
- Apply Well's criteria

Evaluation options

- Chest x-ray
- CBC if fever or tachycardic
- BMP if diabetic or tachycardic
- D-dimer (if negative with Well's criteria 0–1 makes PE unlikely)
- CT chest (see below)
- Apply Well's pulmonary embolism and DVT criteria and chart Well's score as indicated
- Record positive or negative calf tenderness and Homan's sign (Homan's sign useful for malpractice considerations to avoid litigation but has no clinical usefulness)

Evaluation with D-dimer

D-dimer (LIA method) — some methods currently in use not reliable

- Useful if negative at cutoff value to rule out DVT or PE
    - Rare exception is cancer (especially hematological cancer) patients with PE

may have negative d–dimer in small percentage (0.4%)

- Negative D–dimer with low to moderate probability Well's DVT or PE score largely excludes venous thromboembolic disease
- Well's DVT criteria high probability: order ultrasound scan regardless of D-dimer result
- If positive — not as useful as a negative result which usually rules out VTE (venous thromboembolic) disease
- Frequently positive with
    - Hospitalization in past month
    - Chronic bedridden or low activity state
    - Increasingly positive with age without significant acute disease process
        - D-dimer increases 10 mcg/L for every year over 50 years of age if the upper cutoff is 500 mcg/L (80 year old with d-dimer 700 mcg/L would be in the normal range)
        - If another assay used, then 2% increase/year over age 50 may be used to adjust upper limit for age
    - CHF
    - Chronic disease processes
    - Edematous states

Well's DVT criteria

- One point each:
    - Active cancer
    - Paralysis/recent cast immobilization
    - Recently bedridden > 3 days or surgery < 4 weeks
    - Deep vein tenderness
    - Entire leg edema
    - Calf swelling > 3 cm over other leg
    - Pitting edema > other calf
    - Collateral superficial veins
- Two points — alternative diagnosis less likely

High probability: ≥ 3 points

Moderate probability: 1–2 points

Low probability: 0 points

Well's PE criteria score 3 or greater consider D-dimer and CT chest PE protocol

- Suspected DVT = 3
- Alternative diagnosis less likely than PE = 3
- Heart rate > 100 = 1.5
- Immobilization/surgery past 4 wks. = 1.5
- Previous DVT/PE = 1.5
- Hemoptysis = 1
- Cancer past 6 months = 1

Well's score ≥ 6: order CTA chest PE protocol

Document positive or negative Homan's sign and calf tenderness regardless of Well's scores

Document PERC and/or Well's scores when appropriate

Pulmonary Embolism Rule-out Criteria (PERC Rule)
(Reportedly decreases significantly the likelihood of pulmonary embolism if all 8 criteria met — recent studies state not superior to clinical gestalt)

- Age < 50
- Pulse oximetry > 94%
- Heart rate < 100
- No history of DVT or VTE
- No hemoptysis
- No estrogen use
- No unilateral leg swelling
- No recent surgery or trauma hospitalization past 4 weeks

Treatment

- Treat pneumonia/bronchitis per current national recommendations and Sanford Guide or other drug databases
- Pericarditis: NSAID's and/or colchicine (if uncomplicated)
    - Colchicine 1–1.2 mg qday for 3 months
    - Dexamethasone 6 mg qday for 2–4 weeks then slow taper if failure of NSAID's and/or colchicine

- NSAID or hydrocodone, or other narcotics as needed
- Treat chest pain from abdominal causes or other causes as per training, experience, and protocols

Chest Pain that Could Represent Acute Coronary Syndrome (ACS) or Stable Angina

Evaluation

- EKG
- CBC
- BMP
- Chest x-ray
- Troponin

Acute Coronary Syndrome treatment (STEMI, NSTEMI and Unstable Angina) — consult physician promptly

- Aspirin 160–325 mg chew and swallow or Clopidogrel 300 mg PO once
- Nitrates prn (See nitrate contraindications and side-effects below)
- Oxygen — maintain O_2 Sat > 90%
- Morphine 2–5 mg IV q5–15 minutes prn (caution if SBP < 105 mm Hg)

Short-acting nitrates

- NTG 0.3–0.6 SL prn — may repeat × 2 q5minutes prn continued ischemic cardiac pain (caution if SBP < 105–110 mm Hg)
- May use before anginal provoking activities
  - Comes in tablets or spray
  - Tablets need refrigeration and last 3–6 months, and should tingle tongue when used
  - NTG spray lasts 2–3 years

NTG paste if needed

- 0.5–1 inch — caution if SBP < 105 mm Hg

NTG drip if needed

- Start at 10–20 mcg/minute IV and titrate for chest pain and limit SBP decrease to 10% if normotensive and 30% if hypertensive

        - NTG 0.4 mg SL is 400 mcg which reaches peak blood levels in 2 minutes and falls to 50% of peak at 7.5 minutes by comparison, and is gone by 20 minutes, so more vigorous IV dosing can be considered for angina or hypertensive CHF when indicated
- Keep SBP ≥ 90 mm Hg
- See nitrate contraindications and side-effects below

Heparin if needed

- Bolus 60 units/kg IV — NMT 4,000 units
- 12 mg/kg/hour IV drip — initially NMT 1,000 units/hour to be adjusted to PTT 50–75 seconds

OR

Enoxaparin if needed

- 1 mg/kg SQ q12hr
- May give first dose as 30 mg IV along with the SQ dose for STEMI
    - Age > 75 years give 0.75 mg/kg SQ and no IV dose for STEMI
- Dose 30 mg SQ qday for creatinine clearance < 30 ml/minute

Stable angina treatment

Short-acting nitrates

- NTG 0.3–0.6 SL prn — may repeat x 2 q5minutes prn continued ischemic cardiac pain (caution if SBP < 105–110 mm Hg)
- May use before anginal provoking activities
    - Comes in tablets or spray
    - Tablets need refrigeration and last 3–6 months, and should tingle tongue when used
    - NTG spray lasts 2–3 years

Long-acting nitrates for stable angina

- Timing — taken at time of day that anginal symptoms or anginal equivalent symptoms (i.e., dyspnea) are most prevalent
- NTG 2.5 mg or 6.5 mg PO bid
- Isosorbide mononitrate

    - Standard dose — 20 mg PO bid given 7 hours apart
    - Smaller patients start 5 mg PO bid given 7 hours apart and increase to 10–20 mg PO bid given 7 hours apart over 2–3 days
    - Take on empty stomach 30 minutes prior to a meal or 1 hour after a meal
- Isosorbide mononitrate ER (extended release)
    - 30–120 mg PO qday
- Transdermal nitroglycerin (Nitro-Dur)
    - 0.2–0.4 mg/hr. qday — remove for 10–12 hours each day
    - Max dose 0.4–0.8 mg/hr. qday
    - Starts acting in 30 minutes and lasts 8–14 hours

Nitrate side–effects (some)

- Headache
- Hypotension
- Tachycardia
- Nausea

Nitrate contraindications

- Shock or hypotension
- SBP < 90 m Hg or ≥ 30 mm Hg below baseline SBP in ACS
- Bradycardia < 50 beats per minute
- Tachycardia in absence of heart failure (> 100 beats per minute)
- Acute right ventricular myocardial infarction
    - Caution in inferior myocardial infarction
- Use of erectile dysfunction medications (sildenafil, tadalafil, or vardenafil)
- Severe anemia

Beta-blockers for stable angina

- Reduce heart rate, blood pressure and cardiac contractility which decreases cardiac work and oxygen needs
- First choice usually with stable angina
- Prolongs survival and decreases second AMI incidence

Selective beta–1 blocker

- Metoprolol (Lopressor) initially 50 mg PO bid and may be increased to 200 mg PO bid
- Metoprolol (Toprol XL) 100 mg PO qday — NMT 400 mg PO qday
- Atenolol (Tenormin) 50 mg PO qday — NMT 200 mg PO qday

Beta–blocker side effects

- Bradycardia
- Hypotension
- Worsening of asthma and COPD
- Depression
- Heart failure
- Exacerbation of angina and hypertension on abrupt withdrawal (Black Box Warning)
- Worsening of peripheral arterial disease symptoms

Contraindications

- Pre-existing sinus bradycardia (< 60 beats/minutes)
- Moderate to severe left ventricle failure and pulmonary edema
- SBP < 100 mm Hg
- Signs of poor peripheral perfusion
- 2nd and 3rd degree heart block
- Asthma and COPD
- Sick sinus syndrome without pacemaker
- Untreated pheochromocytoma

ACEI or ARB added to a beta-blocker if needed in stable angina

Consult criteria

- Notify physician promptly for ACS (STEMI, NSTEMI and Unstable angina
- Consult physician for suspected stable angina

Heart score (point system)

History

- Highly suspicious 2
- Moderately suspicious 1
- Slightly suspicious 0

EKG

• Significant ST deviation	2
• Nonspecific ST repolarization disturbance	1
• Normal	0

Age

• ≥ 65 years	2
• 45–65 years	1
• ≤ 45 years	0

Risk factors

• ≥ risk factors or hx of atherosclerotic disease	2
• 1 or 2 risk factors	1
• No risk factors known	0

Troponin

• ≥ 3 times normal limit	2
• 1–3 times normal limit	1
• ≤ normal limit	0

Risk factors for atherosclerotic disease

- Hypercholesterolemia
- Hypertension
- Diabetes mellitus
- Cigarette smoking
- Positive family history for CAD
- Obesity

Interpretation

- 0–3 points indicates low risk of MACE (0.9–1.7%)
  - Usually discharged
- 4–7 points indicates moderate risk of MACE (12–16.6%)
  - Usually admitted
- 8–10 points indicates high risk of MACE (50–65%)
  - Admit

MACE defined as Major Adverse Cardiac Event within 6 weeks

- Acute MI
- Requires PCI
- Requires CABG
- Death

Author recommendations

- Do not discharge chest pain patients with elevated troponin until discussed with physician
- If troponin is normal in low risk patient then incidence of MACE at 6 weeks is 1%

- Follow-up for cardiac stress testing in 3 days
- 2 negative troponins 3 hours apart and 2 negative EKG's helpful for disposition and discharge purposes considering parameters of lower risk and chest pain timing
    - ACS pain lasting 20 minutes or so frequently may have negative troponins and nonacute EKG's that cannot be relied on fully for disposition purposes

2015 American College of Cardiology/American Heart Association (ACC/AHA) guideline recommendations on the workup of non-ST-elevation ACSs to assist in maximizing patient outcomes

- Patients with chest pain or other symptoms suggesting acute coronary syndromes (ACS) should have 12-lead electrocardiography (ECG) performed and evaluated within 10 min of arrival at an emergency facility, and serial ECGs should be performed to detect ischemic changes.
- Serial cardiac troponin I or T levels (using a contemporary assay) should be obtained at presentation and at 3-6 hours after symptom onset. Risk scores can help assess prognosis.
- In patients with symptoms consistent with ACS without objective evidence of myocardial ischemia (nonischemic ECG and normal cardiac troponin levels), noninvasive imaging is reasonable before emergency department discharge or within 72 hours after discharge.

General Discharge Criteria for Chest Pain

- Benign noncardiac chest pain
- Chest wall pain
- Pleurisy or pleurodynia
- Adult heart rate < 100
- Herpes zoster
- O_2 Saturation $\geq 95\%$

- Normal cardiac marker lab tests
- Stable and nonacute CBC, BMP and chest x-ray

Discharge instructions

- Chest pain aftercare instructions
- Follow up with primary care provider or cardiologist within 1–3 days as indicated

Consult Criteria

- Suspected angina or acute coronary syndrome
- Suspected anginal equivalent — arm, neck, jaw or epigastric pain, or dyspnea
- Acute chest x-ray abnormalities
- Pulmonary embolism or aortic dissection/aneurysm
- Pericarditis
- Severe pain in Provider's clinical judgment
- Chest pain of uncertain etiology in medium to high risk patient
- Follow General Patient Criteria Protocol (page 22) for care/evaluation not covered in this protocol

Suggested age consult criteria

- Nonspecific chest pain age ≥ 30 with history of
  - Hypertension
  - Diabetes
  - Smoking
  - Coronary artery disease history
  - Hyperlipidemia
  - Family history of coronary artery disease by age of 60

    OR
  - Age ≥ 50 without risk factors

Suggested vital signs and lab consult criteria

- WBC ≥ 15,000
- Elevated troponin
- Bandemia ≥ 15%
- Increased anion gap
- Metabolic acidosis
- Significant electrolyte abnormally (see electrolyte disorders)
- Glucose ≥ 400 mg/dL in diabetic patient
- Glucose ≥ 300 mg/dL in non-diabetic patient
- Hyperglycemia with metabolic acidosis (decreased serum CO_2 or elevated anion gap)

- Chest pain with O_2 Saturation on room air < 95% in non-COPD or non-bronchospasm presentation (see Dyspnea Protocol)
- Adult heart rate ≥ 100
- Developing hypotension or relative hypotension (SBP < 105 with history of hypertension)

Notes

References:

Circulation 2010;122:S787–S817

CHEST October 2011;140(4_MeetingAbstracts):594A-594A. doi:10.1378/chest.1112163

CHEST August 2011;140(2):509–518. doi:10.1378/chest.10–2468

Angina Pectoris Author: Jamshid Alaeddini, MD, FACC, FHRS; Chief Editor: Eric H Yang, MD emedicine.medscape.com/article/150215

Amsterdam EA, Wenger NK. The 2014 American College of Cardiology ACC/American Heart Association guideline for the management of patients with non-ST-elevation acute coronary syndromes: ten contemporary recommendations to aid clinicians in optimizing patient outcomes. *Clin Cardiol*. 2015 Feb. 38(2):121-3

Acute Coronary Syndrome; Author: David L Coven, MD, PhD; Chief Editor: Eric H Yang, MD emedicine.medscape.com/article/1910735

Circulation. 1979 Mar;59(3):585-8; Blood levels after sublingual nitroglycerin. Armstrong PW, Armstrong JA, Marks GS

Age-Adjusted D-Dimer Cutoff Levels to Rule Out Pulmonary Embolism: The ADJUST-PE Study *JAMA.* 2014;311(11):1117-1124. doi:10.1001/jama.2014.2135

JEM, epub, 7/29/16

CCJM;81:233

Emerg Radiology, 2016;23:405

Circulation, Vol. 117, pg. 1897

Harhash AA, et al. *Am J Med*. 2019 Jan 8. [Epub ahead of print]

PT O'Gara, et al. *Circulation*. 2013;127: e362-e425

DJ Engelen, et al. *J Am Coll Cardiol*. 1999;34: 389-395

Tamura A. *World J Cardiol*. 2014;6: 630

Celecoxib Associated With Lower MACE Risk Than Naproxen and Ibuprofen; Brandon May; thecardiologyadvisor.com May 21, 2018

CARDIAC DYSRHYTHMIA PROTOCOL

When using any protocol, always follow the Guidelines of Proper Use (page 18).

Definition

- Disorders of cardiac rhythm

Differential Diagnosis

- Sinus tachycardia
- Atrial tachycardia
- Multifocal atrial tachycardia
- Atrial fibrillation
- Atrial flutter
- Sinus bradycardia
- Junctional bradycardia
- Atrioventricular blocks
- Premature atrial contractions
- Premature ventricular contractions

Considerations

- Unifocal premature ventricular contractions (PVCs) without associated symptoms of acute ischemic disease are usually benign and typically do not warrant treatment
- Premature atrial contractions (PACs) are usually benign
- Sinus bradycardia, without hypotension or presycope/syncope, usually does not warrant acute treatment
- Prolonged QTc interval on the EKG can lead to a serious or life threatening arrhythmia
- PVCs with R wave on the T wave of preceding beat on the EKG or monitor can lead to ventricular tachycardia or death

General evaluation options

- Cardiac history
- Complete physical exam
- Associated symptoms

- Medication history
- EKG; consider monitor if heart rate ≥ 130 (adults) or ≤ 50
- CBC (depending on clinical situation)
- BMP (depending on clinical situation)
- Chest x-ray (depending on clinical situation)
- Troponin for anginal complaints or dyspnea
- BNP for dyspnea if needed (chest x-ray usually suffices)
- Consider D-dimer if PE suspected

Atrial Dysrhythmias

Sinus tachycardia

Definition

- Tachycardia in adults arising from the sinus node with a rate in adults > 100 beats/minute. Sinus tachycardia rates in pediatrics dependent on age

Considerations

- Significant sinus tachycardia (ST) that is unexplained can represent a high risk disease process
- Sinus tachycardia context is important: ST of 120 with influenza may be less concerning than ST at 105 with GI bleeding

Causes

Physiologic

- Pain or exertion

Pharmacologic

- Sympathetic agents; caffeine; bronchodilators

Pathologic

- Fever
- Dehydration
- Anemia
- Hemorrhage
- Pulmonary embolism
- Hypoxemia
- Infarction

- Ischemia
- Hyperthyroidism

Evaluation and treatment are aimed at underlying condition

Discharge instructions

- Sinus tachycardia aftercare instructions
- Follow up within 1–2 days if tachycardia persists
- Return if no improvement or worsening

Consult criteria

- Consult physician for unexplained adult ST ≥ 110 unless otherwise specified in other protocols

Premature atrial contractions

- Commonly benign; can be anxiety provoking
- Fatigue, stress or high adrenergic state can be the cause
- Evaluation is for associated disorders and not for PACs per se
- Usually no treatment needed
- If treatment desired, atenolol 50 mg PO qday or Lopressor 100 mg PO qday can be used (follow up recommended to evaluate response and side effects)

Discharge instructions

- Premature atrial contractions aftercare instructions

Atrial fibrillation

Definition

- Lack of organized atrial electrical activity and contractions – an irregularly irregular rhythm on EKG and cardiac auscultation or pulse palpation

Differential diagnosis

- Multifocal atrial tachycardia
- Wolf-Parkinson-White Syndrome (WPW)
- Atrial flutter
- Atrial tachycardia
- Supraventricular tachycardia

Considerations

- Most common cause of dysrhythmia
- Up to 9% of patients ≥ 80 years of age are affected
- CVA risk increased (do not acutely convert if present > 48 hours without therapeutic anticoagulation)
- BNP usually elevated even without overt CHF
- Recent onset of atrial fibrillation converts spontaneously to normal sinus rhythm in 2–3 days in 2/3 of patients
- Increases mortality 1.5–2 times more than general population without atrial fibrillation
- Risk of stroke 1.5% in age 50–59 years and nearly 30% in age 80–89 years
- Commonly heart rates are 110–140 per minute
- No treatment may be needed if heart rate ≤ 110 per minute and patient is on appropriate stroke prophylaxis
- Standing the patient up may reveal degree of tachycardia
- Loss up to 20% of stroke volume

Causes

- Hypertension
- CHF
- Coronary artery disease
- Carditis
- Sick sinus syndrome
- Alcohol
- Pulmonary embolism
- Hyperthyroidism
- Sympathetic drugs
- Pneumonia
- Hyperthermia
- Hypothermia
- Postoperative
- Hypokalemia, hypomagnesemia and hypocalcemia

Management options

- Medication management to maintain normal sinus rhythm
- Medication management to achieve rate control of atrial fibrillation
- Catheter ablation

- Anticoagulation to prevent thromboembolic disease

Signs and symptoms

- Altered mental status
- Weakness
- Hypotension
- Syncope
- Angina
- CHF
- Emboli
- Digit ischemia
- Neurologic deficits
- Mesenteric ischemia

Evaluation options

- EKG
- CBC
- BMP
- Chest x-ray
- Troponin for anginal complaints or dyspnea
- BNP for dyspnea or suspected CHF (chest x-ray alone may suffice)
- Thyroid function tests if hyperthyroidism suspected
- D-dimer if pulmonary embolism suspected
- Digoxin (digitalis) level if currently prescribed

Treatment options

- IV NS KVO
- Oxygen if dyspneic; O_2 saturation < 92% on room air
- Treatment of fever or hypovolemia if contributing to rapid ventricular response > 110

***Oral rate control medications may be considered if rate not too high or needed for chronic rate control as outpatient** (increased interactions with any of PO medications listed below when used in combination)*

Beta-blockers PO to choose from

- Metoprolol 25–200 mg PO bid
- Atenolol 25–100 mg PO qday (avoid in acute heart failure)

Calcium channel blocker PO

- Cardizem CD 180–360 mg PO qday

- Avoid in heart failure

Amiodarone 200–600 mg PO qday

IV treatment for rapid ventricular response

- **Cardizem** (diltiazem) 0.25 mg/kg IV over 2 minutes (usually 20 mg initial dose) for rate ≥ 120–125/min
  - May be repeated at 0.35 mg/kg IV over 2 minutes after 15 minutes of initial dose if needed (usually 25 mg)
  - Lower dose 0.2 mg/kg may be effective with less hypotension
    - Maintenance is 5–15 mg/hour IV
  - Exercise caution in patients with a pre-existing low ejection fraction **(heart failure)** or low preload - may cause hypotension
    - Probably should use different medication
  - Avoid with wide QRS
  - If high atrial fibrillation rate is from systemic condition, address that condition also (increased rate, if not very excessive, may be needed to compensate for underlying systemic condition)
- **Amiodarone** 150 mg IV over 10 minutes and then drip at 1 mg/minute for 6 hours, followed by 0.5 mg/minute next 18 hours — may repeat bolus if needed (Do not use in atrial fibrillation wide complex WPW QRS
- **Metoprolol** 5 mg IV, may repeat q5 minutes prn × 2 up to 3 doses total
  - May be best choice with atrial fibrillation with angina
  - Do not use if patient hypotensive or decompensated heart failure
  - Do not use in atrial fibrillation wide complex WPW QRS
- **Digoxin** 0.25 mg may be used as adjunct to other medications (slow rate on onset)
  - Repeat dose 0.25 mg IV q2hr. as needed (do not exceed 1.5mg over 24 hr.)
  - Do not use in atrial fibrillation WPW wide QRS complex
- Unstable patients–cardioversion with 120-200J with biphasic waveform device for hypotension

with rapid ventricular response (notify physician immediately for cardioversion if available)
  - May repeat up to 2 times if needed with increasing joules
- If cardioversion unsuccessful and patient still unstable, then amiodarone 300 mg IV over 10-20 minutes may be given
  - If still unstable, another shock may be given, then give amiodarone 900 mg IV over 24 hours
- **Wide complex atrial fibrillation** is potentially a life threatening rhythm — Notify physician immediately
  - Procainamide 10–18 mg/kg IV and infusion of 1–4 mg/minute may be considered
  - May need emergent cardioversion

Anticoagulation

- Aspirin 325 mg PO qday in low risk patients if direct thrombin or factor Xa inhibitors cannot be used or are not indicated
  - Age 60–74 years
  - Female
  - CHA_2DS_2VASc score 0–1
  - High risk of bleeding
- Coumadin (warfarin) 5–10 mg PO qday — (INR target of 2–3) with moderate or high risk factors
  - Age > 75 years
  - CAD
  - CHF
  - Hypertension
  - Diabetes mellitus
  - Mitral stenosis
  - Prior TIA/CVA
  - Mechanical valve
- Lovenox 1 mg/kg SQ q12hr

Stroke prevention in atrial fibrillation

- Should be screened for at age > 65 years
- Aspirin 325 mg PO daily may be used for low risk for stroke — CHA_2DS_2VASc score 0–1
- Treatment with warfarin in post–AMI patients with left ventricular thrombus or akinetic segment is reasonable

Anticoagulation recommendations in patients with nonvalvular atrial fibrillation per American Academy of Neurology

- Inform patients of the benefits of anticoagulation vs. the risks of major bleeding
- TIA/CVA patients with atrial fibrillation should be offered anticoagulation therapy
- Dabigatran, Rivaroxaban or Apixaban, which have a lower risk of intracranial bleeding than warfarin, may be offered to patients who have a higher risk of intracranial bleeding
- Dabigatran, Rivaroxaban or Apixaban may be used in patients unable to undergo frequent INR testing for warfarin therapy
- Dementia patient families or those that fall occasionally should be informed that the risk-benefit ratio is uncertain

CHA_2DS_2–VASc score

- Used to quantify risk of stroke in atrial fibrillation patients
- 2014 AHA/ACC/HRS Guideline for the Management of Patients With Atrial Fibrillation deemphasizes aspirin or use of platelet agents if warfarin (Coumadin), dabigatran (Pradaxa), rivaroxaban (Xarelto) or apixaban can be safely used and are indicated
- Stands for heart failure, hypertension, age ≥ 75 years , diabetes mellitus and prior stroke/TIA, vascular disease (MI, PAD or aortic plaque), age ≥ 65 and sex category (female)
- 1 point each for heart failure, hypertension, diabetes mellitus, age ≥ 65 and sex category (female)
- 2 points for prior stroke/TIA and age ≥ 75 years
    - Low risk = 0 points
    - Moderate risk = 1–2 points
    - High risk = 3–6 points

Long–term anticoagulation for nonvalvular atrial fibrillation recommended with score of ≥ 2, if no significant risk of hemorrhage

- Warfarin (Coumadin), dabigatran (Pradaxa), rivaroxaban (Xarelto) or apixaban
- With warfarin determine INR weekly initially, then monthly when stable
- Direct thrombin or factor Xa inhibitor recommended if unable to maintain therapeutic INR
- Evaluate renal function prior to direct thrombin inhibitors or factor Xa inhibitors and annually
- Adjust dosage per creatinine clearance for each specific drug (warfarin adjusted per INR) per PDR or other references

Warfarin prophylaxis

- CHA_2DS_2VASc score ≥ 2
- Age > 75 years
- Target INR 2.0–3.0
- May be lower (1.8–2) in high risk bleeding patients, or 2.5–3.5 in mechanical artificial valve, rheumatic heart, or recurrent stroke patients
- May be used age 65–75 years at discretion of clinician based on underlying disorders such as valvular disease etc.

Dabigatran (Pradaxa)

- CHA_2DS_2VASc score ≥ 2
- 150 mg PO bid for stroke prevention in nonvalvular atrial fibrillation is indicated in patients > 30 mL/min
- 75 mg PO bid CrCl 15–30 mL/min
- Not recommended if CrCl < 15 mL/min
- Less bleeding risk than warfarin
- Read Physician Desk Reference (PDR) drug or database information

Rivaroxaban (Xarelto)

- CHA_2DS_2VASc score ≥ 2
- 20 mg PO qday for stroke prevention in nonvalvular atrial fibrillation/min for CrCl > 50 mL/min

- 15 mg PO qHS if creatinine clearance (CrCl) 15–50 mL/minute
- Not recommended for CrCl ≤ 15
- Less bleeding risk than warfarin
- Consider PCC (Kcentra prothrombin complex concentrate or recombinant activated factor VII) if Andexxa not available for life threatening bleeding (not a specific antidote)
- Read Physician Desk Reference (PDR) drug or database information

Apixaban (Eliquis)

- CHA_2DS_2VASc score ≥ 2
- 5 mg PO bid for CrCl ≥ 30 mL/min
- 2.5 mg PO for age > 80 years, weight < 60 kg, creatinine ≥ 1.5 mg/dL
- Not recommended in severe liver disease
- Less bleeding risk than warfarin
- Read Physician Desk Reference (PDR) drug or database information

Dabigatran, rivaroxaban, apixaban or warfarin should not be used in the following patients. Aspirin safer

- Poor compliance
- Uncontrollable hypertension
- Aortic dissection
- Bacterial endocarditis
- Alcohol dependency
- Liver disease
- Bleeding lesions
- Malignant tumor
- Retinopathy with bleeding risk
- Advanced microvascular changes in the brain
- Known aneurysm of a cerebral artery
- Previous spontaneous cerebral hemorrhage
- Bleeding diathesis (e.g., coagulopathies, thrombocytopenia)
- Benefit/risk is uncertain in patients with frequent falls

Bleeding risk with warfarin (2 points for history of bleeding, 1 point for the rest) **HEMORR$_2$ HAGES 100 patient years of warfarin**

- Hepatic or renal disease
- Ethanol abuse
- Malignancy
- Old age (>75 y)

- History of bleeding
- Low platelet counts or platelet dysfunction
- Hypertension that is uncontrolled
- Anemia
- Genetic factors
- Elevated fall risk
- Stroke

HEMORR$_2$ HAGES score	Bleeding risk 100 pt./yr.
0	1.9
1	2.5
2	5.3
3	8.4
4	10.4
>5	12.3
Any score	4.9%

Monitor routinely for bleeding

Discharge criteria

- Stable chronic atrial fibrillation with rate ≤ 110 and pre-existing history of atrial fibrillation
    - Standing the patient may clarify degree of tachycardia
- Appropriate stroke prevention treatment in place or initiated
- No other concerning symptoms

Discharge instructions

- Atrial fibrillation aftercare instructions
- See treatment options above
- Adjust Digoxin (digitalis) if needed
- Follow up within 7 days

Consult criteria

- Adult heart rate ≥ 110
- Chest discomfort
- Dyspnea
- Hypotension
- Suspected hyperthyroidism
- Acute neurologic complaints or findings
- New onset atrial fibrillation
- Age > 55
- Digoxin (digitalis) toxicity

- PT/INR not therapeutic on warfarin and not experienced in adjusting dosage
- Anticoagulation therapy
- Antiarrhythmia therapy

Supraventricular tachycardia

Definition

- Tachycardia not involving the sinus node that is maintained by the atria or atrioventricular node

Differential diagnosis

- Atrial fibrillation
- Atrial flutter
- Multifocal atrial tachycardia (commonly in COPD patients)
- Ventricular tachycardia
- Sinus tachycardia

Considerations

- Usually narrow complexes on EKG with rapid and regular rhythm
- Paroxysmal most common
- Can have wide complexes with aberrant or retrograde conduction
- Heart rate usually 150–200/minute in adults
- Higher rates may be present in WPW
- Wide complex SVT can be ventricular tachycardia — notify physician immediately
- Treatment of wide complex SVT with calcium channel blockers, beta-blockers or Digoxin (digitalis) may result in deterioration of rhythm to ventricular fibrillation if antidromic (retrograde conduction) WPW is present — notify physician immediately prior to antiarrhythmia drug treatment

Presenting complaints

- Palpitations
- Dizziness
- Chest pain
- Shortness of breath
- Diaphoresis

Evaluation options

- EKG (may be all that is needed in young healthy patient without concerning complaints or comorbidities)
- CBC
- BMP
- Chest x-ray if respiratory complaints or findings present
- Troponin for anginal complaints
- BNP for dyspnea or suspected CHF (chest x-ray may suffice)
- Digoxin (digitalis) level if taking digoxin

Treatment options

- IV NS KVO or INT
- Oxygen if dyspneic or O_2 saturation < 92% on room air
- Vagal maneuvers in stable patient
- Breath holding
- Bearing down like in having a bowel movement
- Unilateral carotid massage for 10 seconds at a time in young healthy patients
- Face immersion in cold water

Medication treatment options (discuss with physician initially if available)

Narrow complex

- Adenosine 6 mg rapid IVP followed by 10–20 ml of saline — may repeat with 12 mg if needed
- Diltiazem 0.25 mg/kg over 2 minutes (usually 20 mg in adults — may be repeated with 0.35 mg/kg IV over 2 minutes (usually 25 mg in adults)
    - Caution if CHF present
- Metoprolol 5 mg slow IV, may repeat q5min up to total of 15 mg

Wide complex tachycardia (notify physician immediately)

- Amiodarone 150 mg IV over 10 minutes then 1mg/minute infusion x 6 hours, then 0.5 mg/minute infusion for 18 hours

Outpatient PO medications for PSVT prevention with narrow QRS only (select one)

- Metoprolol 25 mg PO bid or propranolol 10–30 mg tid
- Verapamil 240–480 mg/day divided tid–qid or diltiazem
- Digoxin 0.125–0.25 mg qd–q.o.d depending on age and renal function (for patients intolerant of beta–blockers or CCB)
- Recommend cardiology consult

Discharge criteria

- SVT conversion in stable patient without cardiac or other concerning comorbidities

Discharge instructions

- Supraventricular tachycardia aftercare instructions
- Follow up with PCP or cardiologist within 1–7 days

Recommended consult criteria

- Discuss all cases with physician if available before treatment and prior to discharge

Junctional rhythm

Definition

- Heart rhythm arising from AV node

Differential diagnosis

- Second and third degree AV block
- Digoxin (digitalis) toxicity
- Sinus node dysfunction
- AV nodal reentry tachycardia
- Idioventricular rhythm

Evaluation options

- EKG
- CBC
- BMP
- Chest x-ray
- Troponin for anginal complaints
- BNP for dyspnea or suspected CHF

Treatment options

- IV NS KVO or INT

- Oxygen if dyspneic or O_2 saturation < 95% room air
- Dependent on cause of the rhythm

Recommended consult criteria

- Discuss all cases with physician

Sinus bradycardia

Definition

- Sinus rhythm < 50 beats per minute

Causes

Physiologic

- Vagal tone

Pharmacologic

- Calcium channel blockers; beta-blockers; Digoxin (digitalis)

Pathologic

- AMI
- Hypothyroidism
- Sick sinus syndrome
- Carotid hypersensitivity
- High intracranial pressure
- Hypoglycemia

Evaluation

- EKG
- Per other complaints or findings

Treatment

- Usually no treatment needed if heart rate ≥ 40 in healthy patient with normal BP
- IV NS bolus if hypotensive and not in CHF
- Atropine 0.5–1 mg IV if SBP < 90 mmHg and heart rate < 50/minute

Discharge criteria

- Asymptomatic sinus bradycardia ≥ 50 beats/minute

Discharge instructions

- Sinus bradycardia aftercare instructions
- Follow up with PCP or cardiologist within 7 days if new onset

Consult criteria

- Heart rate < 50
- Hypotension
- Dyspnea
- Anginal complaints

Second and third degree AV block

Definition

- Second degree heart block has some of the atrial electrical impulses not conducted to the ventricles
- Third degree heart block has no atrial electrical impulses conducted to the ventricles

Considerations

- Can be caused by AMI or myocarditis
- Can be seen with Lyme disease
- Can occur with structural heart disease

Mobitz type 1 second degree heart block (Wenkebach)

- PR interval progressively lengthens before dropping a ventricular beat
- Can be seen in healthy athletes
- Usually asymptomatic
- May have chest pain if ischemia or myocarditis present
- Rarely have syncope
- May be drug induced — beta–blocker, calcium channel blockers, Digoxin (digitalis), amiodarone

Mobitz type 2 second degree heart block

- Intermittent dropped ventricular beats without progressive lengthening of the PR interval
- Syncope may occur
- AMI or myocarditis more common than mobitz type 1
- May be drug induced
- More serious type of heart block than mobitz type 1

Third degree heart block

- Most patients are asymptomatic

- May be hypotensive or have syncope
- Sudden death can occur
- May be caused by AMI
- Confusion can occur in elderly

Evaluation

- Cardiac monitor
- EKG
- CBC
- BMP
- Chest x-ray
- Troponin
- BNP for dyspnea or suspected CHF

Treatment

- IV NS KVO
- Oxygen if dyspneic; O_2 saturation < 92% on room air
- External pacing if hypotensive and heart rate < 60 (apply external pacing pads to mobitz type 2 and third degree heart block)
- Atropine 0.3–1 mg IV – discuss with physician

Consult criteria

- Notify physician promptly on all heart block patients

Ventricular Dysrhythmias

Premature ventricular contractions

Definition

- A premature ventricular contraction caused by an ectopic cardiac pacemaker in the ventricle usually > 120 msec on EKG

Consideration

- Usually benign and stable
- Usually unifocal and needs no acute treatment

Causes

- Frequently normal finding
- Digoxin (digitalis) toxicity
- Cardiac ischemia
- Cardiomyopathy
- Hypoxemia

- Mitral valve prolapse
- Myocarditis
- Cardiac contusion
- Stimulant medications or drugs (caffeine, cocaine, methamphetamines, tobacco)
- Hypokalemia
- Hypomagnesemia
- Hypercalcemia
- CHF
- Alkalosis

Evaluation

- EKG
- BMP if comorbid conditions present or on diuretics
- Other tests as dictated by symptoms or other findings

Treatment options

- Usually none
- Correction of potassium and magnesium levels if checked
- Treat underlying condition causing PVCs if present
- If antiarrhythmia treatment desired, atenolol 50 mg PO qday or metoprolol (Lopressor) 100 mg PO qday can be used (follow up with primary care provider)

Discharge criteria

- If it is a benign finding without concerning comorbid conditions

Discharge instructions

- PVC aftercare instructions
- Follow up with primary care provider or cardiologist as needed

Consult criteria

- EKG shows R on T phenomenon
- Comorbid conditions of concern: chest pain; dyspnea; syncope; etc.
- Potassium ≤ 2.5 mEq/L
- Digoxin (digitalis) toxicity
- Prolonged QTc interval
- New onset renal insufficiency

PVC couplets or multifocal PVCs

- Consult physician
- Usually needs no treatment
- Treating the cause may be indicated unless benign
- If antiarrhythmia treatment desired, atenolol 50 mg PO qday or metoprolol (Lopressor) 100 mg PO qday can be used (follow up with primary care provider)

Accelerated idioventricular rhythm (AIVR)

Definition

- Wide complex ventricular rhythm
- Rate 40–120 per minute

Considerations

- Associated with reperfusion in AMI

Treatment

- Observe
- Treating with antiarrhythmia drugs can cause asystole — do not treat patient with these drugs

Consult criteria

- Discuss all cases of AIVR with physician promptly

Ventricular tachycardia

Definition

- Tachycardia originating from the ventricles that is ≥ 120/minute and is wide complexed of ≥ 140 msec on EKG

Causes

- Cardiac ischemia
- Hypokalemia, hypomagnesemia, or hypocalcemia
- QT prolonging drugs
- Digoxin (digitalis) toxicity

Symptoms or findings

- May be asymptomatic, especially in nonsustained ventricular tachycardia (30 beat run or less)
- Chest pain
- CHF

- Hypotension
- Altered mental status

Evaluation

- Order EKG; CBC; BMP; chest x-ray; troponin
- Cardiac monitor

Treatment per physician if available

- IV NS KVO
- Oxygen to keep O_2 saturation > 94%
- Amiodarone 150 mg IV over 10 minutes followed by drip of 1 mg/min

  OR
- Lidocaine 1 mg/kg IV up to 100mg — may repeat × 2 up to 3 mg/kg followed by drip of 2–4 mg/min IV
- Have nurse deploy cardiac defibrillation pads on patient
- Activate cardiac code and start CPR and ACLS if no pulse present and patient unconscious

Warning

- Treating **"slow ventricular tachycardia"** (rate ≤120 beats/minute) with an antiarrhythmia drug, may actually be treating accelerated idioventricular rhythm (a life sustaining ventricular escape rhythm), resulting in asystole and death

Notes

References:

Guidelines for the Primary Prevention of Stroke

A Guideline for Healthcare Professionals from the American Heart Association/American Stroke Association

ACC/AHA/ESC Practice Guidelines

ACC/AHA/ESC 2006 Guideline for the Management of Patients with Atrial Fibrillation

2014 AHA/ACC/HRS Guideline for the Management of Patients with Atrial Fibrillation

Am J Emerg Med. 2011 Oct;29(8):849–54. doi: 10.1016/j.ajem.2010.03.021

Anticoagulation After Cardioembolic Stroke: To Bridge or Not to Bridge?
www.ncbi.nlm.nih.gov/pmc/articles/PMC2678170/

[Guideline] January CT, Wann LS, Alpert JS, Calkins H, Cigarroa JE, Cleveland JC Jr, et al. 2014 AHA/ACC/HRS guideline for the management of patients with atrial fibrillation: executive summary: a report of the American College of Cardiology/American Heart Association Task Force on practice guidelines and the Heart Rhythm Society. *Circulation*. 2014 Dec 2. 130 (23):2071-104

medscape.com/viewarticle/858839

HYPERTENSION PROTOCOL

When using any protocol, always follow the Guidelines of Proper Use (page 18).

Definition

- Adult SBP ≥ 140 or DBP ≥ 90
- Age 1 ≥ 104/58
- Age 6 ≥ 115/75
- Age 12 ≥ 125/82
- Age 17 ≥ 138/87

Considerations (acute care settings)

- Most hypertension is acutely asymptomatic
- Care should be exercised in too aggressively over-treating asymptomatic hypertension acutely
- Blood pressure usually comes down with repeated measurements only. Repeat q15 min. prn
- Poor outcomes possible from acutely lowering asymptomatic blood pressure too much
- In ED patients with asymptomatic markedly elevated blood pressure, routine screening for acute target organ injury (e.g., serum creatinine, urinalysis, EKG) is not required
- In certain patient populations (poor follow-up, etc.), checking for an elevated serum creatinine level may identify kidney injury that affects disposition
- In patients with asymptomatic markedly elevated blood pressure, routine ED medical intervention is usually not required.
- In select patient populations (such as poor follow-up), providers may treat markedly elevated blood pressure and/or initiate therapy for long-term control
- Patients with asymptomatic markedly elevated blood pressure should be referred for outpatient follow-up
- 70% ED patients with BP ≥ 140/90 with no prior history of HTN will continue to have elevated BP on follow up

Hypertensive categories

- Hypertensive urgency*:* SBP ≥ 180 or DBP ≥ 115 with cardiac risk factors

- Severe uncontrolled hypertension: SBP ≥ 180 or DBP ≥ 115 without cardiac risk factors
- Hypertensive emergency*:* elevated blood pressure with acute end organ compromise or injury

Evaluation

- Complete history and physical exam
- Detailed cardiopulmonary exam
- Check for peripheral edema
- Asymptomatic hypertension in above hypertensive categories, excluding hypertensive emergency, by itself may require no further acute tests
- BMP and U/A (for protein/blood) can be considered, especially if starting new hypertensive medications or in pregnancy
- Add CBC if pregnant to check platelet count
- EKG, CXR, BNP and troponin for acute signs/symptoms of cardiac disease
- Hypertensive urgency — lab appropriate to address existing risk factor screening

Treatment Options

- Hypertensive urgency — begin treatment within 24–48 hours per primary care provider
- Severe asymptomatic hypertension — begin treatment within 1–7 days per primary care provider
- SBP > 200 or DBP > 120 at discharge can begin treatment as indicated; May need 2 medications or combination medication
- Hypertensive emergency consult physician for treatment options
- Hypertensive emergency blood pressure should not be lowered more than 25% acutely
- IV therapy safer in hypertensive emergency: better control
- See CVA/TIA Protocol for CVA/TIA presentation

Discharge Criteria

- Asymptomatic SBP < 220 or DBP < 120 mm Hg
- No concerning comorbidities

Discharge instructions

- Hypertension aftercare instructions
- Follow up with PCP within 1–2 days if SBP ≥ 200 mm Hg or DBP ≥ 110
- Patient to notify PCP of visit and blood pressure readings within 1–2 days

Consult Criteria

- SBP ≥ 240 or DBP ≥ 140 at presentation (asymptomatic) with preexisting hypertension history
- Asymptomatic SBP > 220 or DBP > 120 at time of disposition with history of hypertension
- Asymptomatic SBP > 195 or DBP > 115 at time of disposition without history of hypertension
- Hypertension in pregnancy or within 6 weeks postpartum
- Hypertensive emergency
- Acute cardiac, neurologic or renal disorder suspected
    - Intracranial hemorrhage, TIA, CVA, CHF, angina, MI, acute renal failure
- New onset renal insufficiency or worsening renal insufficiency
- See General Patient Criteria Protocol (page 22)

Acute care initiation of outpatient treatment options (if desired)

JNC 8 Goals of Therapy

- Age < 60 years initiate treatment for a SBP ≥ 140 mm Hg or DBP ≥ 90 mm Hg to achieve a target SBP of < 140 mm Hg and DBP < 90 mm Hg in patients without diabetes or chronic kidney disease
- Age ≥ 60 years treat SBP ≥ 150 mm Hg or DBP ≥ 90 mm Hg to achieve SBP < 150 mm Hg and DBP < 90 mm Hg
    - If SBP < 140 mm Hg is well tolerated and without adverse effects on quality of life, then medications do not need to be adjusted
- Age ≥ 18 years with diabetes or chronic kidney disease (CKD), initiate treatment if SBP ≥ 140

mm Hg DBP ≥ 90 mm Hg to achieve SBP < 140 mm Hg and DBP < 90 mm Hg

- General nonblack population initiate treatment with either a thiazide diuretic, CCB, ACEI or ARB
- General black population
    - Initial therapy with either a thiazide diuretic or CCB
        - More effective than beta-blockers, ACEIs or ARBs
    - ACEI induced angioedema occurs 2-4 times more frequently than in other groups
        - Treat with FFP (fresh frozen plasma) if needed
- Age ≥ 18 years with CKD, initial or add-on therapy should include an ACEI or ARB
    - Improves renal outcomes
- If blood pressure goal cannot be achieved in 1 month, increase or add a second drug from the list of thiazide diuretic, CCB, ACEI or ARB. If blood pressure control cannot be achieved with 2 drugs from the above list, add and titrate a third drug. If 3 drugs do not control blood pressure, a drug from another class can be added.
    - Do not use an ACEI with an ARB

Stable angina

- Atenolol 50 mg PO qday

Congestive heart failure

- Lisinopril 5-10 mg PO qday
- Lasix (furosemide) 20-40 mg PO qday

Other medications than listed above are acceptable as indicated

Notes

References:

www.nhlbi.nih.gov/guidelines/hypertension/express.pdf
JNC 7 — The Seventh Report of the Joint National Committee on Prevention, Detection, Evaluation and Treatment of High Blood Pressure

Hypertension Treatment & Management
Author: Meena S Madhur, MD, PhD; Chief Editor: David J Maron, MD, FACC, FAHA

2014 Evidence-Based Guideline for the Management of High Blood Pressure in Adults
Report From the Panel Members Appointed to the Eighth Joint National Committee (JNC 8)

ACEP Clinical policy: critical issues in the evaluation and management of adult patients in the emergency department with asymptomatic elevated blood pressure (revised 2013)

Wolf SJ, Lo B, Shih RD, Smith MD, Fesmire FM, American College of Emergency Physicians Clinical Policies Committee. Clinical policy: critical issues in the evaluation and management of adult patients in the emergency department with asymptomatic elevated blood pressure. Ann Emerg Med. 2013 Jul;62(1):59–68

Current Hypertension Reports, April 2016, 18:37

Preston RA, et al. *J Hypertens*. 2018 Dec 4. [Epub ahead of print]

Whelton PK, et al. *Hypertension*. 2018; 71:e13-e115.
Clinical pearl

CONGESTIVE HEART FAILURE PROTOCOL

When using any protocol, always follow the Guidelines of Proper Use (page 18).

This protocol is for acute heart failure decompensation

Definition

- Cardiac dysfunction secondary to decreased ability of the left ventricle (LV) to eject or fill with blood

Systolic dysfunction

- Decreased left ventricular ejection fraction (LVEF) < 50%

Diastolic dysfunction

- Abnormal left ventricular filling
- LVEF > 50%

Differential Diagnosis

- Pneumonia
- COPD
- Bronchitis
- Pulmonary embolism
- Noncardiac pulmonary edema
- Adult respiratory distress syndrome

Considerations

- Main treatment is vasodilatation in nonhypotensive patients
- Isolated right heart failure is without dyspnea or pulmonary congestion
- Troponin can be mildly elevated with CHF alone

BNP

- BNP < 100 rules out CHF if not obese (lower in obese patients: < 50 is cutoff)

- Elevated in renal insufficiency, renal failure or atrial fibrillation (sometimes markedly)
- BNP > 200 CHF likely
- BNP > 500 : acute exacerbation likely

BNP level cutoffs dependent on the assay used

Classification of heart failure

- Class 1 – no limitation of normal physical activity
- Class 2 – slight limitation of activity (fatigue, dyspnea)
- Class 3 – marked limitation of activity
- Class 4 – symptoms at rest

Findings

- Fatigue
- Malaise
- Dyspnea
- Peripheral pitting edema
- Orthopnea and paroxysmal nocturnal dyspnea
- Rales
- Cough
- Hepatomegaly
- Ascites
- Jugular venous distension
- Hypotension
- Cardiac gallop sounds

Chest x-ray

- Cephalization of flow
- Pulmonary vascular congestion
- Cardiomegaly
- Pleural effusion
- Accurate in diagnosis
- Can have delayed findings

Evaluation

- EKG
- Chest x-ray (upright if possible)
- CBC
- BMP (chest x–ray may alone suffice)
- Troponin

- BNP

Treatment Options (Non-hypotensive Patients)

- Oxygen — avoid high flow oxygen
  - Causes coronary and systemic vasoconstriction
  - Avoid high O_2 saturations caused by supplemental oxygen
- IV KVO
- Nitroglycerin (NTG) 0.4 mg SL — may repeat to decrease SBP 15–30% (if initial SBP ≥ 140 mmHg)
  - Keep SBP ≥ 90 mmHg
- IV NTG for refractory significant hypertension (SBP ≥ 180 mmHg) in CHF
  - NTG 0.4 mg SL is 400 mcg which reaches peak blood levels in 2 minutes and falls to 50% of peak at 7.5 minutes by comparison, and is gone by 20 minutes, so more vigorous IV dosing can be considered for angina or hypertensive heart failure when indicated
- Nitroglycerin paste ½–2 inch (if SBP ≥ 110)
- Captopril 25 mg PO (or SL) if NTG not decreasing SBP adequately
  - If SBP ≥ 110 (effects start in 10 minutes and peaks in 30–40 minutes)
  - Chronic ACE inhibitors prolong survival
- Lasix (furosemide) 40–80 mg IV bolus (match home single dose)
- **Preferable to use vasodilators initially if possible**
  - NTG and/or ACEI then Lasix (furosemide) 15 or more minutes later
- Avoid morphine
- Avoid NSAID's and calcium channel blockers

Discharge Criteria

- Good response to treatment for mild chronic CHF
- Back to baseline respiratory function on room air

Discharge instructions

- CHF aftercare instructions
- Follow up with PCP or cardiologist within 1 day

- Return immediately if worse

Consult Criteria

- CHF exacerbation including
  - Inadequate response to treatment
  - New onset congestive heart failure
  - Preferable to discuss all cases with physician prior to discharge
- Normotensive (contact physician for treatment options if SBP < 120)
- Hypotension (notify physician)
- Elevated troponin
- Chest pain or anginal symptoms
- Near syncope or syncope

Notes

Reference:

Cornet AD, et al. *Crit Care* 2013 Apr 18;17:313
emedicine.medscape.com/article/163062

Circulation. 1979 Mar;59(3):585-8; Blood levels after sublingual nitroglycerin. Armstrong PW, Armstrong JA, Marks GS.

SYNCOPE/NEAR SYNCOPE PROTOCOL

When using any protocol, always follow the Guidelines of Proper Use (page 18).

Definitions

- Transient loss of consciousness or near loss of consciousness secondary to decreased perfusion of the brain

Differential Diagnosis

- Cardiac arrhythmia
- Pulmonary embolism
- TIA
- CVA
- Seizures
- Dehydration
- Aortic stenosis
- Hypoglycemia
- Subarachnoid hemorrhage
- Intracranial hemorrhage
- Hemorrhage
    - GI bleeding
    - Ectopic pregnancy
- Adrenal insufficiency
- Sepsis

Causes

Neurally mediated

- Vasodepressor type — loss of upright vasoconstrictor tone
- Cardioinhibitory type — bradycardia
- Mixed type — both occur together

Examples

- Vasovagal
- Situational
- Carotid sinus

***Orthostatic vital signs** (assuming upright from recumbent position)*

- Definition
    - SBP drop 20 mm Hg or DBP 10 mm Hg with assumption of upright posture
    - Sustained HR increase 30 bpm within 10 min of moving from recumbent to nonexertional standing position (or 40 bpm if 12-19 yrs. of age)
    - Orthostatic vital signs are present in up to 40% of asymptomatic patients older than 70 years, and 23% of those younger than 60 years
- Volume depletion or hemorrhage
- Advanced age
- Autonomic dysfunction
- Vasodepressor drugs
- Sepsis (distributive shock)
- Postural blood pressure changes can occur after standing for 10 minutes and so blood pressure should be checked again at 10–15 minutes if low orthostatic blood pressure is suspected as cause of the fall
- Orthostatic measurements do not, in isolation, reliably diagnose or exclude orthostatic syncope, nor do they exclude life-threatening causes of syncope

Cardiac

- Dysrhythmias
    - Heart block — 2nd and 3rd degree types
    - Atrial fibrillation/flutter
    - Ventricular tachycardia
    - Sick sinus syndrome
    - Brugada syndrome (precordial pseudo appearing right bundle branch block with > 2 mm ST coved elevation and negative T wave
        - May have normal EKG in 1/3 patients when initially seen
    - Valvular heart disease
        - Aortic stenosis
        - Mitral stenosis
    - Pulmonary embolism
    - Cardiomyopathy
    - Cardiac tamponade

- Aortic dissection
- Severe heart failure
- Pulmonary hypertension

Other causes

- Unknown etiology
- Psychiatric
- Medications
- Neurologic

Considerations

- EKG recommended in all patients
- Testing for unexplained syncope is based on risk factors
- Near syncope patients experience nearly the same amount of interventions and adverse events as syncope patients
- Vasovagal episode is the most common cause
- Medication can cause syncope or near syncope
- Sharp increase in age > 70 years
- All cause mortality after an ED visit for syncope
    - 30 days — 1.4%
    - 6 months — 4.3%
    - 1 year — 7.6%

Clinical important features suggestive of specific cause

Exertion

- Aortic stenosis
- Mitral stenosis
- Coronary artery disease

Head rotation

- Carotid-sinus syncope

Arm exercise

- Subclavian steal

Mimics

- Seizures (post-ictal and lateral tongue bite helpful, as is prolactin level)
- Vertebrobasilar TIA
- Subarachnoid hemorrhage
- Subdural/epidural hematoma
- Hypoglycemia
- Hypoxia

- Hyperventilation
- Intoxication
- Chemical/drug exposure
- Anxiety/somatization/conversion disorder

Red Flags

- Exertional onset: ischemic coronary disease or aortic stenosis
- Chest pain: ischemic coronary disease
- Severe headache: subarachnoid or cerebral hemorrhage
- Back pain: aortic dissection or aneurysm
- Dyspnea: pulmonary embolism or CHF
- Palpitations: symptomatic arrhythmia
- Neurologic deficits

Evaluation

- Syncope/Near syncope lasting < 20 seconds in healthy patients get an EKG, but may not need further testing if all the following exist:
  - Age < 50
  - Normal physical exam
  - Normal vital signs and O_2 sat on room air
  - No comorbidities
  - Clinically had a vasovagal episode
  - No other complaints
- Perform orthostatic vital signs
- Blood pressure measurements in both arms for comparison (not to be greater than 20 mm Hg difference)
- Record positive or negative calf tenderness and Homan's sign

Apply Well's pulmonary embolism and DVT criteria and Pulmonary Embolism Rule-out Criteria (PERC Rule) as indicated

- Review in Chest Pain or Dyspnea sections
- Document PERC and/or Well's scores when appropriate

All other patients testing options

- CBC
- BMP
- Chest x-ray

- EKG
- UCG if pregnancy possible
- Check stool hemoccult if any of the following
  - Acutely anemic
  - Tachycardic
  - Orthostatic vital signs
  - Melena or rectal bleeding history
  - BUN elevated out of proportion to creatinine level
- Chest pain: order troponin (angina) and D-dimer
- Consider CT head for neurologic complaints, findings or headache (low yield otherwise)

Pulmonary Embolism Rule-out Criteria (PERC Rule)

(Reportedly decreases significantly the likelihood of pulmonary embolism if all 8 criteria met — clinical gestalt as effective in identifying PE)

- Age < 50
- Pulse oximetry > 94%
- Heart rate < 100
- No history of DVT or VTE
- No hemoptysis
- No estrogen use
- No unilateral leg swelling
- No recent surgery or trauma hospitalization past 4 weeks

Treatment Options

- Dehydration — give oral rehydration in nontoxic pediatric or adult patients (see Gastroenteritis protocols)
- IV NS or LR rehydration in all others as needed
- Blood transfusion for symptomatic anemia or hemorrhage prn
- Anti-emetics prn
- Treatment aimed at cause of syncope or near syncope

Discharge Criteria

- Benign cause of syncope or near syncope in healthy patient age < 50 years

Discharge instructions

- Syncope or near syncope aftercare instructions
- Follow up with PCP within 1–2 days
- Consider ambulatory holter monitor

- Return if symptoms recur

Consult Criteria

- Syncope or near syncope > 30 seconds
- Age ≥ 50 (elderly will usually need hospital admission)
- GI bleeding
- Acute anemia, or chronic anemia with hemoglobin < 10 gms or a decrease in hemoglobin > 1 gm from previous levels
- Hypotension or tachycardia
- O_2 sat < 95% on room air (less than patient's baseline) or acute dyspnea
- Relative hypotension (SBP < 105 with history of hypertension or age ≥ 50 years)
- Abnormal EKG
- Cardiac dysrhythmia
- Positive orthostatics (a normal finding occasionally in elderly)
- Unclear cause of syncope or near syncope
- Chest pain or arrhythmia

Comorbid conditions present

- Hypertension
- Diabetes
- Cardiac
- Pulmonary disease
- Pregnancy
- Pulmonary embolism
- DVT
- Neurologic complaints or findings
- Toxic ingestion
- Dehydration
- Fever

ACEP Critical Issues in the Evaluation and Management of Adult Patients Presenting to the Emergency Department with Syncope (April 2007)

Admission to hospital recommended

- Older age and associated comorbidities
- Abnormal EKG
  - EKG abnormalities include acute ischemia, dysrhythmias, or significant conduction abnormalities
- <Hct 30% (if obtained)

- History or presence of heart failure, coronary artery disease, or structural heart disease

Low risk for adverse events

- Younger patients with nonexertional syncope, who have no history or signs of cardiovascular disease, no family history of sudden death and no comorbidities

Lab and x-ray consult criteria

- New onset renal insufficiency or worsening chronic renal insufficiency
- Metabolic acidosis (increased anion gap)
- Hemoglobin decrease > 1 gm or creatinine increased > 0.5 from baseline
- Newly elevated LFT's
- Elevated amylase or lipase
- WBC ≥ 15,000
- Bandemia ≥ 15%
- Significant electrolyte abnormally
- Glucose ≥ 400 mg/dL in diabetic patient
- Glucose ≥ 300 mg/dL in non-diabetic patient
- Hyperglycemia with metabolic acidosis (decreased serum CO_2 or elevated anion gap)
- Acute thrombocytopenia
- New chest x–ray infiltrate(s) or increased interstitial changes

Notes

References:

CHEST August 2011;140(2):509–518. doi:10.1378/chest.10–2468

Grossman SA, Babineau M, Burke, L et al. Do outcomes of near syncope parallel syncope? Am J Emerg Med. 2012;30(1):203–206

Quinn J, McDermott D, Kramer N, et al. Death after emergency department visits for syncope: how common and can it be predicted? Ann Emerg Med. 2008;51(5):585–590

Roos M, Sarkozy A, Brodbeck J, et al. The importance of class-I antiarrhythmic drug test in the evaluation of patients with syncope: unmasking Brugada syndrome. J Cardiovasc Electrophysiol. 2012;23(3):290–295

ACEP Critical Issues in the Evaluation and Management of Adult Patients Presenting to the Emergency Department with Syncope (April 2007)

Circulation, epub, 3/9/17

Ann of EM, Vol.655:622

JEM. 2018;55:780

Annals of EM, Vol. 49, pg. 431

Respiratory

Section Contents

When using any protocol, always follow the Guidelines of Proper Use (page 18).

DYSPNEA PROTOCOL

When using any protocol, always follow the Guidelines of Proper Use (page 18).

Definition

- Subjective perception of shortness of breath

Differential Diagnosis

- COPD
- Asthma
- Bronchitis
- Pneumonia
- CHF
- Angina
- Pulmonary embolism
- Pleural effusion
- Cardiac tamponade
- Pulmonary hypertension

Dyspnea of Uncertain Cause

Evaluation

If CHF suspected order:

- BNP (chest x-ray alone may suffice in lieu of BNP)
- BMP
- CBC
- Troponin
- EKG
- Chest x-ray

Consider pulmonary embolism if Well's PE criteria score 3 or greater

- Order D-dimer (can be frequently positive without DVT/PE in elderly, with history of hospitalization within past month, cancer history, edematous conditions, bedridden — see Chest Pain or Syncope Practice Guides)

Well's Pulmonary Embolism Criteria

- Suspected DVT = 3
- Alternate diagnosis less likely than pulmonary embolism = 3
- Heart rate > 100 = 1.5
- Immobilization/surgery past 4 wks. = 1.5
- Previous DVT = 1.5
- Hemoptysis = 1
- Cancer past 6 months = 1

Well's PE score > 6

- Order CTA chest PE protocol
- Document positive/negative Homan's sign and calf tenderness (documented negative Homan's sign useful for malpractice considerations only)

- If anginal equivalent suspected as complaint in elderly, refer to Chest Pain Practice Guide

Discharge criteria

- Panic disorder or benign hyperventilation
- Benign cause of dyspnea (i.e., mild to moderate asthma or bronchitis responding well to treatment)

Consult physician

- If angina equivalent suspected
- CHF suspected or diagnosed
- Pulmonary embolism suspected
- Uncertain diagnosis as cause of symptoms
- Discuss with physician if D-dimer positive or Well's PE criteria ≥ 3 and DVT and/or PE is considered as possible cause of dyspnea

Pulmonary Embolism (PE)

Definition

- Blocked of pulmonary artery usually by a migrating blood clot from legs (most commonly) or pelvic veins

Differential diagnosis

- Acute coronary syndrome
- Acute pericarditis
- ARDS

- Panic disorder
- Aortic stenosis
- Atrial fibrillation
- Cardiogenic shock
- Cor pulmonale
- Cardiomyopathy
- COPD
- Fat embolism
- Mitral stenosis
- Acute MI
- Pneumothorax
- Pulmonary hypertension
- Sudden cardiac death
- Superior vena cava syndrome
- Syncope or near syncope

Considerations

- Can be either minimally asymptomatic or catastrophic
- Occurs 1 person per 1,000/year
- Commonly a missed diagnosis on initial evaluation
- Present in 60–80% of DVT patients even though one half have on PE symptoms
- More common cause of hospitalized patient death
- One year mortality is 24%
    - Mainly due to cardiac disease, recurrent PE, infection or cancer
- NT-proBNP >500 ng/L associated with central PE and possible predictor of increased death risk (pre–existing conditions such renal failure and atrial fibrillation that have chronic increased NT-proBNP would make this assumption not as useful)
- Elevated troponin is an increased severity risk marker — 19% probability of death during hospitalization
- Massive PE second only to sudden cardiac death as a cause of sudden death
- Majority of deaths from PE occur in the first 1–2 hours of care
- Nonmassive PE defined as a systolic BP ≥ 90 mmHG and accounts for 95.5–96% of patients

- See Well's Pulmonary Embolism Criteria in above section

Pulmonary Embolism Rule-out Criteria (PERC Rule)

(Reportedly decreases significantly the likelihood of pulmonary embolism if all 8 criteria met — not superior to clinical gestalt)

- Age < 50
- Pulse oximetry > 94%
- Heart rate < 100
- No history of DVT or VTE
- No hemoptysis
- No estrogen use
- No unilateral leg swelling
- No recent surgery or trauma hospitalization past 4 weeks

American College of Physicians (ACP) 2015

- Plasma D-dimer tests are more appropriate for those at intermediate risk for a PE, and no testing may be necessary for some patients at low risk
- Use either the Wells or Geneva rules to choose tests based on a patient's risk for PE
- Low risk patients clinicians should use the 8 Pulmonary Embolism Rule-Out Criteria (PERC) and if negative for all 8 criteria then no testing is needed
- Intermediate risk patients or for those at low risk who do not meet all of the rule-out criteria, use a high-sensitivity plasma D-dimer test initially
- In patients >50 years use an age-adjusted threshold age × 10 ng/mL
    - Normal D-dimer levels increase with age
- D-dimer level below the age-adjusted cutoff should not receive any imaging studies
    - Patients with elevated D-dimer levels should receive imaging
- Patients at high risk skip the D-dimer test and proceed to CT pulmonary angiography
    - Negative D-dimer test does not eliminate the need for imaging in these patients

- Obtain ventilation-perfusion scans in patients with a contraindication to CT pulmonary angiography or if CT pulmonary angiography is unavailable
- Use validated clinical prediction rules to estimate pretest probability in patients in whom acute PE is being considered

American College of Emergency Physicians (ACEP) 2011

- Negative quantitative D-dimer assay results can be used to exclude PE in patients with a low pretest probability for PE
- Negative quantitative D-dimer assay results may be used to exclude PE in patients with an intermediate pretest probability for PE
- Low or PE unlikely patients (Wells score 4) pretest probability for PE who require additional diagnostic testing (positive D-dimer result or highly sensitive D–dimer not available), a negative multidetector CT pulmonary angiogram alone can be used to exclude PE
- Intermediate or high pretest probability for PE and a negative CT pulmonary angiogram result in whom a clinical concern for PE still exists and CT venogram has not already been performed, consider additional diagnostic testing (e.g., D-dimer, lower extremity imaging, VQ scanning, traditional pulmonary arteriography) prior to exclusion of VTE disease
- Venous ultrasound
    - May be considered as initial imaging in patients with obvious signs of DVT for whom venous ultrasound is readily available
    - Patients with relative contraindications for CT scan (e.g., borderline renal insufficiency, CT contrast agent allergy)
    - Pregnant patients
    - A positive finding in a patient with symptoms consistent with PE can be considered evidence for diagnosis of VTE disease and may preclude the need for additional diagnostic imaging

Risk factors

Virchow triad

- Endothelial injury
- Stasis or turbulence of blood flow
- Blood hypercoagulability

- Immobilization
- Malignancy
- Inherited or acquired thrombophilia states (hypercoagulable states)
- Acute medical illness
- Surgery past 3 months
- Trauma (mostly lower extremities or pelvis) past 3 months
- Oral contraceptives or estrogen
- Pregnancy
- Prior pulmonary embolism
- COPD
- Heart failure
- Stroke, hemiplegia or paralysis
- Central venous lines within past 3 months

Signs and symptoms

- Tachypnea (respiratory rate >16/min) — 96%
- Rales — 58%
- Accentuated second heart sound — 53%
- Tachycardia (heart rate >100/min) — 44%
- Fever>37.8°C (100.04°F) — 43%
- Diaphoresis — 36%
- S_3 or S_4 gallop — 34%
- Clinical signs and symptoms suggesting thrombophlebitis — 32%
- Lower extremity edema: 24%
- Cardiac murmur — 23%
- Cyanosis — 19%

Presenting complaints and findings

- Dyspnea — 73%
- Pleuritic chest pain — 66%
- Cough — 37%
- Hemoptysis — 13%

- Hypoxia
- Delirium in elderly
- Wheezing
- Productive cough
- Syncope or near syncope
- Hypotension or relative hypotension (for the patient with hypertension history)
- Lung infarction
- New onset atrial fibrillation
- Ventricular arrhythmia
- Pleural effusion
- Pulseless electrical activity

Testing options

- Chest x-ray (may be normal or nonspecific)
    - Westermark sign — decreased vascularity
    - Hampton hump — pleural based triangular density from pulmonary infarction (rare)
- CBC
- EKG
    - Sinus tachycardia most common
    - Nonspecific STT wave changes or with ischemic appearing biphasic T waves in V2 and V3
    - New right bundle branch block
    - S1Q3T3 pattern in 20%
    - Right axis deviation in 5%
    - Left axis deviation in 10%
    - New onset atrial fibrillation
- D-dimer (do not use in high clinical PE probability — scan instead)
    - More useful in eliminating younger healthy patients if negative
- ABG (may be normal or have increased A-a gradient or hypoxemia)
- BNP or NT-proBNP
- Troponin
- Echocardiogram RV strain have 10% mortality, 0% mortality with normal RV function
- Chemistries
- CTA chest pulmonary embolism protocol

- V/Q lung scan if CTA chest not available or contraindicated
  - May be performed in healthy low risk patients (if normal then very useful)
  - Low probability scans can have PE from 4–20% depending whether clinical suspicion is low or high
- Leg venous ultrasound

Treatment guidelines

American College of Chest Physicians (ACCP)

- Dabigatran, rivaroxaban, apixaban, or edoxaban are preferred over vitamin K antagonist (VKA) therapy as long-term (first 3 months) anticoagulant therapy for noncancer patients
- Low-molecular-weight heparin (LMWH) is recommended over VKA therapy, dabigatran, rivaroxaban, apixaban, or edoxaban as long-term (first 3 months) anticoagulant therapy for patients with cancer-associated thrombosis
- Aspirin is recommended over no aspirin to prevent recurrent venous thromboembolism (VTE) in patients who are stopping anticoagulant therapy and do not have a contraindication to aspirin
- In most patients with acute PE not associated with hypotension, systemically administered thrombolytic therapy is not recommended
- Selected patients with acute PE who deteriorate after starting anticoagulant therapy but have yet to develop hypotension and who have a low bleeding risk, systemically administered thrombolytic therapy is preferred over no such therapy
- Thrombolytic therapy is suggested in select patients with acute PE not associated with hypotension and with a low bleeding risk whose initial clinical presentation or clinical course after starting anticoagulation suggests a high risk of developing hypotension

- Thrombolytic therapy is not recommended for most patients with acute PE not associated with hypotension
- First episode of VTE and with a low or moderate risk of bleeding should have extended anticoagulant therapy
- First episode of VTE with a high bleeding risk should have therapy limited to 3 months
- Patients who have PE and preexisting irreversible risk factors, such as deficiency of antithrombin III, proteins S and C, factor V Leiden mutation, or the presence of antiphospholipid antibodies, should be placed on long-term anticoagulation

Treatments

- **Embolectomy** in very unstable patients in centers with CV surgery available and thrombolytics thought not to be adequate therapy or contraindicated
  - Nitric oxide 10ppm inhalation may be tried to temporize condition prior to surgery or thrombolytics

Anticoagulation

- Is a passive anticoagulation—prevents new thrombus formation while body breaks down existing thrombus
- **Enoxaparin** (LMWH) 1mg/kg q12hour SQ or 1.5 mg/kg q24hours SQ
  - Do not use with creatinine clearance <30
  - Do not use with history of heparin induced thrombocytopenia (HIT)
  - No PTT monitoring
- **Heparin** (unfractionated) load 80units/kg IV and 18 units/kg/hour IV
  - Goal is PTT 1.5–2.5 times normal
  - Creatinine clearance <30 increased bleeding risk

Do not use with history of heparin induced thrombocytopenia Stop all heparins if platelet count drops to 100,000, or a 50% decrease in baseline platelet count occurs, or 30% decrease in platelet count with new thrombus formation development (heparin induced thrombocytopenia) — a life threatening immune process

- **Warfarin** 15 mg PO load
  - Overlap with heparin until INR 2-3
  - 2-10mg PO daily (start >6 hours after LMWH)
  - **Contraindicated in pregnancy**

Direct oral anticoagulants (DOACs)

- **Apixaban (Eliquis)** 10 mg PO BID x 7 days, then 5 mg BID
  - Not recommended in severe liver disease
- **Rivaroxaban (Xarelto)** 15 mg PO q12hr for 21 days with food, then 20 mg PO qday

Thrombolytics

- **TPA** 100mg IV over 2 hours
- May give 100mg IVP during CPR in PE or suspected PE coding patients
- Heparin bolus and drip near end to TPA infusion or immediately following

Disposition

Consult criteria

- Discuss all patients with a physician

Admission

- Unstable or severe PE admit to ICU
- Patients not meeting Hestia criteria
- New elevation of troponin and/or NT-proBNP
- Clinical judgment that overrides Hestia criteria

Discharge

Hestia criteria for outpatient PE therapy — A "No" answer to all questions needed to treat outpatient

- Hemodynamically unstable
- Clot busting necessary

    - Bleeding issues
    - Oxygen required
    - Ongoing anticoagulation
    - Severe pain
    - Inpatient status needed
    - Renal failure
    - Liver disease
    - Pregnancy
    - Documented HIT
- Clinical judgment that outpatient therapy is safe for patient
- No tachycardia

Principles of Asthma and COPD Management

- Recognizing severity of exacerbation
- Using correct therapy
- Identify and treat any precipitants
- Make correct disposition

COPD Exacerbation

Evaluation options

- Monitor cardiac and pulse oximetry
- EKG
- Troponin
- CBC
- BMP
- Chest x-ray (check radiology report if and when available)) and view x-ray and compare to prior films
- Consider ABG if severe dyspnea or significant respiratory fatigue
- BNP if CHF is a consideration

Initial Treatment options

- Albuterol with or without atrovent, up to 3 treatments prn 10–20 minutes apart
- Oxygen therapy to keep O_2 Sat ≥ 90%
- Use titrated oxygen instead of high flow oxygen

- Mortality was significantly lower with titrated oxygen
- BiPAP if patient is in severe respiratory distress and/or fatigue (consult physician)

Steroid treatment options useful for moderate to severe exacerbations (caution with diabetes)

- Course 5 days (no taper needed) — evidence B

Methylprednisolone, prednisolone and prednisone

- 40 mg PO qday

Other steroids that can be used instead

- Depomedrol (methylprednisolone acetate) 80–160 mg IM

  OR

- Decadron (dexamethasone) 10 mg IV/PO
  - Onset of action IV is 1 hour. PO onset of action is 1–2 hours
  - Duration of action is 36–54 hours
  - Dexamethasone 6mg =prednisone 40 mg

  OR

- Solumedrol (methylprednisolone) 80–125 mg IV (if being admitted)

Discharge treatment options

- Albuterol or Combivent inhaler with or without spacer q4hr prn
- Rx PO Zithromax or doxycycline × 5 days, or per Sanford Guide or other drug databases
  - Depomedrol (methylprednisolone acetate) 80–120 IM

    OR

  - Decadron (dexamethasone) 6–10 mg PO daily x5 days

Inhaled steroid treatment options for COPD

- Consider inhaled steroid Rx to start only after acute exacerbation has resolved
  - Prescribe double dose if already on single strength dose

    OR

  - Advair diskus bid (combination of long acting beta-agonist and steroid) to be used only after acute exacerbation has resolved

Discharge criteria

- If patient returns to near baseline function with respiratory effort and O_2 saturation level
- Follow up in 1–5 days depending on severity of presentation and response to therapy

Discharge instructions

- Follow up in 1–5 days depending on severity of illness and response to treatments
- Provide COPD exacerbation aftercare instructions
- Return if worse

Consult physician on

- Work of breathing is moderate to severe post-treatment
- Wheezing not resolving satisfactorily
- Patient feels they are too dyspneic to go home
- WBC ≥ 18,000 or < 3,000; Neutrophil count < 1,000
- Acute thrombocytopenia
- Bandemia ≥ 15%
- Anion gap > 18
- Significant electrolyte abnormality
- Glucose ≥ 400 mg/dL in diabetic patient
- Glucose ≥ 300 mg/dL new onset diabetic patient
- Hyperglycemia with metabolic acidosis (decreased serum CO_2 or elevated anion gap)
- Heart rate ≥ 110 after all treatment are completed

Acute Asthma and Bronchitis

Peak flow % of predicted

- Mild disease > 70%
- Moderate disease 40–69%
- Severe disease < 40%

Initial Treatment Options

- Albuterol with or without atrovent up to 3 treatments prn: 15–20 minutes apart
- Nebulized lidocaine solutions 1cc of a 1% solution in 4mL of saline to give 0.25% solution after albuterol treatment for intractable cough may be tried
    - Nebulized lidocaine solutions 1cc of a 1% solution in 4mL of saline to give 0.25% solution after albuterol treatment for intractable cough may be tried
- Oxygen therapy to keep O_2 Sat ≥ 92%
- Monitor pulse oximetry
- Be careful to not suppress respiratory effort with benzodiazepines or sedating medications

Steroid treatment options useful for moderate to severe exacerbations (caution with diabetes)

- Effectiveness starts around 6 hours after dosing
    - Prednisolone or prednisone 0.5–1 mg/kg PO (NMT 60 mg)

      OR
    - Decadron (dexamethasone) 0.6 mg/kg IV/IM/PO (NMT 20 mg) — preferred in children (see Pediatric Asthma section)
        - Onset of action IV is 1 hour. PO onset of action is 1–2 hours
        - Duration of action is 36–54 hours
        - Dexamethasone 6mg =prednisone 40 mg

Additional treatment options for severe exacerbations

- Terbutaline 0.25 mg SQ prn q15–20 minutes up to 3 as needed for age ≥ 12 years
    - Caution if history of coronary artery disease
- Terbutaline 0.005–0.01 mg/kg SQ q15–20 minutes up to 3 — age < 12 years (NMT 0.4 mg per dose)
- Epinephrine 0.3 mg SQ for adults
    - Caution if history of coronary artery disease

- Epinephrine 0.01 mg/kg in children not to exceed adult dose
- MgSO4 (magnesium sulfate) 1–2 gms IV over 20 minutes in adults per physician
- MgSO4 (magnesium sulfate) 25–50 mg/kg IV over 10–20 minutes per physician (NMT 2 gm) for children
- MgSO4 (magnesium sulfate) 125–250 mg in 0.3 ml NS aerosol q 20 minutes up to 4 doses as needed (off label use)
    - May combine with albuterol
- Heliox 70:30 — do not use if > 30% oxygen needed to maintain O_2 saturation

Discharge treatment options

- Albuterol or Combivent inhaler with or without spacer q4hr prn
- If bacterial infection suspected: Rx PO Zithromax (azithromycin) or doxycycline (age > 8 years) × 5 days, or per Sanford Guide or other drug databases
- Viral infection (most healthy patients) = no antibiotics

Discharge systemic steroid treatment options (caution with diabetes)

- Prednisone 20–60 mg qday for 5 days (no taper needed) age ≥ 12 yrs.

  OR

- Depomedrol (methylprednisolone acetate) 80–120 mg IM age ≥ 12 yrs.

  OR

- Decadron (dexamethasone) 10 mg IV/IM/PO for adults or 0.6 mg IV/IM/PO for children not to exceed 20 mg/dose — recommended in children over prednisolone or prednisone (see Pediatric Asthma section)

  OR

- Pediatrics: prednisolone 1–2 mg/kg PO qday for 5 days (NMT 60 mg per day)

Discharge inhaled steroid options

- Consider inhaled steroid Rx to start only after acute exacerbation has resolved

- Prescribe double dose if already on single strength dose

  OR

- Advair discus bid – age > 3 years (combination of long acting beta–agonist and steroid) to be used only after acute exacerbation has resolved

Discharge Criteria

- Good response to therapy
- If patient returns to near baseline function with respiratory effort and O_2 saturation level
- Wheezing resolution or significant improvement, and no significant respiratory distress
- Peak flow ≥ 70% predicted if checked
- O_2 saturation > 93% on room air
- Good follow up and compliance
- Primary care provider to follow up within 1–3 days if symptoms persist

Discharge instructions

- Follow up in 1–5 days depending on severity of illness and response to treatments
- Provide asthma or bronchitis aftercare instructions

Consult Criteria

- Severe respiratory distress on presentation (notify physician immediately)
- Insufficient response to treatment
- Wheezing not resolving adequately
- Patient or family feels they are too dyspneic to go home
- Cardiac cause of dyspnea suspected or confirmed
- Immunosuppression
- Peak flow < 70% predicted if measured after treatment is finished
- O_2 saturation < 94% on room air post treatments
- O_2 Sat < 92% in COPD patient on room air or lower than baseline O_2 Sat concentrations

- Significant comorbid conditions
- Heart rate ≥ 110 post treatment in adults
- Hypotension develops or relative hypotension SBP < 105 with history of hypertension
- Return visit for same acute dyspnea episode
- Immunosuppression
- Age ≥ 60

Vital signs and age consult criteria

- Age < 6 months
- Adult heart rate ≥ 110
- Pediatric heart rate
  - 0–4 months ≥ 180
  - 5–7 months ≥ 175
  - 6–12 months ≥ 170
  - 1–3 years ≥ 160
  - 4–5 years ≥ 145
  - 6–8 years ≥ 130
  - 9–11 years ≥ 125
  - 12–15 years ≥ 120
  - 16 years or older ≥ 115
- Developing hypotension or relative hypotension (SBP < 105 with history of hypertension)
- O_2 Sat < 94% on room air in non-COPD patient

Notes

References:

CHEST August 2011;140(2):509–518. doi:10.1378/chest.10-2468

Austin MA, et al. *BMJ* 2010, 341:c5462

Chronic Obstructive Pulmonary Disease Author: Zab Mosenifar, MD; Chief Editor: Zab Mosenifar, MD

emedicine.medscape.com/article/297664

Vestbo J, et al. *Am J Respir Crit Care Med* 2013;187(4):347–65

Pediatr Emerg Care. 2018 Jan:34:53

Udezue E Lidocaine inhalation for cough suppression *Am J Emerg Med* 2001;19(3):206-7

Unlabeled Uses of Nebulized Medications
Mary Beth Shirk; Kevin R. Donahue; Jill Shirvani
Am J Health Syst Pharm. 2006;63(18):1704-171
Medscape .com/viewarticle/545484 _8

PNEUMONIA PROTOCOL

When using any protocol, always follow the Guidelines of Proper Use (page 18).

Definition

- Infection of pulmonary parenchymal tissue

Differential Diagnosis

- Pulmonary embolism
- COPD
- Asthma
- CHF
- Bronchitis
- Adult Respiratory Distress Syndrome
- Fluid overload from ESRD
- Bronchopulmonary dysplasia in children with history of prematurity

Considerations

- Number one leading cause of death from infectious disease
- Community acquired causes
    - Strep pneumoniae
    - Mycoplasma pneumoniae
    - H. influenzae
    - Legionella pneumophilia
    - Klebsiella pneumoniae
    - Influenza
- Comorbid conditions
    - Advanced age
    - Smoking
    - COPD
    - Diabetes
    - Alcoholism
    - CHF
    - HIV
    - Immunosuppression
- Signs and Symptoms

  - Cough
  - Sputum production
  - Fever
  - Chills
  - Rigors
  - Dyspnea
  - Chest pain
- WBC ≥ 15,000 suggests bacterial infection
- Very high or very low WBC predicts increased mortality

Evaluation

- CBC
- Chest x-ray (may be negative even if pneumonia is present)
- ABG if moderate to severe respiratory distress or fatigue
- See Dyspnea Protocol
- Blood cultures if toxic or hypotensive and/or patient is to be admitted

Treatment Options

- Oxygen for O_2 saturation < 93% (in COPD patient < 91%) or in respiratory distress
- Viral pneumonia needs no treatment unless immunosuppressed
- IV NS/LR or oral rehydration if dehydrated (see Gastroenteritis Protocols for rehydration therapy)

Nontoxic patient treatment that is to be discharged

No chronic cardiopulmonary disease

- Zithromax PO

  OR

- Doxycycline 100 bid PO x 10 days

Chronic cardiopulmonary disease present

- Second or third generation cephalosporin PO x 10 days

  OR

- Augmentin (amoxicillin/clavulanate)875mg bid x 10 days PO PLUS Zithromax PO

OR

- Levaquin (levofloxacin) PO as a single agent x 10 days
- May use Sanford Guide or other drug databases

CURB-65 scoring system and estimated 30–day mortality

Scoring system (One point is given for each component)

- **C**onfusion (change from baseline or less than alert and oriented x 3)
- **U**remia (BUN > 19 mg/dl)
- **R**espiratory rate ≥ 30
- **B**lood pressure (< 90 mm Hg systolic or ≤ 60 mm Hg diastolic) and
- Age ≥ **65** years
- One point is given for each component met by the patient and they are assigned a total score of 0–5 points

Estimated 30 day mortality

- 1 point: 3.2% mortality
- 2 points: 13.0% mortality
- 3 points: 17.0% mortality
- 4 points: 41.5% mortality
- 5 points: 57.0% mortality

CURB-65 points and suggested disposition

- 0 points: Outpatient
- 1 point: Outpatient
- 2 point: Observation as inpatient
- 3 points: inpatient; consider ICU
- 4 points: Strongly consider ICU
- 5 points: Strongly consider ICU

Pneumonia Severity Index for community acquired pneumonia may also be used

For patients with significant respiratory distress, hypoxemia, toxicity, or are to be admitted:

- IV NS
- IV Zithromax and Rocephin (ceftriaxone) (non-ICU)

- IV piperacillin/tazobactam (Zosyn) 4.5 gms — ICU or nursing home patient
- Consult physician

Discharge Criteria

- Nontoxic patient
- No respiratory distress
- O_2 saturation >93%
- CURB–65 discharge criteria above

Discharge instructions

- Pneumonia aftercare instructions
- Follow up with primary care provider within 1–3 days
- Return if worse

Consult Criteria

- See CURB–65 points and suggested disposition
    - Clinical judgment may override decision rules
- Significant pneumonia
- Patients that the Provider feels need admission
- Significant respiratory distress
- High fever ≥ 104°F (40°C)
- Temperature < 96°F (35.5°C)
- Appears ill or toxic
- Metabolic or respiratory acidosis
- Immunosuppression
- See Dyspnea Protocol

Vital signs and age consult criteria

- Age > 65 or < 3 months
- Adult heart rate ≥ 110
- Pediatric heart rate
    - 0–4 months ≥ 180
    - 5–7 months ≥ 175
    - 8–12 months ≥ 170
    - 1–3 years ≥ 160
    - 4–5 years ≥ 145
    - 6–8 years ≥ 130
    - 9–11 years ≥ 125
    - 12–15 years ≥ 120

  - 16 years or older ≥ 115
- Developing hypotension or relative hypotension (SBP < 105 with history of hypertension)
- O_2 Sat < 94% on room air in non-COPD patient; O_2 Sat < 92% in COPD patient on room air or home O_2 Rx

Lab and x-ray consult criteria

- New onset renal insufficiency or worsening renal insufficiency
- WBC ≥ 15,000 or < 4,000; Neutrophil count < 1,000
- Bandemia ≥ 15%
- Acute thrombocytopenia
- Anion gap > 18
- Significant electrolyte abnormally
- Glucose ≥ 400 mg/dL in diabetic patient
- Glucose ≥ 300 mg/dL in new onset diabetic patient
- Hyperglycemia with metabolic acidosis (decreased serum CO_2 or elevated anion gap)
- Pleural effusion
- Cavitary changes on chest x–ray

Notes

References:

Aujesky D, Auble TE, Yealy DM, et al. Prospective comparison of three validated prediction rules for prognosis in community-acquired pneumonia. *Am J Med* 2005; 118:384–92

Mandell LA, Wunderink RG, Anzueto A, et al. Infectious disease society of America/American Thoracic Society consensus guidelines on the management of community-acquired pneumonia. *Clin Infect Dis* 2007: 44(2):S27–72

Bacterial Pneumonia Author: Nader Kamangar, MD, FACP, FCCP, FCCM, FAASM; Chief Editor: Zab Mosenifar, MD emedicine.medscape.com/article/300157

INFLUENZA PROTOCOL

When using any Protocol, always follow the Guidelines of Proper Use (page 18).

Definition

- Infection by a single–stranded RNA virus

Differential diagnosis

- Viral URI
- Mononucleosis
- SARS
- Pneumonia
- Encephalitis
- Meningitis
- HIV infection
- Dengue
- Hantavirus Pulmonary Syndrome

Considerations

- One of the most common infectious diseases
- Airborne spread
- During peak flu season, clinical judgement may be as good as rapid testing, making rapid testing less necessary
- Rapid testing may be more beneficial in times of lower disease prevalence
- Empiric treatment of critically ill patients should be considered even if rapid testing is negative
- Baloxavir marboxil is a new single-dose antiviral agent and is effective for treatment of influenza type A and type B strains
- In children, the most common presenting symptoms are fever, cough, and rhinitis
- Vomiting and diarrhea are more common in children than adults
- Early treatment of within 2 days of symptom onset was associated with a reduction in mortality risk when compared to later treatment in adults
- Neuraminidase inhibitor therapy in children aged < 12 years found that symptoms was reduced by 36 hours among previously healthy children taking oseltamivir and by 30 hours among those taking zanamivir

- >23,000 US deaths annually
- Incubation period usually 2 days, but can range from 1–4 days

Vaccination

- Children 6–59 months
- Pregnancy or postpartum, or who may become pregnant
- Immunocompromised
- Caregivers of high risk patients
- Age ≥65 years
- Chronic kidney disease
- COPD and chronic pulmonary disease patients
  Patients with egg allergy may be given any recommended influenza vaccine as appropriate for their health status

Signs and symptoms

- Fever (2–5 days duration)
- Sore throat (3–5 days duration)
- Myalgias
- Frontal or retro-orbital headache
- Nasal discharge
- Weakness and severe fatigue
- Cough and other respiratory symptoms
- Tachycardia
- Red, watery eyes

High risk patients

- Age ≥ 65 years
- Age < 2 years
- Chronic pulmonary disease — asthma or chronic obstructive lung disease
- Chronic cardiovascular, renal, and/or hepatic disease
- Hematologic disease (e.g., sickle cell disease)
- Metabolic disorders (e.g., diabetes mellitus)
- Immunosuppression secondary to either disease or a medication
- Compromised respiratory function or other conditions that increase risk of aspiration
- Pregnancy and up to 2 weeks post-partum
- Long-term aspirin therapy for chronic medical conditions in patients aged < 19 years

- Neuromuscular disorders, seizure disorders, or other cognitive dysfunction that may compromise handling of respiratory secretions

Complications

- Acute bronchitis
- Primary viral pneumonia (uncommon)
- Secondary bacterial pneumonia (occurs 4–5 days after onset of illness)
  - Staphylococcus aureus, Streptococcus pneumoniae and Haemophilus influenzae
- EKG abnormalities
- Otitis media

Testing

- In epidemics in healthy patients with typical symptoms, no testing may be indicated
- Testing is appropriate in times of low disease prevalence
- Nasopharyngeal swab
  - Depending on the test, generally accurate 60–80%
- Chest x–ray in high risk patients or when diagnosis is unclear
- CBC and chemistries may be ordered for toxic patients or with concerning comorbidities and signs/symptoms

Treatment considerations

- Supportive care may suffice in healthy patients
- Prescribe antiviral medications for patients who are more severely ill or at high risk for a more severe disease course
- Nursing homes, etc. the CDC further recommends that antiviral chemoprophylaxis should be given for a minimum of 2 weeks and should continue for at least 7 days after the last known case was identified.
  - May be considered or offered to healthcare personnel who care for patients at high risk for complications

Medications

Oseltamivir (Tamiflu)

- Oseltamivir 75 mg bid for adults x 5 days
- Pediatric dosing
    - ≤15 kg 30 mg PO bid x 5 days
    - 15.1–23 kg 45 mg PO bid x 5 days
    - 23.1–40 kg 60 mg PO bid x 5 days
    - >40 kg same as adult
- Currently approved for the treatment of influenza in patients of all ages

Zanamivir (Relenza)

- Adult inhalation 5 mg bid x 5 days
- Pediatric >10 mg inhaled q12hr x 5 days

Permivir (Rapivab)

- 600 mg IV as a single dose
- For patients aged ≥2 years who have been symptomatic for no more than 2 days
    - CrCl 30-49 mL/min: 200 mg IV as a single dose
    - CrCl 10-29 mL/min: 100 mg IV as a single dose

Baloxavir marboxil (Xofluza)

- 40 to <80 kg: 40 mg PO x 1
- ≥80 kg: 80 mg PO as a single dose

Prophylaxis

- Oseltamivir and zanamivir one dose daily for 10 days
- May be extended to 2 weeks in high risk patients
- May be extended for community outbreaks to 6 weeks for oseltamivir and 28 days for zanamivir

Admission Criteria (consult physician)

- Exacerbations of underlying disease
- Elderly with signs of pneumonia
- Elderly with dehydration
- Significant respiratory compromise

Discharge Criteria

- Most healthy patients without concerning comorbities or signs/symptoms

Notes

References:

cdc. gov/flu/professionals/infectioncontrol/ltc-facilityguidance.htm

ebmedicine.net/topics.php?paction=showTopic&topic_id=591

emedicine.medscape.com/article/219557

Stein J, Louie J, Flanders S, et al. Performance characteristics of clinical diagnosis, a clinical decision rule, and a rapid influenza test in the detection of influenza infection in a community sample of adults. Ann Emerg Med. 2005;46(5):412-419

Prevention and Control of Seasonal Influenza with Vaccines: Recommendations of the Advisory Committee on Immunization Practices—United States, 2018–19 Influenza Season

Recommendations and Reports / August 24, 2018 / 67(3);1–20

Adult Asthma/Acute Bronchitis Protocol

When using any protocol, always follow the Guidelines of Proper Use (page 18).

This protocol is for acute exacerbations

Definition

- Reversible acute bronchospasm and airway resistance secondary to infectious, allergic, environmental or internal causes

Differential Diagnosis

- Panic disorder
- Pneumonia
- Bronchitis
- CHF
- COPD
- Pulmonary embolism
- Anaphylaxis
- URI
- Vocal cord dysfunction
- Laryngospasm
- Epiglottitis
- Croup
- Retropharyngeal abscess

Considerations

- Cough is commonly the first symptom
- Viral URI, allergens or environmental factors are frequently precipitants
- Severe episode may have decreased breath sounds without wheezing
- Inability to speak more than 2–3 words at a time indicates a severe episode
- Steroids very useful — both PO, IM/IV and inhaled (inhaled steroids are for prophylaxis)

    - Cochrane review found that inhaled corticosteroids are superior to anti-leukotrienes when used as monotherapy in adults and children with persistent asthma
- Usually there is pre-existing asthma or bronchitis history

Peak flow % of predicted

- Mild disease > 70%
- Moderate disease 40–69%
- Severe disease < 40%

Risk Factors

- Prior intubation
- Visit in the last month for asthma
- Hospitalization > 1 time
- Two emergency visits past year
- Current or recent systemic steroid use
- Concomitant disease
- Illicit drug use

Evaluation

- Complete history and physical exam
- Assess respiratory effort
- Monitor O_2 saturation
- Consider peak flows before and after aerosols
- CBC and/or BMP for significant tachycardia and fever
- Check radiology interpretations prior to discharge if available

Chest x-ray

- If pneumonia suspected
- Significant respiratory distress
- If CHF considered as possible cause of dyspnea
- Respiratory distress not responsive to aerosols
- Age ≥ 50
- Cardiac history

If CHF suspected

- BNP may be ordered though chest x–xay usually suffices
- Troponin

- EKG

Treatment Options

- Supplemental oxygen for O_2 Sat < 92% room air or significant respiratory distress
- Albuterol with or without atrovent aerosol every 15–20 minutes prn — up to 3 treatments total

Steroid treatment options useful for moderate to severe exacerbations in adults (caution with diabetes)

- Prednisone 40–60 mg PO

  OR

- May give Decadron (dexamethasone) 0.6 mg/kg IM instead (NMT 10 mg) if PO route not usable (caution with diabetes)
  - Onset of action IV is 1 hour. PO onset of action is 1–2 hours
  - Duration of action is 36–54 hours
  - Dexamethasone 6mg =prednisone 40 mg

  OR

- Depomedrol (methylprednisolone acetate) 120–160 mg IM (caution with diabetes)

Additional treatment options if needed for severe exacerbations

- Epinephrine 0.3 mg SQ (caution with coronary artery disease history)
- Terbutaline 0.25 mg SQ prn q15–20 minutes up to 3 treatments as needed (caution with coronary artery disease history)
- MgSO4 (magnesium sulfate) 1–2 gms IV over 20 minutes in adults per physician
- MgSO4 (magnesium sulfate) 25–50 mg/kg IV over 10–20 minutes per physician (NMT 2 gm) for children
- MgSO4 (magnesium sulfate) 125–250 mg in 0.3 ml NS aerosol q 20 minutes up to 4 doses as needed (off label use)
  - May combine with albuterol
- Heliox 70:30 — do not use if > 30% oxygen needed to maintain O_2 saturation

Discharge medications

- Albuterol MDI with or without spacer prn
  - May direct up to 6 puffs per treatment if needed
- Antibiotics are not usually needed
  - Consider antibiotics in smokers
  - If bacterial infection suspected, may use Sanford Guide or other drug databases
    - Zithromax PO

Discharge systemic steroid treatment (caution with diabetes)

- Prednisone 40–60 mg PO × 5 days (NMT 60 mg qday)

  OR
- Decadron (dexamethasone) 0.6 mg/kg IV/IM/PO (NMT 10 mg) instead of prednisone may be used

Discharge inhaled steroids for asthma only

- Consider inhaled steroid Rx only after the acute exacerbation has resolved
  - Prescribe double dose if already on single strength dose

    OR
  - Advair diskus bid for asthma or COPD only (combination long acting beta-agonist and steroid) to be used only after acute exacerbation has resolved

Discharge Criteria

- Good response to therapy
- Wheezing resolution and no significant respiratory distress
- Peak flow ≥ 70% predicted if checked
- O_2 saturation > 93% on room air
- Good follow up and compliance
- Primary care provider to follow up within 1–3 days if symptoms persist

Discharge instructions

- Follow up with primary care provider in 1–5 days depending on severity of illness and response to treatments
- Provide asthma or bronchitis aftercare instructions

Consult Criteria

- Severe respiratory distress on presentation (notify physician immediately)
- Insufficient response to treatment
- Family or patient feels they are too ill to go home
- Peak flow < 70% predicted if measured after treatment is finished
- Moderate or severe respiratory distress post treatment
- O_2 saturation < 94% on room air post treatments if O_2 saturation normal on room air in past
- Significant comorbid conditions
- Heart rate ≥ 110 post treatment
- Hypotension develops or relative hypotension SBP < 105 with history of hypertension
- Return visit for same acute episode
- Immunosuppression
- Age ≥ 60

Lab and x-ray consult criteria

- New onset renal insufficiency or worsening renal insufficiency with creatinine increase ≥ 0.5
- WBC ≥ 15,000 or < 3,000; Neutrophil count < 1,000
- Bandemia ≥ 15%
- Acute thrombocytopenia
- Anion gap > 18
- Significant electrolyte abnormally
- Glucose ≥ 400 mg/dL in diabetic patient
- Glucose ≥ 300 mg/dL in new onset diabetic patient
- Hyperglycemia with metabolic acidosis (decreased serum CO_2 or elevated anion gap)
- Pleural effusion
- New chest x–ray infiltrate(s) or increased interstitial changes

Notes

References:

Asthma Author: Michael J Morris, MD, FACP, FCCP; Chief Editor: Zab Mosenifar, MD

emedicine.medscape.com/article/296301

Chauhan BF, Ducharme FM. Anti-leukotriene agents compared to inhaled corticosteroids in the management of recurrent and/or chronic asthma in adults and children. Cochrane Database Syst Rev. May 16 2012;5:CD002314

Unlabeled Uses of Nebulized Medications

Mary Beth Shirk; Kevin R. Donahue; Jill Shirvani

Am J Health Syst Pharm. 2006;63(18):1704-171

Medscape .com/viewarticle/545484 _8

VENTILATOR PROTOCOL

When using any management guideline, always follow the Guidelines of Proper Use (page 18).

For clinical settings that permit the practitioner to perform ventilator management and they are trained and experienced to perform those duties

Considerations

- Mechanical ventilation after intubation is a common lifesaving therapy in critically ill patients
- Potential benefits of mechanical ventilation
  - Improved oxygenation with increased FiO_2 and the application of positive end-expiratory pressure (PEEP)
  - Improved ventilation through manipulation of the tidal volume and respiratory rate
  - Decreased work of breathing
- Optimization of ventilation parameters may decrease complications and hospital length of stay
  - Low tidal volume ventilation (6 mL/kg ideal body weight) decreases barotrauma
  - Weaning FiO_2 to target an O_2 saturation of 90–93 percent. Prolonged hyperoxia promotes inflammation and contributes to tissue injury
- Checking an ABG 30 minutes after ventilator adjustments may help the clinician assess the adequacy of oxygenation and ventilation
  - A reliable pulse oximeter waveform is generally as useful as checking serial ABGs to monitor oxygenation.
  - Manipulate one parameter at a time when changes are needed (respiratory rate, tidal volume, PEEP, FiO_2 etc.)
- If the practitioner feels that intubation is needed, then it most likely is needed
- No absolute contraindications to intubation exist
  - Extreme caution is needed in cervical spine injuries or with cervical spine rheumatoid arthritis or ankylosing spondylitis

- Clinicians should anticipate precipitous drops in BP in hypotensive patients at the time of intubation, and medications (vasopressors) and IVFs should be available for administration

Common disease processes requiring intubation when severe

- Asthma
- Heart failure
- COPD exacerbation
- Sepsis
- ARDS
- Pneumonia
- Trauma
- Neuromuscular disorders
- Drug overdose

Complications

Pulmonary

Barotrauma – high peak pressures > 40 cm H20

- Pneumothorax
- Pneumomediastinum
- Development of bronchopleural fistula
- Interstitial emphysema

High oxygen concentration

- Free radical cellular damage
- Absorption atelectasis from nitrogen washout

Other

- Nosocomial pneumonia

Cardiovascular effects

- From high PEEP (high intrathoracic pressures)
    - Decreased venous preload and cardiac output
    - Right ventricular dysfunction
- Decreased cardiac output effects
    - Decreased renal, hepatic, and other end-organ blood flow leading to impaired functioning

Indications for mechanical ventilation

Clinical indications

- Bradypnea or apnea
- Severe or advanced respiratory fatigue
- Coma
- Obtundation
- Loss of protective airway reflexes (cough and gag reflexes)
- Acute lung injury or ARDS with inability to oxygenate or ventilate by non-invasive means
- Shock, particularly with metabolic acidosis and inadequate respiratory compensation

Clinical conditions

Hypercapneic respiratory failure

- COPD
- Status asthmaticus
- Neuromuscular disease
- Severe chest wall trauma (flail chest)

Hypoxemic respiratory failure

- Pneumonia
- Non-cardiogenic pulmonary edema (ARDS, neurogenic pulmonary edema, other conditions)
- Cardiogenic pulmonary edema
- Diffuse lung disease
    - Interstitial fibrosis or inflammation
    - Pulmonary hemorrhage
- Extreme work of breathing with developing respiratory fatigue
- Protect or ensure patency of airway and control secretions with impaired cough reflex
    - CVA
    - Drug overdose
    - Cervical spine injury
    - Anaphylaxis or other causes of airway edema

Laboratory indications

- $PaCO_2$ > 50 mm Hg with a pH < 7.25

- PaO_2 < 55 mm Hg on maximal supplementary oxygen (usually either a 100 percent non-rebreather, CPAP, or BiPAP)

Pulmonary function test abnormalities which suggest impending respiratory failure

- Vital capacity < 15mL/kg in adults
- Vital capacity < 10 mL/kg in children
- Negative inspiratory force < -20 cm H20 (normal -65 to -75 cm H20
- Forced expiratory volume (FEV1) < 5 mL/kg

Basic modes of mechanical ventilation

Volume-cycled

- Delivers a set tidal volume during a specified time (which is determined by the respiratory rate)
- Delivers constant inspiratory flow rate
- Airway pressures vary with changes in pulmonary compliance and resistance
- When paired with a set respiratory rate, volume-cycled modes guarantee a minimum minute ventilation
- High airway pressures can occur in non-compliant lungs resulting in barotrauma and potentially pneumothorax. This can be seen with:
    - ARDS or other diffuse lung disease with decreased lung compliance
    - Right mainstem intubation
    - Increased intra-abdominal pressure
    - Chest wall rigidity
    - "Fighting the ventilator" due to patient agitation

Pressure-cycled

- Delivers a set pressure until a specified time (pressure control) or flow (pressure support) is met
- Useful in situations with non-compliant lungs (ARDS) because they guarantee a set peak pressure will not be exceeded; however this may be at the expense of the tidal volume

- Changes in lung compliance may result in varying tidal volumes which is a disadvantage and requires close monitoring
- Some ventilators allow for volume assured pressure-cycled ventilation with breath-to-breath adjustments in pressure as needed to deliver a desired tidal volumes

Specific modes of mechanical ventilation

There are many modes of mechanical ventilation, some of which are quite complex. It should be noted that no mode has been proven to be superior to another mode in the general population of mechanically ventilated patients.

Assist-controlled ventilation

- Patient is guaranteed to get a preset tidal volume (volume-cycled) or pressure (pressure-cycled) at a set respiratory rate. Ventilator cycles with patient respiratory effort above the set rate and will deliver additional tidal volumes or pressure for extra breaths.
- Tachypnea can lead to breath stacking and air trapping, particularly in patients with COPD.

Synchronous intermittent mandatory ventilation

- Patient is guaranteed to get a preset tidal volume or pressure at a set respiratory rate. Additional patient respirations are allowed but not supported.
- Typically, additional breaths above the set respiratory rate are pressure supported.

Airway pressure release ventilation and Bivent

- A type of pressure control ventilation delivering a high pressure (P_{high}) for a longer interval (T_{high}) and low pressure (P_{low}) for a shorter interval (T_{low}). This contrasts other modes where the inspiratory phase is shorter than the expiratory phase.
- Improves oxygenation by maximizing mean airway pressures
- Ventilation can worsen in some patients and the pH and PCO_2 must be monitored carefully
- Most commonly employed in patients with ARDS
- Clinician should be trained in the use of this complex mode of ventilation

Pressure support ventilation

- For spontaneously breathing patients
- Level of pressure support is set to assist spontaneous respirations
- Can be useful in determining readiness for extubation
- May improve patient comfort

Noninvasive ventilation

- Positive pressure ventilation through a mask
- Useful in specific types of respiratory failure
    - Good evidence for decreased mortality and decreased hospital length of stay in patients with COPD exacerbations, cardiogenic pulmonary edema, and in immunocompromised patients with acute respiratory failure
    - Also may benefit patients with severe asthma exacerbations, neuromuscular disease, and post-extubation for patients with COPD
    - Conflicting evidence for benefit in other causes of hypoxic respiratory failure
- Generally, patients must be able to follow commands and protect their airway to attempt non-invasive positive pressure ventilation
- Full mask preferred in acute settings
- Complications
    - Barotrauma (rare)
    - Pressure necrosis of facial tissues
    - Gastric dilation, vomiting, and aspiration
    - Patient intolerance

Continuous positive airway pressure (CPAP)

- Most commonly used in the setting of cardiogenic pulmonary edema in conjunction with diuresis
- Initial settings
    - CPAP pressure 4–12 cm H_2O

Bilevel positive airway pressure (BPAP)

- Similar to CPAP but BPAP may improve ventilation and is therefore most useful to treat COPD with acute hypercapneic respiratory acidosis
- Initial settings:

- Inspiratory pressure (IPAP) 8–12 cm H_2O
- Expiratory pressure (EPAP) 3–5 cm H_2O

Commonly used ventilation parameters

- **Tidal volume** (TV)
  - Amount of air delivered in a single breath, typically 4–12 mL/kg
  - Mortality benefit with low tidal volumes (6 mL/kg) in patients with ARDS, and this ventilation strategy is generally applied to most ventilated patients with respiratory failure
- **Respiratory rate** (RR)
  - Generally set at 8–24 breaths per minute
  - Respiratory rates that are too fast rate can cause air trapping (auto–PEEP) in patients with obstructive lung disease
- **Minute ventilation** is amount of air delivered in a minute, and this equals the TV x RR (5–10 L/min)
- **Peak inspiratory pressure** (PIP)
  - Highest level of pressure applied by the ventilator, which is only partially transmitted to the distal airways
  - In a volume cycled mode, this depends on the size of the tidal volume and on airway resistance. This is specified in a pressure cycled mode.
  - Barotrauma can occur at higher pressures
  - Generally aim to keep PIP < 35 cm H_2O
- **Plateau pressure**
  - The pressure applied to the small airways and alveoli. This is a function of lung compliance.
  - Checked by performing an inspiratory hold maneuver
  - Plateau pressure > 30 cm H_20 may lead to increased barotrauma
- **Positive end expiratory pressure** (PEEP)
  - Usually set between 5–15 cm H_2O
  - Can improve oxygenation by recruitment of alveoli to participate in gas exchange
  - High levels of PEEP can have complex effects on the cardiovascular system through decreased RV and LV preload, increased RV afterload, and decreased LV afterload. The cardiac output is

typically increased in hypervolemic patients and decreased in euvolemic and hypovolemic patients
    - Generally wean PEEP along with FiO_2 to lowest tolerated levels
- **Fraction of inspired oxygen** (FiO_2)
    - Start at 100 percent, and titrate down to maintain a p_aO_2 > 60 mm Hg or an O_2 saturation > 90 percent
    - Prolonged use of an FiO_2 > 60 percent may be harmful
- **Inspiratory:expiratory ratio** (I:E ratio)
    - Most patients are set at 1:1.5 - 1:4
    - Inadequate expiratory time may lead to air trapping (auto-PEEP)
- **Inspiratory flow rate**
    - The amount of gas given during inspiration (40–100 L/minute)
    - Adjusting the flow rate will affect the I:E ratio

Suggested Initial Ventilator Settings

Volume-cycled assist control – "Volume control"

- Respiratory rate 10–12/minute
    - A low RR allows the patient to breathe above the set rate and therefore determine their own respiratory rate, which is generally ideal
    - A higher RR might be needed in paralyzed patients who cannot breath spontaneously
- Tidal volume 6–8 mL/kg ideal body weight
    - Goal should be 6 mL/kg in ARDS
- PEEP 5–10 cm H_2O
    - Severely hypoxic patients will need more PEEP
- FiO_2 — start at 100 percent
    - Decrease as permitted to maintain pO_2 > 60 or an O_2 saturation > 90 percent)
- I:E ratio 1:2

Monitoring ventilator support

- Obtaining ABGs after a ventilator parameter change can be helpful, particularly for patients who are not breathing above the set RR. If a patient has a functioning pulse oximeter and they are breathing above the set RR, frequent ABGs are less like to be useful.

- Maintain pH > 7.3 and < 7.45
    - pH > 7.45 decrease ventilator rate
    - pH 7.15–7.30 increase ventilator rate
    - In patients with ARDS, we tolerate lower tidal volumes, and therefore less minute ventilation and a lower pH/higher pCO_2 (pH as low as 7.20), to minimize barotrauma. This is termed "permissive hypercapnia."
- Maintain pO_2 60–90 mm Hg
- Maintain pCO_2 35–45 mm Hg unless pH indicates patient is a chronic pCO_2 retainer
    - For example a pH > 7.45 with pCO_2 35–45 mm Hg indicates that the patient may normally have a higher resting pCO_2 from COPD or another condition causing chronic ventilatory impairment

- Cardiac monitoring
- Blood pressure monitoring
- Pulse oximetry (maintain O_2 saturation > 90%)
- Peak pressures < 40 cm H_2O
- Plateau pressures < 30 cm H_2O
- Increase PEEP in 2 cm H_2O increments as needed for hypoxia with assessing vital signs for several minutes afterward

High pO_2 with high FiO_2

- Decrease FiO_2 in 5–10% increments
- Once the FiO_2 < 60%, lower PEEP by 2cm H20 increments
- After each change, allow 5–10 minutes for equilibration to occur
- A stepwise weaning protocol has been developed by the ARDS network investigators (see reference)

High or low pCO_2

- Must be interpreted in the context of the pH
- A high pCO_2 and a near normal pH suggests a chronic respiratory acidosis and no adjustment may be needed

- A high pCO_2 and a low pH indicates increased ventilation is necessary, and the RR or TV should be increased
- With metabolic acidosis, the pH will be low and the pCO_2 should be < 40 to compensate for the primary metabolic process. If the pCO2 is > 40, the RR or TV should be increased

Reducing risk of ventilator-associated pneumonia

- Shorten the duration of mechanical ventilation
    - Protocolized daily spontaneous breathing and spontaneous awakening trials have been shown to result in fewer days on the ventilator
- Chlorhexidine oral rinse
- Diligent hand hygiene
- Elevating head of bed 30–45° when possible
- Note: Stress ulcer prophylaxis is recommended in patients on mechanical ventilation > 48 hr. However, agents that increase pH (PPIs and H2 receptor antagonists) may increase the risk of ventilator associated pneumonia.

Sedation

- Most patients need sedation and/or analgesia by continuous infusion or scheduled dosing
- Daily interruption of sedation allows for less days of mechanical ventilation
- Most patients should be started on a propofol or fentanyl infusion with a RASS (Richmond Agitation Sedation Scale) goal of 0 to -1
- For a comprehensive and up to date approach to sedation in mechanically ventilated patients, please review the information at www.icudelirium.org

Troubleshooting

Sudden respiratory distress

- Disconnect patient from ventilator
- Manually ventilate with an bag valve mask
- Suction the patient to remove secretions that could be obstructing the airway

- If no improvement, check to see if the patient is adequately sedated (tube biting, ventilator dyssynchroncy, etc.)
- Obtain a CXR and have the respiratory therapist evaluate the patient

Ventilator problems

- Should improve with manual bagging
- Check tubing for obstruction
- Check for circuit disconnect
- Perform an inspiratory hold to evaluate for a resistance or compliance issue
- Check an expiratory hold to evaluate for auto-PEEP

Endotracheal tube problems

Low resistance check for:

- Endotracheal tube (ET) placement
    - Esophageal location
- Cuff leak if low resistance or low peak inspiratory pressure develops
- Internal tube leak if low resistance or low peak inspiratory pressure develops

High resistance (high peak pressures)

- Right mainstem intubation
- Pneumothorax
- Patient biting ET
- Check tubing for obstruction (suction tube)
- Kinked ET tube
- Anything causing reduced lung compliance – ARDS, pneumonia, pulmonary edema, alveolar hemorrhage, etc.

Hypotension treatment options

- IV fluid bolus if pulmonary edema absent
- Think about auto-PEEP. Disconnect ventilator circuit if high levels of auto-PEEP are present on expiratory hold maneuver. Then resume ventilation with a lower RR or lengthen the expiratory time.
- Decrease PEEP as high levels of PEEP may impair cardiac output

- Consider evaluating for pneumothorax or pulmonary embolism

Liberation from mechanical ventilation

- Evaluate patients daily to determine candidacy for a spontaneous breathing trial

Criteria for extubation

- Can patient oxygenate and ventilate independent of mechanical ventilation?
  - O_2 saturation > 90 percent and PaO_2 > 60 mm Hg on FiO_2 < 40% and PEEP < 5 cm H_2O
  - Patient breathing spontaneously
- Mental status and ability to protect airway
  - Patient should be able to follow commands and have strong cough and gag reflexes
- Hemodynamic stability
  - Should be on no or minimal dose vasopressors
- Acid-base and electrolyte balance
  - pH > 7.25.
- Thyroid and adrenal function sufficient

Spontaneous breathing trial (SBT)

- Place on pressure support (PS) mode with a PS above PEEP at 5, PEEP 5, and FiO_2 40 percent
- Observe patient for 30–120 minutes
- Assess respiratory rate/tidal volume ratio (RSBI)
  - RSBI < 105 is predictive of successful extubation
  - Age > 70 years with RSBI < 130 may be acceptable
- If patient fails SBT, resume mandatory ventilation for the next 24 hours
- Another option for an SBT is to disconnect the patient from the ventilator and utilize a T-piece. Patient is monitored in a similar fashion and assessed for readiness to extubate at 30–120 minutes.

Consult criteria

- Management under physician's direction
- Requiring mechanical ventilation > 24 hours

- More complicated ventilator or oxygenation problem
- Complex critical illness

Notes

References:

Clinical practice guidelines for the use of noninvasive positive-pressure ventilation and noninvasive continuous positive airway pressure in the acute care setting. *CMAJ February 22, 2011 vol. 183 no. 3* First published February 14, 2011, doi: 10.1503/cmaj.100071

Ventilator Management
Author: Allon Amitai, MD; Chief Editor: Zab Mosenifar, MD
emedicine medscape.com/article/810126

Non-invasive positive pressure ventilation for treatment of respiratory failure due to exacerbations of chronic obstructive pulmonary disease.. Cochrane Database Syst Rev. 2004; (3):CD004104.

Noninvasive ventilation in acute cardiogenic pulmonary edema: systematic review and meta-analysis. Masip J et al. JAMA. 2005; 294(24):3124–30

Ventilation with Lower Tidal Volumes as Compared with Traditional Tidal Volumes for Acute Lung Injury and the Acute Respiratory Distress Syndrome. ARDSNet Investigators. N Engl J Med 2000; 342:1301–1308

Marini, John J., and Arthur P. Wheeler. *Critical Care Medicine: The Essentials*. Philadelphia: Lippincott Williams & Wilkins, 2009. Print.

"ARDSNet." *NHLBI ARDS Network*. Web. 16 June 2014. www.ardsnet.org

"ABCDEFs of Prevention and Safety." *ICU Delirium and Cognitive Impairment Study Group*. Web. 16 June 2014. <http://www.icudelirium.org/>.

Efficacy and safety of a paired sedation and ventilator weaning protocol for mechanically ventilated patients in intensive care (Awakening and Breathing Controlled trial): a randomised controlled trial. Girard TD et al. Lancet. 2008; 371:126–34

ALLERGY PROTOCOL

When using any protocol, always follow the Guidelines of Proper Use (page 18).

This Protocol is for an acute episode

Definition

- Systemic reaction to chemical mediator release secondary to IgE sensitization from allergen

Considerations

- Most reactions are minor with itching with localized or generalized urticaria
- Anaphylaxis is due to IgE antibody release of histamine and vasoactive mediators
- Most common causes of allergies are food allergy
  - Milk and egg allergies are seen more commonly in younger children, while allergies to shellfish and fin fish are more frequent in teens
  - Peanut allergy has a high incidence and is consistent across all ages
- Symptom presentation possibilities
  - Occurs within 30 minutes usually
  - Can be mild
  - Wheezing
  - Dyspnea
  - Shock
  - Airway obstruction
  - Death
  - Can occur on long-term medication
- Urticaria
  - Etiology unknown usually
  - Usually self-limited
- True opioid allergy rare — usually GI upset or pseudoallergy
- Anaphylactoid reactions to contrast
  - Direct stimulation of mast cells and basophils
  - Seafood allergic patients are not allergic to radiographic contrast material

    - Related to high osmolarity of contrast materials
    - Narcotics can also cause anaphylactoid reactions

        No link between seafood allergy and iodinated contrast allergy

        - There is an increase in nonallergic contrast reactions in any type of allergy history (small increase)
        - Iodine is not an allergen
        - Reactions almost always non–IgE mediated

- Angioedema (may appear with urticaria)
    - Bradykinin mediated usually
    - May be histamine mediated
    - Commonly from ACE inhibitors
        - Decreased metabolism of bradykinin
    - Hereditary C1 esterase deficiency
        - Leads to increased bradykinin
        - Positive family history
    - Caution using steroids in diabetic patients

Evaluation

- Vital signs
- Oropharyngeal and respiratory distress assessment
- Pulmonary and cardiac exam
- Skin examination
- Chest x-ray for significant respiratory distress or O_2 saturation < 93% on room air
- Soft tissue neck films for hoarseness or complaints/findings of throat swelling
- CBC and BMP for moderate to severe systemic reactions

Urticaria

- Vascular reaction of the skin with transient wheals, soft papules and plaques usually with pruritus

Treatment options

Benadryl (diphenhydramine)

- Adult: 25–50 mg PO/IM/IV
- Pediatrics: 1–2 mg/kg PO or IM (NMT 50 mg)

- May continue for 5–7 days PO qid prn

Pepcid (famotidine)

- Adult: 20 mg IV or 40 mg PO
- Pediatric: 0.25 mg/kg IV or 0.5 mg/kg PO (not to exceed maximum adult dose)

Epinephrine

- If urticaria part of anaphylaxis reaction (see below sections)

Consider steroids (caution if diabetic)

- Prednisone 40–60 mg PO qday for 5–7 days (> 40 kg)
- Prednisone/prednisolone 1 mg/kg PO qday for 5–7 days (< 40 kg)
- May give Decadron (dexamethasone) 0.6 mg/kg IM/PO/IV instead (NMT 10 mg)

Discharge criteria

- Discharge with good resolution of rash and itching

Discharge instructions

- Follow up with primary care provider within 7 days
- Avoid offending agent if known
- Provide urticaria aftercare instructions

Angioedema

- Non-life threatening presentation treated same as urticaria
- Less responsive to treatment than urticaria
- Evaluate for airway compromise or significant oropharyngeal swelling
- Oxygen prn
- Consult promptly for posterior oropharyngeal angioedema, stridor or hoarseness
- Discharge mild lip or non-oropharyngeal angioedema with normal vital signs and no distress
- Stop ACE inhibitors if currently taking
    - 4 times more common in African–Americans
    - May develop years after taking current ACE inhibitors
- May involve GI tract mimicking acute abdomen

Types of angioedema

- Histamine mediated
  - Allergic/immunogenic
- Bradykinin mediated
  - ACE inhibitors
  - Hereditary
    - Decreased C1 inhibitor (or poorly functioning C1 inhibitor) allowing overproduction of bradykinin
  - Acquired
  - Bradykinin metabolized mainly by angiotensin converting enzyme
- Physically induced
- Idiopathic

Additional treatments if needed

Histamine mediated angioedema (allergic)

- Epinephrine
  - Caution if history of coronary artery disease
  - Adult: 0.3 mg SQ; (if respiratory distress notify physician promptly)
  - Pediatrics: 0.01 mg/kg SQ not to exceed adult dose; give IV or IM (anterior thigh) if significant respiratory distress (notify physician promptly)
- Antihistamines (diphenhydramine 50 mg IV/IM) helpful in IgE/histamine mediated (may have pruritus)
- Pepcid (famotidine) 20 IV
- Dexamethasone 10 mg IV
  - Onset of action IV is 1 hour. PO onset of action is 1–2 hours
  - Duration of action is 36–54 hours
  - Dexamethasone 6mg =prednisone 40 mg

Bradykinin mediated (ACE inhibitor induced most common)

- May respond to fresh frozen plasma or C1 esterase inhibitor concentrate

Mild Anaphylaxis

- Urticaria/angioedema
- O_2 saturation > 94% room air
- No respiratory distress
- Normotensive
- No tachycardia

Treatment options

Benadryl (diphenhydramine)

- Adult: 50 mg PO or IM
- Pediatric: 1–2 mg/kg PO or IM (NMT 50 mg)
- Continue for 5–7 days PO qid prn

Pepcid (famotidine)

- Adult: 20–40 mg IV/PO
- Pediatric: 0.25 mg/kg IV/PO (NMT 40 mg)

Consider steroids

- Prednisone 40–60 mg PO qday for 5–7 days (> 40 kg)
- Prednisone/prednisolone 1 mg/kg PO qday for 5–7 days (< 40 kg)
- May give Decadron (dexamethasone) 0.6 mg/kg IV/IM/PO instead for 5–7 days daily or every other day (NMT 10 mg/dose)

Additional treatment if needed

Epinephrine

- Caution if history of coronary artery disease
- Adult: 0.3 mg SQ
- Pediatrics: 0.01 mg/kg SQ not to exceed adult dose

Moderate Anaphylaxis

(Notify physician)

- Urticaria/angioedema
- Wheezing
- O_2 saturation 90–94% room air
- Moderate respiratory distress
- No hypotension

Treatment options

Oxygen: nasal or mask (≥ 5 liters/minute if mask used)

Epinephrine (drug of choice)

- Caution if history of coronary artery disease
- Adult: 0.3 mg SQ/IM (thigh) — notify physician promptly
- Pediatric: 0.01 mg/kg SQ/IM (thigh) not to exceed adult dose — notify physician promptly

Benadryl (diphenhydramine)

- Adult: 50 mg IV or IM
- Pediatric: 1–2 mg/kg IV or IM (NMT 50 mg)

Pepcid (famotidine)

- Adult: 20–40 mg IV
- Pediatric: 0.25 mg/kg IV (NMT 40 mg)

Albuterol aerosol

- With or without atrovent
- Repeat q15 min × 2 additional treatments prn
- Continuous prn (for severe dyspnea)

Additional treatments if needed

Glucagon

- 1–2 mg IV if on beta-blocker or resistant to epinephrine

Steroids

- Adult: Solumedrol (methylprednisolone) 125 mg IV
- Pediatric: 1–2 mg/kg IV
- Prednisone 40–60 mg PO qday for 5–7 days (> 40 kg) if discharged
- Prednisone/prednisolone 1 mg/kg (NMT 60 mg) PO qday for 5–7 days if discharged (pediatrics)
- May give Decadron (dexamethasone) 0.6 mg/kg IV/IM instead (NMT 10 mg) and continue PO up to 5–7 days if needed

Severe Anaphylaxis

(Notify physician immediately)

- Urticaria/angioedema
- Wheezing
- O_2 saturation < 90% room air
- Severe respiratory distress
- Oropharyngeal airway swelling or compromise
- Hypotension
- Intubation if impending respiratory failure — notify physician immediately
- Observation for 6 hours if to be discharged by physician
- Usually admitted

Treatment options

Oxygen: nasal or mask (> 5 liters/minute if mask used)

Epinephrine (drug of choice)

- Adult: 0.3–0.5 mg IV (if in shock) or IM anterior lateral thigh if no IV/IO access
    - 1 mg IV/IO if no pulse
        - Activate ACLS and call a code
- Pediatric: 0.01 mg/kg IV (if in shock) or IM anterior thigh (do not exceed adult doses)
- Caution with history of coronary artery disease

For shock

- IV NS 1–2 liters rapidly if hypotensive adult
- 20 cc/kg IV NS if hypotensive pediatric patient — may repeat × 2 prn

Benadryl (diphenhydramine)

- Adult: Benadryl (diphenhydramine) 50 mg IV (preferred) or IM
- Pediatric: 1–2 mg/kg IV (preferred) or IM (NMT 50 mg)

Pepcid (famotidine)

- Adult: 20–40 mg IV
- Pediatric: 0.25 mg/kg IV (NMT 40 mg)

Albuterol aerosol

- With or without atrovent

- Repeat q10–15 min × 2 prn
- Continuous aerosol prn for severe dyspnea

Steroids

- Adult
    - Solumedrol (methylprednisolone) 125 mg IV
    - Prednisone 40–60 mg PO qday for 5–7 days (> 40 kg) if discharged
- Pediatric
    - Solumedrol (methylprednisolone) 1–2 mg/kg IV (NMT 125 mg)
    - Prednisone/prednisolone 1 mg/kg (NMT 60 mg) PO qday for 5–7 days if discharged (pediatrics)
    - May give Decadron (dexamethasone) 0.6 mg/kg IM/IV instead (NMT 10 mg)

Additional treatment if needed

Glucagon

- 1–2 mg IV if on beta–blocker or resistant to epinephrine (consult physician if possible)

Discharge Criteria

- Good resolution of rash and itching in urticaria
- Discharge patients presenting with mild symptoms that have observation post-treatment for 2–4 hours without symptoms

Discharge instructions

- Follow up with primary care provider within 7 days
- Avoid offending agent if known
- Provide allergy aftercare instructions
- Return if worse

Consult Criteria

- Hypotension
- O_2 saturation < 95% on room air after treatments
- Moderate to severe anaphylaxis or respiratory distress on presentation or during stay
- Altered mental status

- Oropharyngeal or throat swelling, complaints of throat swelling, hoarseness or dyspnea
- Wheezing not resolved
- Adult heart rate ≥ 110 post treatment
- Pediatric heart rate post treatment
    - 0–4 months ≥ 180
    - 5–7 months ≥ 175
    - 8–12 months ≥ 170
    - 1–3 years ≥ 160
    - 4–5 years ≥ 145
    - 6–8 years ≥ 130
    - 9–11 years ≥ 125
    - 12–15 years ≥ 120
    - 16 years or older ≥ 110

Notes

References:

Beaty AD, Lieberman PL, Slavin RG. Seafood allergy and radiocontrast media: are physicians propagating a myth? Am J Med 2008 Feb;121(2):158.e1–4.doi: 10.1016/J amjmed.2007.08.025

Seidmann MD. Christopher AL. Sarpa JR. Potesta E. Angioedema related to angiotensin converting enzyme inhibitors. Otolaryngology – Head & Neck Surgery. 102:727–31, 1990.

Brown NJ. Ray WA. Snowden M. Griffin MR. Black Americans have an increased rate of angiotensin converting enzyme inhibitor-associated angioedema. Clinical Pharmacology & Therapeutics. 60(1):8–13, 1996 Jul

World Allergy Organization Guidelines for the Assessment and Management of Anaphylaxis
World Allergy Organ J. Feb 2011; 4(2): 13–37

Am J Med, Vol. 127: S17World Allergy Organization Guidelines for the Assessment and Management of Anaphylaxis

World Allergy Organization Guidelines for the Assessment and Management of Anaphylaxis

World Allergy Organization Guidelines for the Assessment and Management of Anaphylaxis

Acute Care Ultrasound

Section contents

When using any protocol, always follow the Guidelines of Proper Use (page 18).

ACUTE CARE ULTRASOUND

When using any protocol, always follow the Guidelines of Proper Use (page 18).

Definition

- Limited bedside point of care ultrasound performed by the medical provider directly performing patient care

This is a brief introduction

Ultrasound exams

FAST (trauma) — overlaps with RUSH exam

RUSH (shock)

FOCUS ON THE INFERIOR VENA CAVA (IVC)

PULMONARY (DYSPNEA)

PULMONARY EMBOLISM CASE

CARDIAC

GALLBLADDER

RENAL

DEEP VENOUS THROMBOSIS

SOFT TISSUE

Considerations

- Attended ultrasound course
- Practice needed to attain ultrasound pattern recognition
- Credentialing with 25+ exams with quality review in each area
- Limited bedside ultrasounds does not compete with or preclude complete ultrasounds performed and/or read by radiology, cardiology or specific specialties in their area of expertise

- Structures at the top of the image are closest to the probe
- B mode is most commonly used
- M mode is used for imaging over a time window
- PW (Doppler) is pulse wave to determine if vessel is a vein or artery or if there is any flow in a structure
- Orientation of probe — marker on side of probe and corresponding icon on upper side of screen

Types of probes

Curved (low frequency for deeper structures)

- Abdomen
  - Gallbladder
  - Renal – check for hydronephrosis and possibly stones
  - Shock (or hypotension) RUSH exam
  - FAST for trauma
  - Subcostal cardiac imaging

Linear (high frequency for superficial structures)

- Starting central lines (usually internal jugular or femoral)
- Skin abscess determination
- DVT exam
- Pneumothorax (pleura sliding determination)
- Ocular (do not perform if globe rupture present or suspected)
  - Select ophthalmology exam setting (and then reduce power to 25%)
    - May be safer to avoid prolonged scan times
  - Retinal detachment
  - Papilledema of optic nerve
  - Lens dislocation in trauma without globe rupture

Phased array (mid-lower frequency)

- Cardiac
- Abdomen
- Lung

FAST (Focused assessment with Sonography in Trauma)

Curved probe

- Orientation of probe (marker) to patient's right or toward head

Areas to scan

- **Epigastrium** to view heart for pericardial effusion
  - Phased array probe (if used) with marker pointed to right shoulder and probe in the 4-5th area intercostal space (long parasternal view)
- **Right lateral flank** with marker to head to view Morrison's pouch (potential space between right kidney and liver) for fluid (black area represents blood or fluid) – may see with ruptured ectopic pregnancy also
  - May detect as little as 200 mL
- **Left lateral flank** to view left kidney and spleen for bleeding (not as good as CT for extent of injury)
- **Bladder** for surrounding fluid in pelvis (marker to right)
- Both costophrenic angles for pleural effusion
- **Linear probe** bilateral upper chest that detects presence of pleural movement and comet tail artifacts (lung fluid) = no pneumothorax

FAST Indications

- Hemodynamically unstable patients
- Patients who need an emergent bedside procedure and a rapid trauma exam needed
- Patients at a community hospital who require transfer to a trauma center
- Blunt trauma in unconscious or paralyzed patient, or who has altered mental status, or about to be anesthetized for other injuries
- Intoxicated patients who can be observed and re-examined
- Blunt trauma with suspected intraperitoneal injury
- Patients with penetrating trauma, especially with wounds in upper abdomen or lower chest

- Patients with a concerning mechanism of injury but no definitie indication for CT
  - Consider a period of observation and serial FAST exams

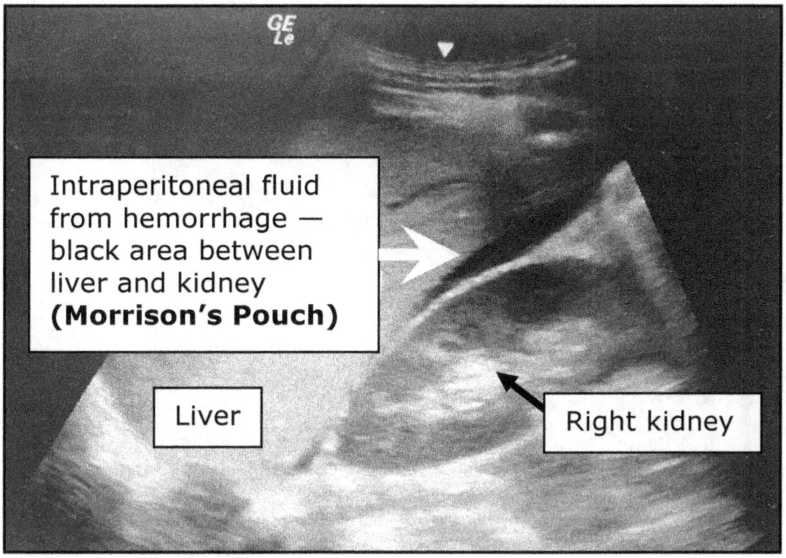

Rapid Ultrasound for Shock (RUSH) – undifferentiated shock (overlaps with FAST exam)

Use all probes

HIMAP

- **H** – Heart for pericardial effusion (with phased array probe 4-5th ICS area with marker pointed to right shoulder)
  - LV contractility (ballpark guestimate)
  - RV size should be 2/3 LV size (if > 2/3 LV may indicate PE, COPD, pulmonary HTN etc.
- **I** – IVC for size and inspiratory collapse
  - > 50% inspiratory collapse and < 1.5 cm diameter may need IV fluid (epigastrum view)
  - Little respiratory phascitiy and > 2.5 cm diameter may need pressor
  - See below
- **M** –Morrison's pouch for intraperitoneal bleeding
- **A** – Aortic aneurysm (> 3 cm diameter)

- Aorta bifurcates at the umbilicus
- Find spine and its shadow – IVC top right side and aorta top left side of spine
- Use transverse and longitudinal views

- **P** – Pleural effusion and pneumothorax (linear probe for pneumothorax evaluation)

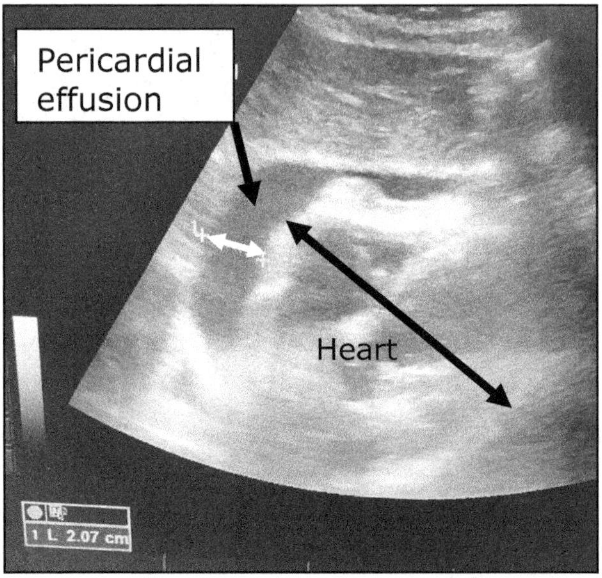

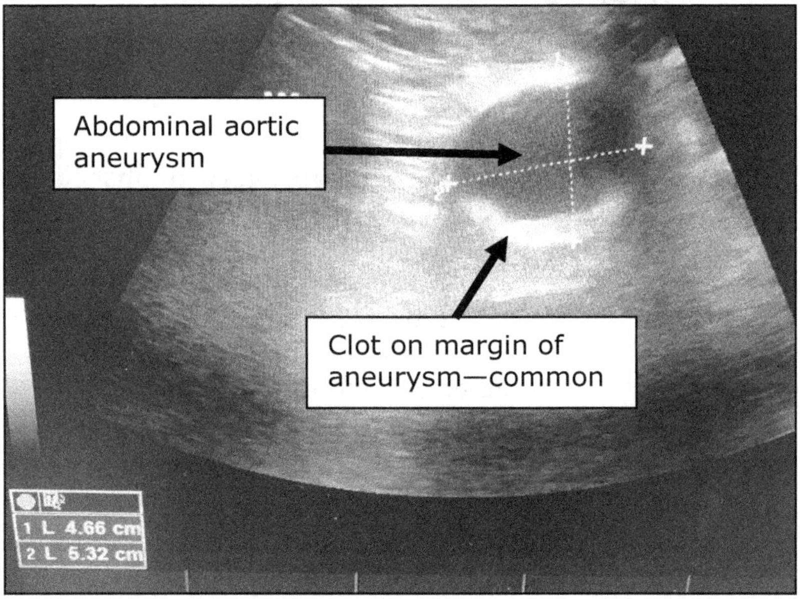

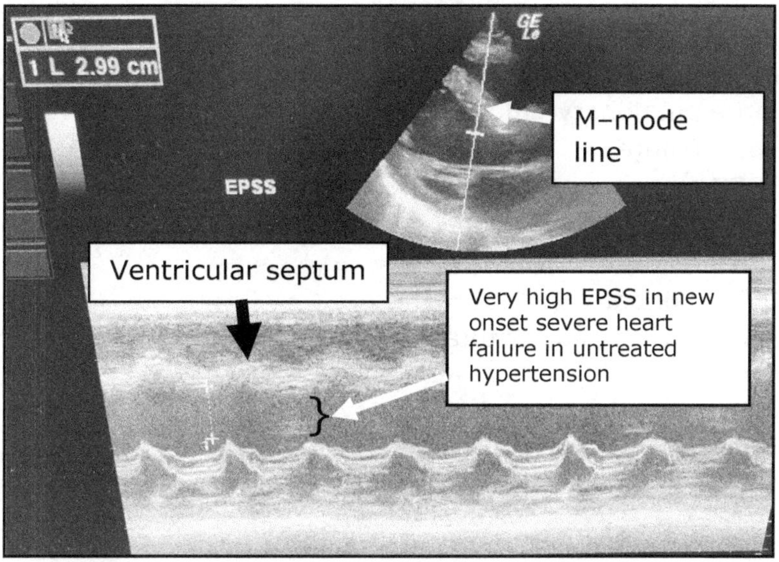

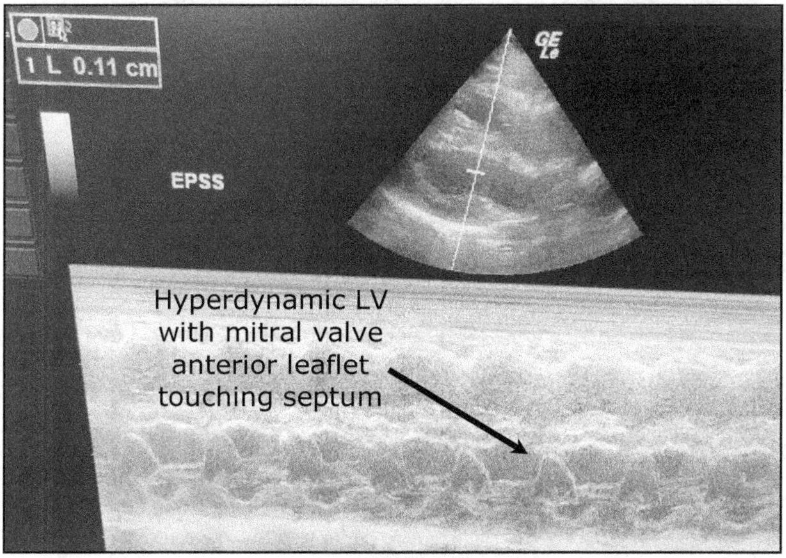

M–mode measures movement over time and is displayed as second image at bottom

Focus On Inferior Vena Cava (IVC)

- If dilated with little to no inspiratory change may have
  - Large pulmonary embolism burden
  - Heart failure
  - COPD
  - Pulmonary hypertension
  - Renal failure
  - Fluid overload
- If small size with near or total inspiratory collapse may have
  - Dehydration
  - Sepsis
  - Hemorrhage

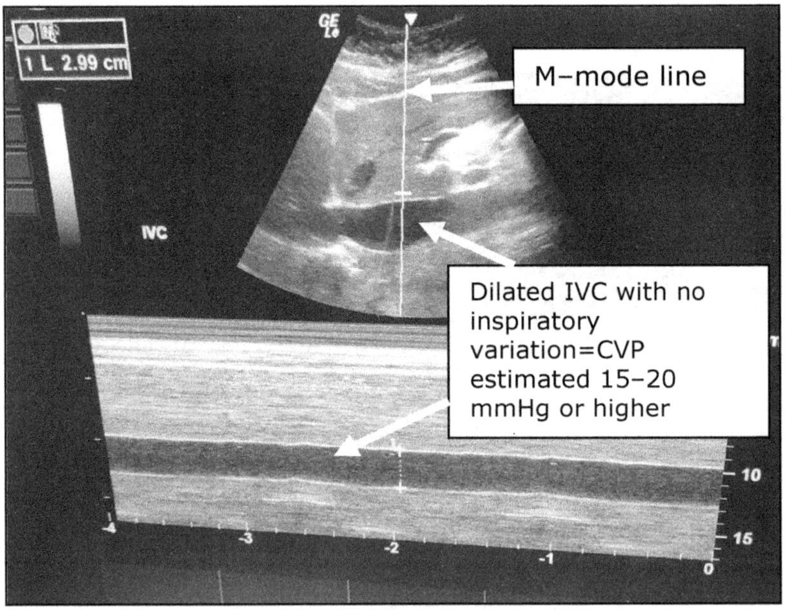

M-mode measures movement over time and is displayed as second image at bottom

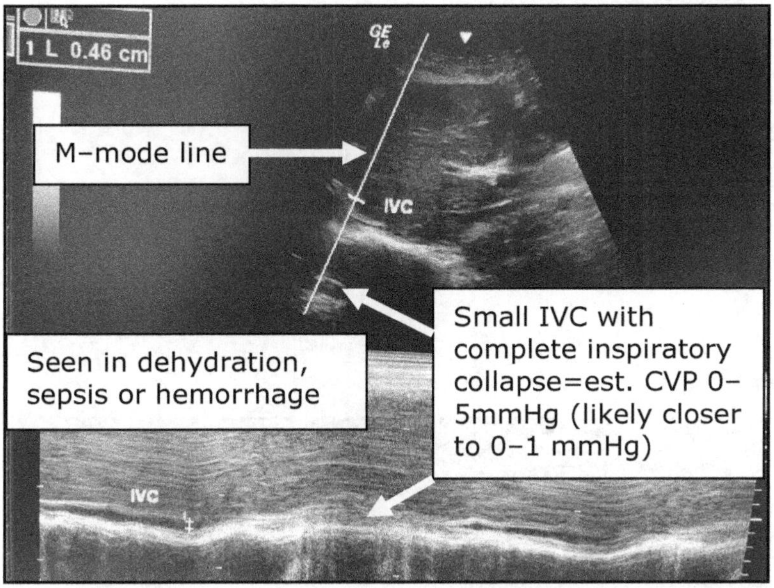

CVP (central venous pressure) estimation

IVC measured	% collapse during inspiration	CVP (mmHg)
< 1.5 cm	>50%	0–5
1.5–2.5 cm	>50%	5–10
1.5–2.5 cm	<50%	10–15
>2.5 cm	Little phasicity	15–20

Pulmonary (Dyspnea)

(see RUSH exam also)

Evaluate for

- Systolic cardiac contractility (guestimate)
- Diastolic dysfunction if able
- Right and left ventricular size

- Pericardial effusion

Lungs

Evaluate for

- Pleural effusion(s)
- Pulmonary parenchymal fluid (B lines)
- A lines
- Pneumothorax

Pleural effusion

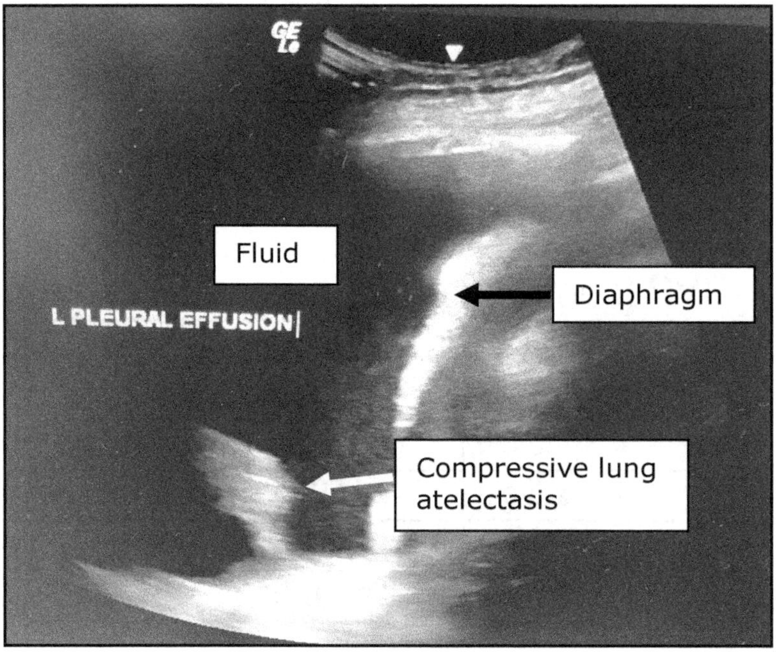

B Lines

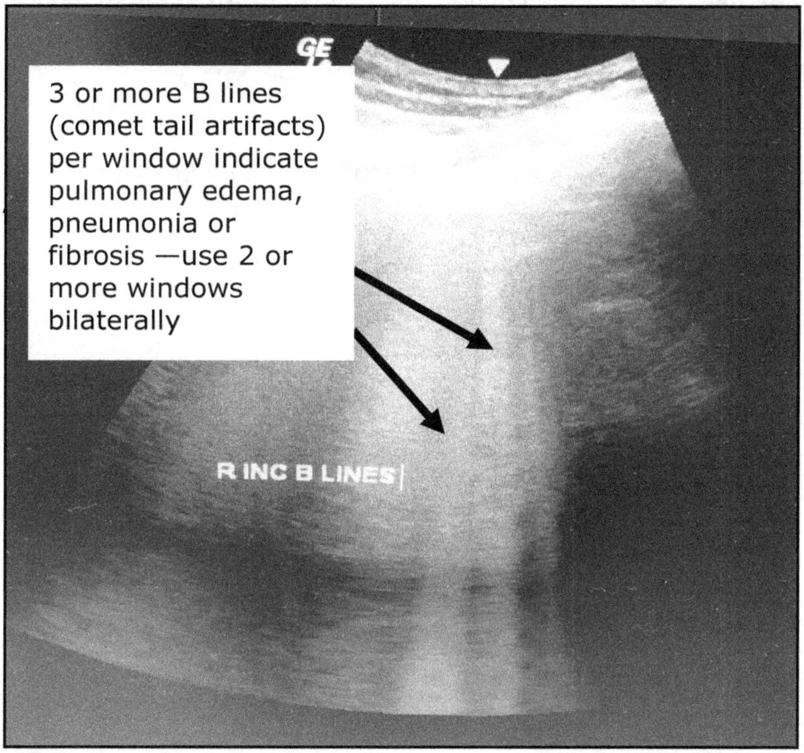

A Lines

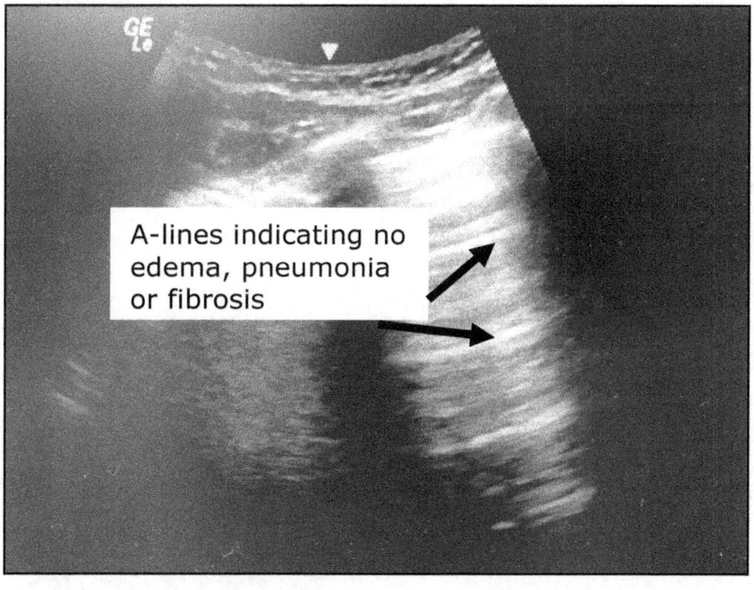

“A–Lines” when present are horizontal and indicate no pulmonary edema, and can be taken usually with other clinical indicators to infer that the patient is at least IV fluid tolerant. Does not establish fluid responsiveness.

“B–Lines” indicate interstitial thickening — 94% sensitivity, 92 % specificity

Pulmonary embolism case ultrasound

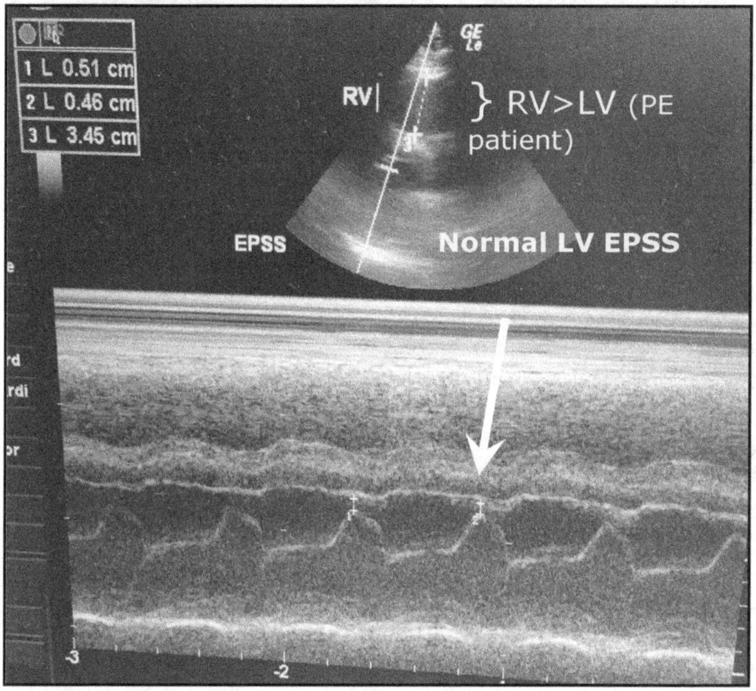

This patient required open thrombolectomy

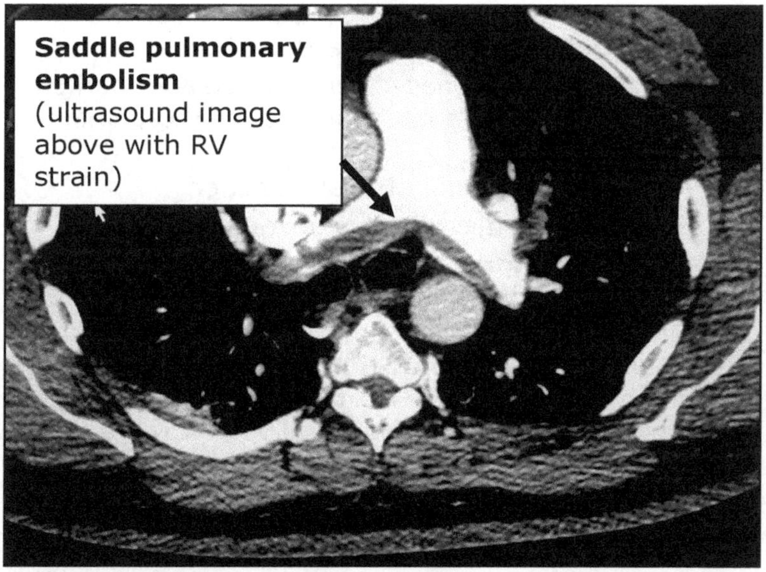

Right ventricular enlargement (Should normally be around 60% or 2/3 size of left ventricle)

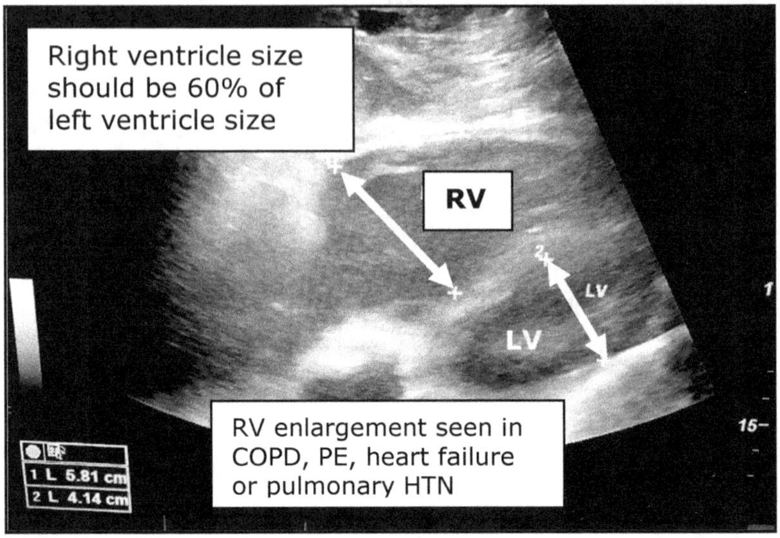

Cardiac Exam (see FAST, RUSH and Pulmonary Exams for representative images)

Windows

- **Subxiphoid (subcostal)** with phased array or curvilinear to view heart and IVC/aorta
  - Evaluate RV and LV size, contractility, wall thickness and for pericardial effusion
- **Apical** area with phased array probe and marker pointed to patient's left slightly angled cephalad 20 degrees
  - Visual inspection of heart function
  - Assess for diastolic dysfunction if able
- **Parasternal long axis** on left sternal border near 4th intercostal space with probe marker aimed at right shoulder
- **E Point Septal Separation** is the distance from the anterior leaflet of the mitral valve, (which is the first deflection of the mitral valve toward the interventricular septum), and the septum seen in parasternal long axis view
  - Elevated in systolic failure — usually > 0.6 cm

    - Decreased in hyperdynamic states such as dehydration, sepsis and high sympathetic states
- **Parasternal short axis** is long axis rotated 90° cephalad
    - Observe wall motion

Gallbladder

Curved probe

- Subcostal sweep with marker toward head
- RUQ – 7 cm medial to xiphoid
- Flatten probe as needed with transverse view
- Gallbladder wall normally is < 4 mm – measure in the short axis
- Gallstones or sludge have shadows
- If gallbladder difficult to visualize, try lateral view looking above the right kidney
- Pericholecystic fluid presence may indicate inflammation or cholecystitis

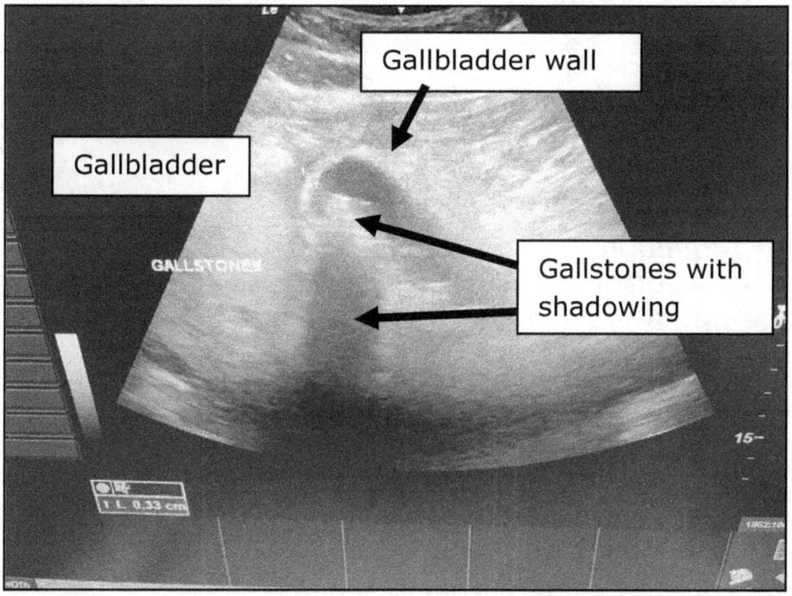

Renal

Curved probe

- Right kidney in midclavicular line inferior ribs
- Left kidney in posterior clavicular line inferior ribs
- Look for dilated collecting system and stones
- Marker probe pointed to head

Hydronephrosis

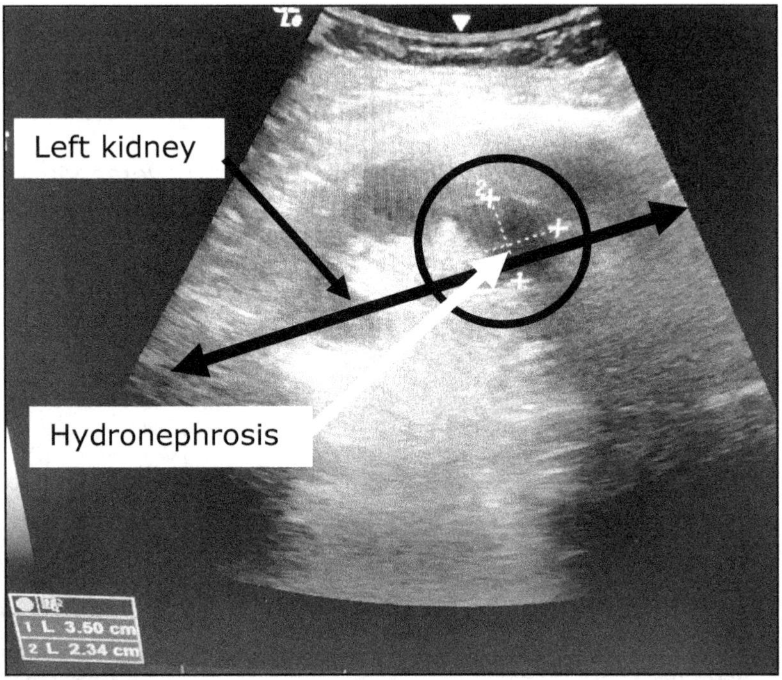

Definition

- Distention of the renal calyces and pelvis as a result of obstruction of the outflow of urine distally

Causes

- Pregnancy
- Bladder outlet obstruction
- Ureteral calculus
- Benign prostatic hypertrophy
- Post-surgical complication
- Vesicoureteral reflux

Considerations

- Permanent of loss renal function by 6 weeks of obstruction

DVT

- **Linear probe** with transverse orientation
- Position thigh externally rotated up to 30 degrees with knee flexed 10 degrees may help with exam
- Start at inguinal ligament and identify common femoral artery and vein
- Compress down anterior thigh 10–20 cm from inguinal ligament
- Blood clot prevents vein from being compressed fully
- Color flow is sometimes absent with DVT
- Popliteal fossa 12 cm above and 5 cm below is compressed
- If negative, then 98% have no DVT
- Sensitivity 95% (95% CI 87-99%) and specificity 96% (95%CI 87-99%)

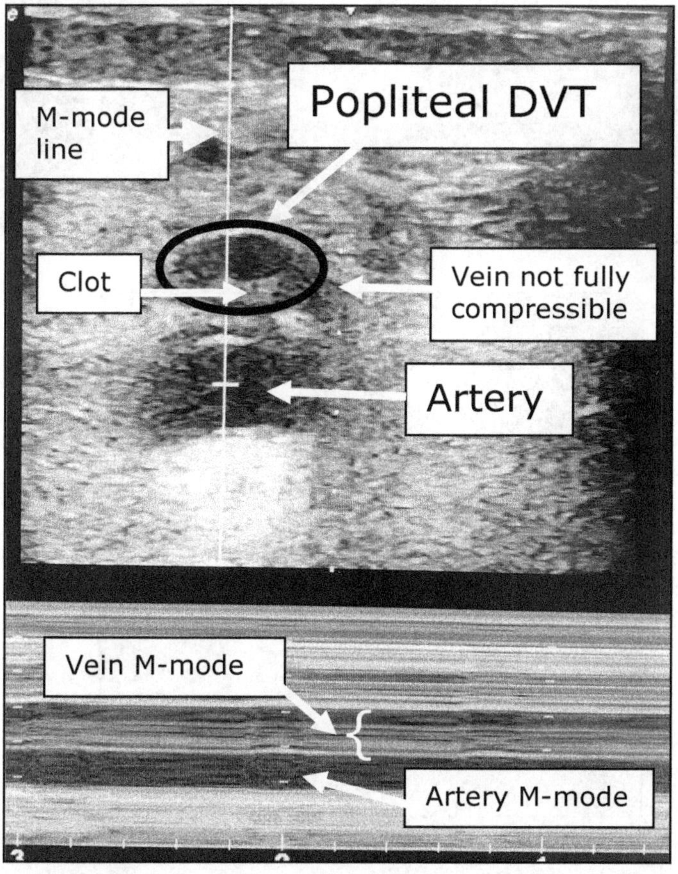

Soft tissue

Linear probe

- Abscess is a black space with white scattered debris
- Cellulitis has cobblestone appearance of the fat globules

Abscess

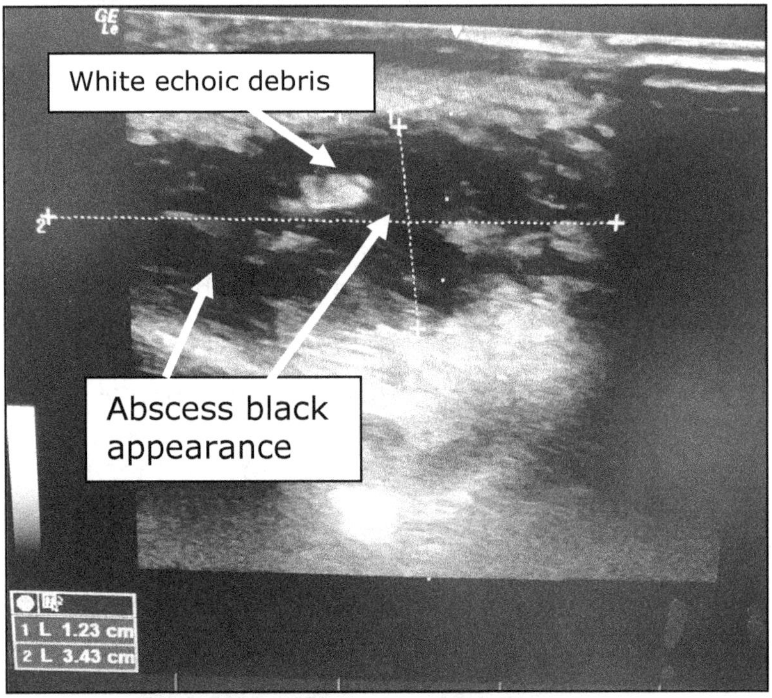

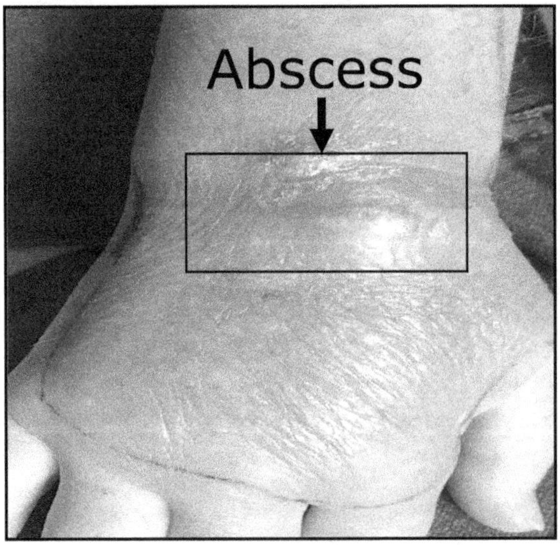

Conclusion

- Ultrasound provides important bedside point of care data that may assist in critical patient management
- Practice is critical in achieving competency
- Ultrasound is an important adjunct and needs to be combined with clinical evaluation and other data

Notes

References:
Sonoguide.com

Ultrasound Volume Assessment
R. Starr Knight, MD

Emedhome.com feature article: Rapid Ultrasound for Shock and Hypotension (RUSH) Scott D Weingart, MD, RDMS Assistant Professor of Emergency Medicine

emergencyultrasoundteaching.com/assets/us_billing_summary

ultrasonix.com/webfm

https://sinaiem.org/accuracy-of-bedside-dvt-study

World Allergy Organization Guidelines for the Assessment and Management of Anaphylaxis

Endocrine

Section Contents

When using any protocol, always follow the Guidelines of Proper Use (page 18).

DIABETES AND HYPOGLYCEMIA PROTOCOL

When using any protocol, always follow the Guidelines of Proper Use (page 18).

This Protocol is mostly for acute diabetic presentations

Definition

- Defect in glucose regulation secondary to inadequate secretion of insulin or resistance to insulin

Considerations

Types

- Type 1: dependent on exogenous insulin to live
- Type 2: does not need insulin to live (peripheral insulin resistance and insulin-secretory defect)
- Type 2 can present initially as DKA (diabetic ketoacidosis) in African-Americans or Hispanic descent patients
    - "Ketosis-prone type 2 diabetes mellitus (KPD)"
        - Usually obese, present with DKA as their first manifestation of diabetes but are subsequently found to have type 2 diabetes
        - African-Americans, or are of African, Hispanic or Caribbean descent
        - KPD has been reported to account for up to 60% of cases of new onset-diabetes with DKA in US African-American and Hispanic patients
- Hospital therapy for DKA in type 2 diabetes is the same as for type 1 diabetes.
- Gestational — appears with pregnancy only

Complications

- Increased infections

- Peripheral arterial insufficiency
- Skin ulcers and gangrene of lower legs and feet
- Hyperglycemic and hypoglycemic emergencies
- Pediatric cerebral edema with hyperglycemic emergencies

Vascular

- Retinopathy
- Renal insufficiency and failure
- Coronary arteries occlusion
- Aortic atherosclerosis
- Stroke

DKA

Definition

- Plasma glucose > 250 mg/dL (usually is > 350 mg/dL)
- Serum bicarbonate < 15 mEq/L
- Anion gap over 12
- Arterial pH <7.3 with moderate ketonemia

Common causes

- Secondary to stress
    - Infection most common
    - AMI
    - Pregnancy
    - Surgery

Differential Diagnoses

- Alcoholic ketoacidosis
- Appendicitis
- Hypophosphatemia
- Hypothermia
- Lactic acidosis
- Metabolic acidosis
- Myocardial infarction
- Pneumonia
- Salicylate toxicity
- Hyperosmolar Coma
- Pancreatitis
- Septic shock

- Sepsis
- UTI

Considerations

- Average adult fluid deficit is 6–10 liters (osmotic diuresis)
- Adjustment to serum Na (sodium) levels — each additional 100 mg% over plasma glucose of 100 add 1.6 mEq/L to serum Na levels to determine actual Na serum level
- Potassium body deficit can be severe despite initial normal serum level (a decrease of 0.3–0.7 mEq/L for each decrease of pH of 0.1)
    - Total body potassium deficit may be 3–5 mEq/kg
- IV PO4 (phosphorous) may be needed if respiratory failure occurs
- Venous pH add 0.03 to estimate arterial pH — if used instead of ABG to measure pH
- Serum osmolarity > 320 mOsm/L
- The overall mortality rate for DKA is 2% or less
    - Presence of deep coma at the time of diagnosis, hypothermia, and oliguria are signs of poor prognosis

Symptoms and findings (some or all)

- Polyuria
- Polydipsia (increased thirst)
- Weakness
- Weight loss
- Mental status changes
- Dry mucous membranes
- Tachycardia
- Nausea and vomiting
- Abdominal pain
- Kussmaul respirations (deep rapid breathing to partially compensate for metabolic acidosis)
- Peripheral vasodilatation can cause normothermia or hypothermia despite infection

Evaluation

- CBC
- BMP

- Accucheck
- Chest x-ray
- U/A
- ABG or venous pH (add 0.03 to adjust to arterial pH)
- Blood, urine or infected site cultures if infection suspected

Serum osmolality

- If < 320mOsm/L, look for another cause of altered mental status
- Osmolol gap > 10–20; suspect substance ingestion (normal < 10)
  - Gap = Osmolality measured – Osmolality calculated (Osmolality calculation equation: 2(Na+K) + glucose/18 + BUN/2.8; normal 280–300mOsm/L)
  - Ethanol mg%/4.6 is added to osmolol gap equation if present
  - Gap > 50 carries high specificity for toxic alcohol such as methanol, ethylene glycol, or isopropyl alcohol (treatment for toxic alcohol is fomepizole and may need emergent hemodialysis – check lactic acid level)

Fluid therapy

Adult

- IV NS infused 15–20 cc/kg/hour (1–1.5 liters average)
- Continue NS if corrected Na is low
- 0.45% NS at 4–14 cc/kg/hour after bolus infusion if "corrected" Na is normal or high
- Add potassium 20–30 mEq/L when serum K reaches < 5.3 mEq/L (if urine output 0.5–1 cc/kg/hour)

Pediatric (< 16 years of age)

- Initial fluid NS IV bolus 20 ml/kg
- May repeat IV fluid boluses if insufficient improvement in circulatory status
- Continued IV with 0.45% or NS after initial fluid therapy

  - Replace estimated fluid deficit over 24 - 36 hours
  - If altered mental status acutely occurs, suspect cerebral edema (treatment 1–2 gms/kg mannitol IV — per physician) — cerebral edema should not occur with IV fluids within proper fluid ranges

Insulin therapy

- Start after IV fluids given for one hour
- If patient is on an insulin pump, it should be stopped
- Check K^+ level first (can cause K^+ to drop; can be dangerous if already low; should be at least 3.3 mEq/L)
- 2011 JBDS guideline recommends the intravenous infusion of insulin at a weight-based fixed rate until ketosis has subsided
  - Should blood glucose fall below 14 mmol/L (250 mg/dL), 10% glucose should be added to allow for the continuation of fixed-rate insulin infusion

Adults

- Bolus 0.15 units/kg IV and/or continuous infusion 0.1 unit/kg/hour (up to 5–7 units/hour)
- Should decrease plasma glucose 50–75 mg%/hour (if not, check hydration status)

Pediatrics

- Insulin bolus not recommended
- Continuous infusion same as adult

Potassium

- Add potassium 20–40 mEq to each liter of IV fluids when serum $K^+ < 5.3$ if urine output 0.5–1 cc/kg/hour or initial potassium < 3.3 mEq/L
  - Serum K^+ 4.5–5.2 mEq/L give 10 mEq/hour IV
  - Serum K^+ 3.0–4.5 mEq/L give 20 mEq/hour IV
  - Serum K^+ initially < 3.0 mEq/L hold off starting insulin and give potassium IV

Consult criteria

- All DKA patients after initial assessment

Hyperglycemic Hyperosmolar Syndrome (HHS)

- Develops over days or weeks
- Plasma glucose > 600
- Serum osmolality > 320 mOsm
- Profound dehydration: adult 8–12 liters fluid deficit
- Small amount of ketonuria; small or absent ketonemia
- Serum bicarbonate > 15
- Arterial pH > 7.3
- Some alteration of consciousness
- Higher mortality than DKA

Associated medications contributing to HHS

- Diuretics
- Propranolol
- Calcium channel blockers
- Dilantin
- Cimetidine
- Corticosteroids

Evaluation

- Same as for DKA

Treatment options

- IV NS 10–20 cc/kg/hour; may repeat prn; should not exceed 50 cc/kg total over 4 hours
- Continued IV with $^{1}/_{2}$NS or NS at 5 cc/kg/hour after initial fluid therapy
- Add D5$^{1}/_{2}$NS or D5NS when plasma glucose reaches 300 mg/dL
- Start insulin infusion 0.1 unit/kg/hour (up to 5–7 units/hour) after first hour of IV fluid therapy
    - Insulin doses often lower than used in DKA

Potassium treatment

- Add potassium 20–40 mEq to each liter of IV fluids when serum K^+ < 5.3 mEq/L if urine output 0.5–1 cc/kg/hour or initial potassium < 3.3 mEq/L

- Serum K^+ 4.5–5.2 mEq/L give 10 mEq/hour IV
- Serum K^+ 3.0–4.5 mEq/L give 20 mEq/hour IV
- Serum K^+ initially < 3.0 mEq/L hold off starting insulin and give potassium IV

Consult criteria

- Notify physician on all HHS patients

Hypoglycemia

Definition

- < 50 mg/dL in men
- < 45 mg/dL in women
- < 40 mg/dL in infants and children

Differential diagnosis

- CVA
- TIA
- Epilepsy
- Multiple sclerosis
- Psychosis

Considerations

Caused by:

- Accidental or intentional overdose of diabetic medications
- Sepsis
- Alcohol use
- Decreased caloric intake

Symptoms

- Severity of symptoms depends on glucose level and rate of glucose decline
- Symptoms may be masked by beta-blockers
- Altered and decreased mental status
- Sweating
- Shaking
- Anxiety

Evaluation

- ABCs (*A*irway, Breathing, Circulation)

- IV
- Oxygen if hypoxic (avoid hyperoxia)
- Monitoring
- Accucheck
- History and physical exam
- Medication and food intake history
- Accucheck every 30 minutes × 2 hours or longer until stable glucose levels achieved
- BMP
- CBC if infection suspected
- Chest x-ray if pneumonia or aspiration suspected, or hypoxic
- U/A if infection suspected

Treatment options

- Awake and alert: complex calorie intake PO
- Altered mental status: IV D50W 1 amp adults (100 calories)
- D25W — 1 gm/kg in pediatrics not to exceed adult dose
- D12.5W for neonates (1 gm/kg)
- D10W drip at 75–100 cc/hour (adult) if repeat D50W boluses needed for recurrent hypoglycemia or hypoglycemic agent overdose
- Glucagon 1 mg IM if no IV access
    - May not work with depleted glycogen stores in malnutrition
        - Liver disease
        - Alcoholics
        - Neonates
- Octreotide can be used in sulfonylurea refractory hypoglycemia
- Hydrocortisone IV for adrenal insufficiency

Discharge criteria

- Stable glucose levels in diabetic patients on preexisting insulin therapy
- Good home support
- Reliable patient

Discharge instructions

- Hypoglycemia aftercare instructions

- Follow up with primary care provider within 12–24 hours

Consult criteria

- Oral hypoglycemia therapy (usually need admission)
- Fasting hypoglycemia not on diabetic medication
- Intentional insulin overdose
- Poor home situation
- Abnormal vital signs
- Continued altered mental status
- Significant comorbidities (cancer, hepatic disease, malnutrition, etc.)

Hyperglycemia without DKA or HHS

Considerations

- Most diabetic patients with elevated glucose levels are asymptomatic
- High glucose levels can affect body water balance
- Acute treatment for levels up to 400 mg/dL usually not needed unless there is a concurrent disease process

Common symptoms

- Polyuria
- Polydipsia (increased thirst)
- Weakness
- Blurred vision

Evaluation

- Glucose < 400 mg/dL without other disease processes or symptoms may not need further testing acutely in patient with history of poor control (if vital signs normal and mentation changes or comorbidities absent)
- Tests are directed to disease processes that may be elevating glucose levels
- BMP
- CBC if infection or inflammatory process suspected
- U/A if UTI suspected

Discharge criteria

- If new onset DM in obese adult patient without DKA or HHS and glucose ≤ 400
- Diabetic history with glucose ≤ 400 mg/dL
- No metabolic acidosis
- No dehydration
- Normal vital signs and no mentation changes

Discharge instructions

- Hyperglycemia aftercare instructions
- Follow up with primary care provider within 1–5 days
- Return if patient develops symptoms

Consult criteria

New onset

- New adult onset DM with glucose > 400 mg/dL
- New onset pediatric DM with glucose ≥ 200 mg/dL
- Hyperglycemia with metabolic acidosis (decreased serum CO_2 or elevated anion gap)

Diabetic patient with

- Significant comorbid symptoms
- Metabolic acidosis
- Vomiting
- Dehydration
- Tachycardia
- Hypotension
- Relative hypotension SBP < 105 with history of hypertension
- Orthostatic vital sign changes
- Progressive renal insufficiency creatinine increase > 1
- Adult heart rate ≥ 110
- Pediatric heart rate
    - 12–15 years ≥ 120
    - 16 years or older ≥ 115

Treatment for Type 2 Adult Diabetes If desired at discharge from acute care facility

Obese

Monotherapy

- Metformin 500 mg PO bid with or after meals × 1 week, increase weekly by 500 mg to achieve 1000 mg PO bid
  - Decreases HbA1c approximated 1.5%

Second drug if needed

- Glipizide (Glucotrol) 5 mg PO qday with breakfast (elderly 2.5 mg PO)

OR

- Consider GLP-1 agonist such as Exenatide (Byetta) 5 mcg SQ bid x 1 month and then may increase as needed to 10 mcg SQ bid
  - Give 1 hr. before AM and PM meals

OR

- Consider SLGT2 inhibitor such as Empagliflozin (Jardiance) 10 mg PO daily

Third drug if needed

- Insulin glargine 10 units SQ (or 0.2 units/kg) −adjust by 1 unit/day to achieve fasting glucose < 100 mg/dL

OR

- Sitagliptin (Januvia) 50 or 100 mg qday

Non-obese

Monotherapy

- Metformin 500 mg PO bid with or after meals × 1 week, increase weekly by 500 mg to achieve 1000 mg PO bid

OR

- Glipizide (Glucotrol) 5mg PO qday (elderly 2.5 mg PO)

Second drug if needed

- Metformin 500 mg PO bid with or after meals × 1 week, increase weekly by 500 mg to achieve 1000 mg PO bid

OR

- Glipizide 5mg (Glucotrol) PO qday (elderly 2.5 mg PO)

Third drug if needed

- Consider DLP-1 Agonist such as Exenatide (Byetta) 5 mcg SQ bid x 1 month and then may increase as needed to 10 mcg SQ bid
  - Give 1 hr. before AM and PM meals

OR

- Insulin glargine 10 units SQ – adjust by 1 unit/day to achieve fasting glucose < 100 mg/dL

Elderly

Monotherapy

- Metformin 500 mg bid with or after meals x 1 week, increase weekly by 500 mg to achieve 1000 mg PO bid
- If unable to tolerate metformin, consider repaglinide (Prandin) 0.5–4 mg PO up to qid ac (not to exceed 16 mg daily)

Monotherapy failure

- Consider DPP–4 inhibitor such as Januvia (Sitagliptin) 50 mg PO daily

OR

- Consider switch to long acting insulin 10 units SQ bedtime

Asians

Monotherapy

- Pioglitazone (Actos) 30 mg PO qday — do not use in bladder cancer, history of bladder cancer, moderate or severe hepatic disease or symptomatic heart failure (NYHA class 3 or 4)

Second drug if needed

- Metformin 500 mg PO bid with or after meals × 1 week, increase weekly by 500 mg to achieve 1,000 mg PO bid

Third drug if needed

- Glipizide or glimepiride

  OR

- Exenatide (Byetta) 5 mcg SQ bid x 1 month and then may increase as needed to 10 mcg SQ bid (not FDA approved with Actos)
  - Give 1 hr. before AM and PM meals

  OR

- Insulin glargine 10 units SQ — adjust by 1 unit/day to achieve fasting glucose < 100 mg/dL

Symptomatic patients

- Repaglinide (Prandin) 0.5–4 mg PO up to qid ac (not to exceed 16 mg qday) or insulin to decrease glucose at start of monotherapy initiation

Diabetic medications, mechanism of actions and clinical effects

Biguanides

- Metformin is the only biguanide in clinical use
- Initial drug of choice
- Decreases hepatic gluconeogenesis production
- Decreases intestinal absorption of glucose
- improves insulin sensitivity by increasing peripheral glucose uptake and utilization
- Unlike oral sulfonylureas, metformin rarely causes hypoglycemia
- Significant improvements in hemoglobin A1c and lipid profile
- Only oral diabetes drug that reliably facilitates modest weight loss
- Probably improves macrovascular risk
- Lactic acidosis during metformin use is very rare

Sulfonylureas

- Glyburide, glipizide and glimepiride
- Stimulate insulin release from pancreatic beta cells
- Indicated for use as adjuncts to diet and exercise in adult patients with type 2 diabetes mellitus
- Generally well-tolerated, with hypoglycemia the most common side effect
- Glyburide had highest cardiovascular mortality (7.5%) compared with other sulfonylureas, such as gliclazide and glimepiride (2.7%) and raises question of whether it should be used

Meglitinide derivatives

- Repaglinide and nateglinide
- Much shorter-acting insulin secretagogues (stimulate insulin release) than the sulfonylureas
- Can be used as monotherapy
- If adequate glycemic control is not achieved, then metformin or a thiazolidinedione may be added

Alpha-glucosidase inhibitors

- Acarbose (Precose) and Miglitol (Glyset)
- Delay sugar absorption and help to prevent postprandial glucose surges
- Induction of flatulence greatly limits their use

Thiazolidinediones (TZDs)

- Pioglitazone (Actos) and rosiglitazone (Avandia)
- Insulin sensitizers and require presence of insulin to work
- May be used as monotherapy or in combination with sulfonylurea, metformin, meglitinide, DPP-4 inhibitors, GLP-1 receptor agonists, or insulin
- Only antidiabetic agents that have been shown to slow the progression of diabetes (particularly in early disease)
- Edema (including macular edema) and weight gain may be problematic adverse effects

- May induce or worsen heart failure in patients with left ventricular compromise and occasionally in patients with normal left ventricular function
- Food and Drug Administration (FDA) currently recommends not prescribing pioglitazone for patients with active bladder cancer and using it with caution in patients with a history of bladder cancer
- In women with type 2 diabetes, long-term (i.e., 1 y or longer) use of TZDs doubles the risk of fracture
- Elevated risk of myocardial infarction in patients treated with rosiglitazone (FDA limits to patients already being successfully treated with this agent and to patients whose blood sugar cannot be controlled with other antidiabetic medicines and who do not wish to use pioglitazone)

Glucagonlike peptide–1 (GLP-1) agonists

- Exenatide, liraglutide, albiglutide and dulaglutide
- Stimulate glucose-dependent insulin release
- Reduce glucagon and slow gastric emptying
- GLP-1 in addition to metformin and/or a sulfonylurea may result in modest weight loss

Dipeptidyl peptidase IV (DPP-4) inhibitors

- Sitagliptin, saxagliptin and linagliptin
- Prolong the action of incretin hormones (stimulate insulin secretion)
- May be added, if inadequate diabetic control, to metformin and sulfonylurea combination improving glycemic control
- Saxagliptin and alogliptin may increase heart failure risk, especially in patients with preexisting heart or renal disease

Selective sodium-glucose transporter-2 (SGLT-2) inhibitors

- Canagliflozin, dapagliflozin (Farxiga) and empagliflozin
- Increased urinary glucose excretion

- Adjunct to diet and exercise to improve glycemic control
- Renal dosing adjustments and warnings
- Dapagliflozin is indicated as monotherapy, as initial therapy with metformin, or as an add-on to other oral glucose-lowering agents, including metformin, pioglitazone, glimepiride, sitagliptin, and insulin

Insulins

- Many patients with type 2 diabetes mellitus become markedly insulinopenic
- Most patients are insulin resistant
- Small changes in insulin dosage may make no difference in glycemia in some patients
- Therapy must be individualized in each patient
- For lowering postprandial glucose, premixed insulin analogues are more effective than either long-acting insulin analogues alone or premixed neutral protamine Hagedorn (NPH)/regular human insulin 70/30
- For lowering HbA1c, premixed insulin analogues are as effective as premixed NPH/regular human insulin 70/30 and more effective than long-acting insulin analogues
- The frequency of hypoglycemia reported with premixed insulin analogues is similar to that with premixed human insulin and higher than that with oral antidiabetic agents

Amylinomimetics

- Pramlintide
- Mimics the effects of endogenous amylin, which is secreted by pancreatic beta cells
- Delays gastric emptying, decreases postprandial glucagon release, and modulates appetite

Bile acid sequestrants

- Colesevelam
- Developed as lipid-lowering agents for the treatment of hypercholesterolemia but were subsequently found to have a glucose-lowering effect

- Adjunctive therapy to improve glycemic control
- Favorable, but insignificant, impact on FPG and HbA1c levels

Dopamine agonists

- Bromocriptine mesylate (Cycloset)
- Adjunct to diet and exercise to improve glycemic control in adults with type 2 diabetes mellitus
- May be considered for obese patients who do not tolerate other diabetes medications or who need only a minimal reduction in HbA1c to reach their glycemic goal
- Can cause orthostatic hypotension and syncope

Agency for Healthcare Research and Quality

- AHRQ concluded that although the long-term benefits and harms of diabetes medications remain unclear, the evidence supports the use of metformin as a first-line agent
- On average, monotherapy with many of the oral diabetes drugs reduces HbA1c levels by 1 percentage point (although metformin has been found to be more efficacious than the DPP-4 inhibitors), and 2-drug combination therapies reduce HbA1c about 1 percentage point more than do monotherapies

Other AHRQ findings included the following:

- Metformin decreased LDL cholesterol levels more relative to pioglitazone, sulfonylureas, and DPP-4 inhibitors
- Unfavorable effects on weight were greater with TZDs and sulfonylureas than with metformin (mean difference of +2.6 kg)
- Risk of mild or moderate hypoglycemia was 4-fold higher with sulfonylureas than with metformin alone; this risk was more than 5-fold higher with sulfonylureas plus metformin than with a TZD plus metformin
- Risk of heart failure was higher with TZDs than with sulfonylureas

- Risk of bone fractures was higher with TZDs than with metformin

Notes

References:

Umpierrez, GE, et al. Narrative review: ketosis-prone type 2 diabetes mellitus *Ann Intern Med* 2006;144: 350

Type 2 Diabetes Mellitus Treatment & Management
Author: Romesh Khardori, MD, PhD, FACP; Chief Editor: George T Griffing emedicine.medscape.com/article/117853

Type 1 Diabetes Mellitus Author: Romesh Khardori, MD, PhD, FACP; Chief Editor: George T Griffing, MD
emedicine.medscape.com/article/117739

Diabetic Ketoacidosis Author: Vasudevan A Raghavan, MBBS, MD, MRCP(UK); Chief Editor: Romesh Khardori, MD, PhD, FACP
emedicine.medscape.com/article/118361

Savage MW, Dhatariya KK, Kilvert A, Rayman G, Rees JA, Courtney CH, et al. Joint British Diabetes Societies guideline for the management of diabetic ketoacidosis. *Diabet Med*. May 2011;28(5):508–15

Acute Hypoglycemia Author: Frank C Smeeks III, MD; Chief Editor: Erik D Schraga, MD
emedicine.medscape.com/article/767359

Effectivehealthcare.ahrq.gov/ehc/products/155/644/CER27_OralDiabetesMeds_20110623.pdf

Ped Emerg Care;31:376

Diabetic ketoacidosis; Davie E. Trachtenbarg, M.D., *University of Illinois College of Medicine, Peoria, Illinois*
Am Fam Physician. 2005 May 1;71(9):1705-1714

Kuppermann N, et al. *N Engl J Med*. 2018;378(24): 2275-2287.

Glaser N, Kuppermann N. *Pediatr Diabetes*. 2018 Nov 11

HYPOTHYROIDISM PROTOCOL

When using any protocol, always follow the Guidelines of Proper Use (page 18).

Definition

- Deficiency or lack of thyroid hormone that causes slowing of metabolic processes

Differential Diagnosis

- Hypothermia
- Sepsis
- Depression
- Constipation
- Addison's disease
- Chronic fatigue syndrome
- Dysmenorrhea
- Goiter — lithium induced
- Nontoxic goiter
- Hypopituitarism
- Subacute thyroiditis
- Iodine deficiency
- Ovarian insufficiency
- Prolactin deficiency

Considerations

- Deficiency of thyroid hormone
- Develops over months to years
- Primary hypothyroidism 95% of cases
- Secondary hypothyroidism 5% of cases
- Postpartum thyroiditis is 5% and usually occurs 3–6 months after delivery
- Myxedema coma is a rare, life threatening condition usually of elderly women
  - Precipitated by environmental stress, infection and medications
  - Frequently a clinical diagnosis initially

Signs and symptoms

- Goiter

- Cold intolerance
- Hypothermia
- Bradycardia
- Lethargy
- Depression
- Hair loss
- Dry coarse skin
- Weight gain
- Constipation
- Headache
- Husky voice
- Deep tendon ankle jerk reflex with prolonged recovery phase
- Ataxia

Causes

- Idiopathic
- Iodine deficiency (most common cause worldwide)
- Hashimoto's thyroiditis (most common cause in U.S.)
- Radioiodine treatment for hyperthyroidism (Grave's disease)
- Thyroid resection
- Lithium
- Amiodarone
- Dilantin
- Carbamazepine
- Iodides
- Pituitary or hypothalamic disorders: tumor, radiation, surgery, sarcoidosis
- Postpartum

Evaluation

- Complete history and physical examination

Testing options depending on history and findings

- CBC (may be anemic)
- BMP (reversible increases in creatinine)
- Chest x-ray for pericardial effusions and cardiomegaly
- ABG if respiratory insufficiency present

- EKG
- U/A
- Thyroid stimulating hormone (TSH) is elevated with low FTI (free thyroxin index) or T4
    - Mild disease if FTI or T4 normal
- Thyroid function tests if available
- Routine screening at age 35 and every 5 years after that
    - Closer attention to pregnant females or females > age 60, type-1 diabetes or autoimmune disease, or with history of neck irradiation

Treatment Options

- Preferable for primary care provider to start thyroid hormone replacement
- Clinical benefits occur in 3–5 days
- Adjust levothyroxine every 6–8 weeks until reference range of TSH achieved
- May take months to achieve target TSH reference range
    - Levothyroxin (Synthroid) 0.1 mg PO qday — age ≤ 60 years
    - Levothyroxin (Synthroid) 0.025–0.05 mg PO qday — age > 60 years (1/4–1/2 of this dose if there is history of heart disease)

Myxedema coma — notify physician immediately

- End of spectrum of hypothyroidism
- IV NS/LR as needed for hypotension
- Levothyroxine 400 mcg IV slow infusion
- May need intubation
- Hydrocortisone sodium succinate (Solu–Cortef) 100 mg IV
- Treat any infection
- Passive rewarming

Discharge Criteria

- Mild disease

Discharge instructions

- Hypothyroidism aftercare instructions

- Follow up with primary care provider within 7 days if seen in acute care facility
- Return if worse

Consult Criteria

- Unstable patient
- Altered mental status
- Hypothermia
- Metabolic or respiratory acidosis
- Respiratory insufficiency
- Refer to General Patient Criteria Protocol (page 22)

Notes

References:

Kreisman SH, Hennessey JV. Consistent reversible elevations of serum creatinine levels in severe hypothyroidism.*Arch Intern Med*. Jan 11 1999;159(1):79–82

Ladenson PW, Singer PA, Ain KB, Bagchi N, Bigos ST, Levy EG, et al. American Thyroid Association guidelines for detection of thyroid dysfunction. *Arch Intern Med*. Jun 12 2000;160(11):1573–5

Hypothyroidism
Author: Philip R Orlander, MD; Chief Editor: George T Griffing, MD emedicine.medscape.com/article/122393

HYPERTHYROIDISM PROTOCOL

When using any protocol, always follow the Guidelines of Proper Use (page 18).

Definition

- Condition from excess thyroid hormone

Differential Diagnosis

- Panic disorder
- Septic shock
- Delirium tremens
- Neuroleptic malignant syndrome
- Serotonin syndrome
- Withdrawal syndromes
- Heat illness
- Cocaine toxicity
- Sympathomimetic drug overdose
- Congestive heart failure
- Pheochromocytoma
- Pregnancy

Considerations

- Grave's disease most common form — autoimmune disease
- 1–2% of patients progress to thyroid storm
- Thyroid storm is potentially fatal
- Normal TSH usually excludes hyperthyroidism

Treatment considerations

- Counteracting the peripheral effects of thyroid hormones
- Inhibition of thyroid hormone synthesis
- Treatment of systemic complications
- These measures should bring about clinical improvement within 12–24 hours
- Cardiopulmonary failure mostly likely cause of death, particularly in the elderly
- Beta blockage can cause collapse

Signs and Symptoms

- Tachycardia
- Weight loss
- Heat intolerance
- Fever
- Diaphoresis
- Dehydration
- Diarrhea
- Goiter
- Hypotension
- Atrial fibrillation
- Exophthalmos and lid lag (Grave's disease only)
- Fine tremor

Causes

- Grave's disease — most common
- Idiopathic — second most common (toxic multinodular goiter)
- Subacute thyroiditis
- Postpartum thyroiditis
- Overdose of thyroid hormone
- Iodine induced
- Amiodarone (high iodine content or induces autoimmune thyroid disease)

Thyroid storm

- Normal TSH usually excludes thyroid storm
- Is a clinical diagnosis initially and start treatment early
- Thyroid function tests do not differentiate between thyrotoxicosis and thyroid storm
- LFT's elevated and hyperglycemia may be present

Severe symptoms

- Shock (use isotonic fluid resuscitation) — avoid norepinephrine as it can worsen symptoms
- Fever
- Altered mental status
- Psychosis
- CHF

- Jaundice

Precipitated by

- Stress
- Infection
- Surgery
- Cardiovascular events
- Preeclampsia
- DKA or HHS
- Stopping antithyroid medication
- Vigorous palpation of thyroid

Evaluation

- Complete history and physical examination

Testing

- CBC
- BMP
- Calcium
- LFT's
- EKG
- Thyroid function tests
- TSH

Treatment Options

- O_2 supplemental
- Tylenol for fever (no aspirin)

Mild hyperthyroidism

- Methimazole 15 mg/day PO divided q8hr initially (drug of choice)

Moderate thyrotoxicosis

- Methimazole 30–40 mg/day PO divided q8hr initially (drug of choice)
- PTU 150–450 mg/day PO or NG tube (second–line drug to methimazole)
- Propranolol 20–40 mg PO q4hr until tachycardia controlled (also blocks conversion of T4 to T3)
- Decadron (dexamethasone) 2 mg PO or IV q6h to q8hr in adults
- Decadron (dexamethasone) 0.15 mg/kg/dose PO or IV q6hr in pediatrics (not to exceed adult dose)

Thyroid storm treatment options

- IV NS 100–200 cc/hr in adults or higher if needed for vital sign findings
- IV NS 1–3 times daily fluid maintenance prn for pediatrics
- IV LR/NS hydration usually needed for volume contraction

Propylthiouracil (PTU)

- Adult: 600–1,000 mg PO or 200–300 mg q4–6h PO/NG (preferred over methimazole in thyroid storm)
- Pediatric: 5–7 mg/kg/day

Methimazole

- 20–30 mg q6–12hr for short term, then reduce dosage to maintenance (5–15 mg/day) or reduce frequency to q12hr or q24hr

SSKI

- 1–5 drops PO 1–2 hours after PTU
    - Earlier than this can increase release of thyroid hormone from the thyroid

Decadron (dexamethasone)

- Adult: 2 mg IV q6hr
- Pediatric: 0.15 mg/kg IV

Propranolol

- 1–2 mg IV; repeat q 10–15 min. prn (caution with CHF and DKA)

Outpatient treatment (Graves disease)

- Methimazole 10–20 mg/day PO (drug of choice)
    - After euthyroidism is achieved, reduce dosage by 50% and administer for 12–18 months
- PTU can be used if pregnant in 1st trimester or contraindications/allergy to methimazole
    - Initiate PTU 150 mg PO qday divided q8h (second-line drug to methimazole)
    - Taper and discontinue if euthyroidism restored (TSH) is normal

Discharge Criteria

- Mildly symptomatic patients that respond to therapy

Discharge instructions

- Hyperthyroidism aftercare instructions
- Follow up with primary care provider or endocrinologist within 1–2 days

Consult Criteria

- Moderate thyrotoxicosis
- Fever
- Thyroid storm — notify physician immediately
- Adult heart rate ≥ 110
- Pediatric heart rate
  - 0–4 months ≥ 180
  - 5–7 months ≥ 175
  - 8–12 months ≥ 170
  - 1–3 years ≥ 160
  - 4–5 years ≥ 145
  - 6–8 years ≥ 130
  - 9–11 years ≥ 125
  - 12–15 years ≥ 115
  - 16 years or older ≥ 110

Notes

References:

Dtsch Med Wochenschr. 2008 Mar;133(10):479–84. doi: 10.1055/s-2008–1046737. Thyroid storm--thyrotoxic crisis: an update

Hyperthyroidism, Thyroid Storm, and Graves Disease Author: Erik D Schraga, MD; Chief Editor: Romesh Khardori, MD, PhD, FACP emedicine.medscape.com/article/767130

Toxic Ingestions

Section Contents — one protocol

When using any protocol, always follow the Guidelines of Proper Use (page 18).

TOXICOLOGY PROTOCOL

When using any protocol, always follow the Guidelines of Proper Use (page 18).

Considerations

Principles of toxicology

- Reduce exposure (remove from skin and environment)
- Reduce absorption
- Increase elimination
- Supportive care
- Give specific therapy and antidotes when appropriate

Pearls

- Most pediatric accidental ingestions of common OTC medications are of low dose and may require only observation for 2–4 hours
- Intentional ingestions require acute psychiatric intervention
- Ascertain types and amount of ingestions

Syrup of Ipecac not usually recommended

Activated charcoal

- Usually of no benefit
- Can be used if no aspiration risk < 1 hour post ingestion with serious ingestions
- May be considered > 1 hour post serious ingestion with agents that delay absorption or GI transit

Orogastric lavage use indications

- Presentations approximately within one hour post-ingestion
- No known antidote
- Substance does not bind activated charcoal

Whole bowel irrigation indications and considerations

- With lithium and iron ingestion
- In "body stuffers"
- Beware of aspiration risk

- Avoid with decreased bowel sounds, surgical abdomen, hypotension

Toxidromes (causes and symptoms)

Opioids

Agents

- Narcotics

Findings

- CNS depression
- Respiratory depression
- Miosis

Sympathomimetics

Agents

- Cocaine
- Amphetamine

Findings

- Agitation
- Pupil dilation
- Diaphoresis
- Tachycardia
- Hypertension
- Hyperthermia

Cholinergic

Agents

- Insecticides

Findings

- Salivation
- Lacrimation
- Diaphoresis
- Nausea
- Vomiting
- Urination
- Defecation
- Muscle fasciculations
- Weakness
- Bronchorrhea

Anticholinergic

Agents

- Antihistamines
- Atropine
- Scopolamine

Findings

- Altered mental status
- Dilated pupils
- Dry/flushed skin and mucous membranes
- Urinary retention
- Decreased bowel sounds
- Hyperthermia

Salicylates

Agents

- Aspirin
- Oil of wintergreen (1 tsp lethal in child weighing < 10 kg; 1 cc has 14 gms of salicylate)

Findings

- Tachypnea
- Respiratory alkalosis
- Metabolic acidosis
- Altered mental status
- Tinnitus
- Tachycardia
- Nausea
- Vomiting
- Diaphoresis

Hypoglycemia

Agents

- Oral hypoglycemia agents
- Insulin

Findings

- Altered mental status
- Diaphoresis
- Tachycardia
- Hypertension

Serotonin syndrome

Agents

- Meperidine or dextromethorphan + MAOI
- SSRI (selective serotonin reuptake inhibitor) + tricyclic antidepressant
- SSRI + amphetamine
- Tricyclic antidepressant + amphetamine
- MAOI + amphetamine
- SSRI overdose

Findings

- Altered mental status
- Increased muscle tone
- Hyperreflexia
- Hyperthermia

Evaluation

- Complete history and physical exam
- Contact Poison Control Center or consult physician
- Monitoring and EKG with potentially toxic ingestions
- Send someone to patient's home to obtain ingestants if necessary
- CMP
- Specific drugs levels if available
- Calculate anion gap: Na – Cl – HCO3
- CT head for altered mental status not clearly attributable to toxin/overdose/ingestion
- Evaluate for comorbid conditions
- ASA and acetaminophen nomograms as indicated

Anion gap mnemonic — A CAT MUDPILES

A – Alcoholic ketoacidosis
C – Cyanide; carbon monoxide
A – Aspirin; other salicylates
T – Toluene
M – Methanol; metformin
U – Uremia
D – DKA
P – Paraldehyde; phenformin
I – Iron; INH
L – Lactic acidosis
E – Ethylene glycol
S – Starvation

Osmolol gap ≥ 10–20 suspect substance ingestion (Normal < 10)

- Gap = Osmolality measured – Osmolality calculated (calculation equation: 2(Na+K) + glucose/18 + BUN/2.8; normal 280–300mOsm/L)
- Ethanol mg%/4.6 is added to osmolol gap equation if present
- Gap > 50 carries high specificity for toxic alcohol such as methanol, ethylene glycol, or isopropyl alcohol
- Normal gap < 10

Treatment Options

- Nontoxic ingestions: observation and discharge with instructions and follow up
- Suspected toxic ingestions: refer to previous Considerations section and contact Poison Control Center or consult physician
- IV NS
- Hypotension
    - Adult IV NS 500–1000 cc bolus if hypotensive (consult physician), may repeat if needed
    - Pediatrics 20 cc/kg IV NS bolus, may repeat × 2 prn (consult physician)
- Specific antidotes per physician (or poison control center)
- Coma cocktail

- Dextrose
- Naloxone (Narcan)
- Thiamine
- Flumazenil (Is thought to increase seizure in benzodiazepine overdose or chronic users—this is controversial)
    - Recent data suggest low risk of seizure
    - Seizure patients may have keppra or valproic acid treatment with flumazenil

Hemodialysis indications for severe ingestions

- Ethylene glycol or methanol (fomepizole should be given also as treatment)
- Salicylate
    - Level > 90 in acute ingestion
    - Level > 60 in chronic ingestion
    - Severe symptoms
    - Unable to alkalinize urine in a less severe ingestion
    - Large ingestion (death may result if not hemodialyzed promptly)
- Phenobarbital
- Theophylline
- Lithium
- Valproic acid level > 750 or severe symptoms
- Diethylene glycol
- Massive acetaminophen ingestion > 1000 mg/kg if early post-ingestion

Seizures

- Adult: lorazepam 2–6 mg IV; may repeat q10–15 minutes prn
- Pediatric: lorazepam 0.05–0.1 mg/kg IV; may repeat q10–15 minutes prn (NMT 10 mg)
- If no IV available in children, use Diastat (diazepam rectal gel)
    - Age up to 5 years: 0.5 mg/kg
    - Age 6–11 years: 0.3 mg/kg
    - Age > 12 years: 0.2 mg/kg
    - Round up to available dose: 2.5, 5, 7.5, 10, 12.5, 15, 17.5, 20 mg/dose

- Midazolam IV/IM/PR/ET/intranasal 0.1–0.2 mg/kg/dose; not to exceed a cumulative dose of 10 mg)

Antidotes (if clinically indicated)

- Acetaminophen: N-acetylcysteine
  - Give if ingestion suspected with elevated ALT
  - Give even if acetaminophen induced hepatic failure present and acetaminophen no longer measurable
- Anticholinergic: physostigmine
- Benzodiazepines: flumazenil (thought to increase seizure potential — controversial)
  - Recent data suggest low risk of seizure
  - Seizure patients may have keppra or valproic acid treatment with flumazenil
- Beta-blockers: glucagon
- Calcium channel blockers: calcium chloride, insulin
- Calcium channel blocker severe toxicity
  - CaCl 1–3 gms (10–30 mg/kg) q30 min. prn up to 8 doses
  - High dose insulin therapy
    - Bolus of 0.5–1 Unit/kg, followed by a drip with a rate of 0.5–1 Unit/kg/hr
    - If blood glucose < 250 give supplemental IV glucose (D10)
    - Accucheck q15 min. to avoid hypoglycemia
  - Levophed IV if hypotensive per physician
- Carbon monoxide: 100% FiO_2
  - Consider immediate transfer to hyperbaric facility
    - Levels above 40%
    - Cardiovascular or neurologic impairment
    - Persistent impairment after 4 hours of oxygen therapy necessitates transfer to a hyperbaric facility
    - Pregnant patients with lower carboxyhemoglobin levels (above 15%)
- Coumadin (warfarin): vitamin K, FFP
- Cyanide: cyanide antidote kit

- Digoxin (digitalis): digibind
- Ethylene glycol and methanol: fomepizole
    - Osmolol gap ≥ 10 = treatment indicated
    - Large ingestion is indication for stat hemodialysis
- Iron: deferoxamine
- INH: pyridoxine (vitamin B6)
- Methemoglobinemia: methylene blue
- Organophosphates: atropine and/or PAM, atrovent aerosol for bronchospasm
- Tricyclic antidepressants: NaHCO3 IV
- Opiates: narcan (naloxone) for toxic narcotic overdose
    - For adults: 0.4–2 mg IV or IM
    - For pediatrics: narcan (naloxone) 0.1 mg/kg IV or IM (NMT 2 mg)
    - Reports and animal data available only

Lipid Emulsion Therapy

- Start ACLS
- Mainstream therapy
- Safe
- Used in cardiac arrest due to a single agent
    - Bupivacaine (intra-arterial injection)
    - Verapamil
    - Amitriptyline
    - An unknown agent
- An initial bolus of 20% lipid emulsion at a dose of 1.5 mL/kg
    - Bolus could be repeated 1–2 times for persistent asystole
- Followed by an infusion at a rate of 0.25 ml/kg/min for 30–60 minutes
- Infusion rate could be increased if the BP declines
- Interferes with some laboratory measurements
    - Serum glucose concentrations when determined by colorimetric testing
    - Serum magnesium
    - Creatinine, lipase, ALT, CPK and bilirubin become unmeasurable

Discharge Criteria

- Psychiatrically cleared
- No toxicity present or is totally detoxified
- Hemodynamically stable
- Good follow up and home situation

Discharge instructions

- Drug or substance ingestion aftercare instructions
- Refer for substance abuse treatment as indicated
- Follow up with PCP within 1 days as needed
- Return if worse

Consult Criteria

- Notify physician immediately for potentially dangerous ingestions or toxicity
    - Unstable vital signs
    - Metabolic acidosis
    - Osmolol gap ≥ 10
    - Altered mental status
- Acetaminophen ingestion
    - Pre-school child of 200 mg/kg or greater
    - Older child and adult > 150 mg/kg or total dose of 7.5 gms
    - Nomogram positive for toxicity
    - Liver function abnormalities
    - Delayed presentation
- Aspirin 150 mg/kg or serum level > 40 mg%
    - Lethal dose 300 mg/kg
- Discuss toxic ingestions with physician

Notes

References: Lipidrescue.org recommended as reading for those interested in this therapy

Christian MR, et al. *J Med Toxicol* 2013 May 10

Grunbaum AM, et al. *Clin Toxicol (Phila)* 2012;50:812–7

Carbon Monoxide Toxicity Treatment & Management
Author: Guy N Shochat, MD; Chief Editor: Asim Tarabar, MD
emedicine.medscape.com/article/819987

Flumazenil Revisited Williams JS, Lee MA, Schauben J, Nasca L, Kalynynch C/University of Florida, Jacksonville, FL

Neurology

Section Contents

When using any protocol, always follow the Guidelines of Proper Use (page 18).

HEADACHE PROTOCOL

When using any protocol, always follow the Guidelines of Proper Use (page 18).

Definition

- Cephalic pain disorder

Differential Diagnosis

- Tension headache
- Migraine headache
- Cluster headache
- Sinusitis
- Otitis media
- Trigeminal neuralgia
- Brain tumor
- Subarachnoid hemorrhage
- Subdural hematoma
- Epidural hematoma
- Temporal arteritis
- Chronic daily headache
- Thunderclap headache
- Analgesic rebound headache
- CVA
- Meningitis
- Encephalitis
- Normal pressure hydrocephalus
- Ventricular peritoneal shunt malfunction
- Temporal mandibular joint disorder

Considerations

- "Functional" or "Primary" headache
  - No detectable cause (common)
  - Migraine
  - Cluster
  - Headache tension type
- "Organic" or "Secondary"
  - From pain sensitive structures; vessels; periosteum
  - Post-concussion headaches
  - Spinal tap headaches

- History is one of the more important tools in headache evaluation
- New headache type in elderly is suggestive of a higher risk process
- Do not use response to therapy to judge seriousness of headache
- Subarachnoid hemorrhage (SAH) up to 1% of all headaches in ED
    - Sudden onset and reaching maximal intensity in seconds to minutes
    - 1/3 not exertional
    - May awake with SAH
    - Sentinel leak in SAH headache may improve over time

Lumbar puncture for possible SAH evaluation

- Xanthochromia is formed by the breakdown of hemoglobin and can take 2-12 hours to develop
- Xanthochromia will be present in up to 20% of patients with SAH who have an LP within 6 hours of headache onset
- Xanthochromia approaches 100% after 12 hours

Historical red flag headaches

- Sudden onset or onset with exertion
- New, progressive, frequent headaches
- Trauma
- Cancer history
- Immunosuppression/HIV
- Clotting disorders
- First headache
- Worst headache
- Fever

Evaluation

- Complete history and physical exam
- Check gait, motor and sensory exam
- Funduscopic exam

Lab (usually not needed in most headaches)

- CBC
- ESR (age > 50 years: temporal arteritis) — not needed with no changes in chronic headache pattern
- Carbon monoxide level prn

- UCG prn

Benign Headaches — Tension, Migraine, Cluster

General treatment options for all types of benign headaches

- Decadron (dexamethasone) 10 mg IV or IM for adults may be ordered, when not contraindicated, to decrease return visits for same headache
- O_2 therapy can be given for all types of headaches
- Lidocaine 1 cc of a 4% solution placed on a swab in each nostril for 5 minutes is potentially helpful
    - May repeat in 15 minutes

Tension headache

- Pressing or tightening (nonpulsatile quality)
- Frontal-occipital location
- Bilateral: mild/moderate intensity
- Not aggravated by physical activity

Treatment

- NSAID's PO prn
- Tylenol prn
- Fiorinal 1–2 PO q4hr prn not to exceed 6 per 24 hour period
- Midrin 1–2 caps qid PO prn
- Decadron 10 mg IV/IM decreases recurrence of headache at 48–72 hours

Migraine

Associated with:

- Photophobia
- Phonophobia
- Nausea and vomiting
- May be unilateral or bilateral
- Aura occurs 20%
    - Scotoma (blind spots)
    - Fortification (zigzag patterns)
    - Scintilla (flashing lights)
    - Unilateral paresthesia/weakness

  - Hallucinations
  - Hemianopsia
- The unilateral motor weakness associated with a hemiplegic migraine typically lasts from 5 minutes to 72 hours

Migraine risk factors

- Increased levels of C-reactive protein
- Increased body weight
- High blood pressure
- Hypercholesterolemia
- Impaired insulin sensitivity
- High homocysteine levels
- Stroke
- Coronary heart disease

Evaluation

- Don't perform neuroimaging studies in patients with stable headaches that meet criteria for migraine
- Don't perform computed tomography imaging for headache when magnetic resonance imaging is available, except in emergency settings

Indications for neuro imaging

- See related section below

Treatment options

- Compazine (prochlorperazine) 5–10 mg IV or IM
- Thorazine (chlorpromazine) 75 mg with Benadryl (diphenhydramine) 25 mg IM
- Ergots DHE 1 mg IV or IM
- Reglan (metoclopramide) 10 mg IV or IM
- Sumatriptan 6 mg SQ (do not use with history of coronary artery disease) — read drug information
- Maxalt (rizatriptan) 5–10 mg PO q2h prn for headache not to exceed 30 mg/d (do not use with history of coronary artery disease) — read drug information
- Midrin 2 caps PO initially then 1 cap PO q1hr prn not to exceed 5 caps/day
- Toradol (ketorolac) 30–60 mg IM (do not use if creatinine is elevated)

- Compazine suppository (prochlorperazine) 25 mg PR bid prn
- Don't prescribe opioid or butalbital-containing medications as first-line treatment for recurrent headache disorders
- Don't recommend prolonged or frequent use of over-the-counter pain medications for headache
- Narcotic prn (not as preferred)
- Decadron 10 mg IV/IM decreases recurrence of headache at 48–72 hours

Intractable migraine (lasting > 72 hours)

- IV valproate up to 1 gm IV
- Dihydroergotamine 1 mg IV/IM/SQ
- May need hospital admission

Cluster

- Lancinating and severe
- Sudden onset — peaks in 10–15 minutes
- Unilateral facial
- Duration: 10 minutes to 3 hours per episode
- Character: boring and lancinating to eye
- Distribution: first and second divisions of the trigeminal nerve (approximately 18–20% of patients complain of pain in extratrigeminal regions)
- Frequency: may occur several times a day for 1–4 months (often nocturnal)
- Periodicity: circadian regularity in 47%
- Remission: long symptom-free intervals occur in some patients 2 months to 20 years

Treatment options

- O_2 8 LPM face mask or 100% nonrebreather mask
- Sumatriptan 6 mg SQ (do not use with history of coronary artery disease) — read drug information
- Lidocaine 1 cc of a 10% solution placed on a swab in each nostril for 5 minutes is potentially helpful
- Capsaicin applied intranasally (has a burning sensation side effect)

Trigeminal neuralgia

- Commonly idiopathic

- Shock like severe pains in the distribution of trigeminal nerve
- Onset usually around age 60–70 years of age
- Pains last seconds to less than 2 minutes
- Can be triggered by specific activities such as eating, talking, brushing teeth, etc.
- No associated neurologic deficits
    - A sensory deficit excludes the diagnosis

Glossopharyngeal neuralgia

- Pain is over the distribution of glossopharyngeal nerve triggered by coughing, yawing, swallowing cold liquids

Occipital neuralgia

- Pain is in the posterior scalp region

Treatment options of cranial neuralgias

- Carbamazepine 200 mg PO bid to start (DOC)
    - Titrate increasing dose every 3 days by 200 mg
    - Effective dose is usually 600–1200 mg qday
    - Instruct patient they will need monitoring for aplastic anemia and severe leucopenia
- Dilantin (phenytoin) for carbamazepine failures (lower rate of success in treating neuralgia)
    - Dose of 300–600 mg PO qday (levels need monitoring)
    - Cerebyx (fosphenytoin) 250 mg IV for severe attack
- Lamictal (lamotrigine) 100–400 mg PO qday (NMT 250 mg PO qday in children)

Discharge criteria

- Uncomplicated cases

Discharge instructions

- Trigeminal neuralgia aftercare instructions
- Follow up with PCP or neurologist in 7–10 days

Consult criteria

- Complicated cranial neuralgias

Temporal arteritis

- True emergency of the elderly

    - Age of onset 50–70 years of age
    - Six times more common in females than in males
- Headache localized over eye or to scalp
- Fever, malaise and weight loss are associated symptoms
- Jaw claudication is important associated symptom
- Frequently associated with polymyalgia rheumatica (joint and muscles aches)
- ESR 50–100
    - 15% of temporal arteritis patients have normal ESR
- C-reactive protein elevated usually
- Vision loss can occur early in course of disease

Treatment

- Prednisone 40–80 mg PO bid for several months to one year
    - In suspected temporal with normal ESR, treat with steroids

Discharge criteria

- Minimal symptoms can be treated as outpatient
- Severe symptoms or question of eye involvement should be admitted with IV high dose steroid treatment and ophthalmology consultation obtained
- Discuss all temporal arteritis cases with physician

Discharge instructions

- Temporal arteritis aftercare instructions
- Follow up with PCP within 1 day
- Return for visual changes

Consult criteria

- Discuss all temporal arteritis cases with physician

Headaches Prompting CT Brain Scan Consideration

- Worst headache of life — Consider lumbar puncture if CT negative
    - CT in first 6 hours of headache onset with high accuracy of detecting cerebral hemorrhage

- First headache
- New daily or persistent headache
- Change in headache from previous headache symptoms/patterns
- Neurologic complaints
- New onset seizure with headache
- Complaints of altered mental status
- Migraine aura that is sensory or motor
- Change in migraine aura
- Focal deficits
- Headache > 24 hours
- Thunderclap headache
- Headache in elderly
- Posterior headache, especially in children but also in adults
- Historical Red Flag Headaches
- Recommend that all CT brain scan patients prior to discharge should be discussed with physician

Indications for lumbar puncture include

- First or worst headache of a patient's life
- Severe, rapid-onset, recurrent headache
- Progressive headache
- Unresponsive, chronic, intractable headache

Consider Following "Don't Miss Diagnoses"

(Perform testing for possible diagnoses when suspected)

- Subarachnoid hemorrhage
- Meningitis and encephalitis
- Temporal arteritis
- Acute narrow angle closure glaucoma
- Hypertensive emergencies
- Carbon monoxide poisoning
- Cerebral venous sinus thrombosis (seen for example with OCP use or with women with coagulopathy)
- Trigeminal neuralgia
- Pseudotumor cerebri
- Acute strokes
- Mass lesions

Discharge Criteria

- Benign headache diagnosis and prognosis

- Trigeminal or cranial neuralgias refer to neurologist (website: tna.support.org)

Discharge instructions

- Headache aftercare instructions
- Follow up with PCP or neurologist within 7–10 days as needed
- Return if headache persists > 24 hours

Consult Criteria

- Headache with fever unless consistent with a benign process
- Neck/nuchal rigidity
- Headaches where CT brain scan performed
- Follow General Patient Criteria Protocol (page 22) for care/evaluation not covered in this protocol
- Possible High Risk Headache
- Acute neurologic complaints or findings
- Above diagnosis suspected in the "Don't miss diagnosis" section
- Return visit for same headache
- Age ≥ 60 unless known chronic headache patient without pattern change
- Questionable diagnosis
- Status migrainosus (> 24 hours; dehydration)
- "Historical Red Flags" headache

Lab consult criteria

- Adult WBC ≥ 14,000 or < 1,000 neutrophils
- Pediatric WBC ≥ 15,000 or < 1,000 neutrophils
- Bandemia
- Thrombocytopenia — acute
- Metabolic acidosis
- Significant electrolyte abnormality
- Glucose ≥ 400 mg/dL in diabetic patient
- Glucose ≥ 300 mg/dL in new onset diabetes
- Hyperglycemia with metabolic acidosis (decreased serum CO_2 or elevated anion gap)

Notes

References:

Brennan KC, Farrell CP, Deough GP, Baggaley S, Pippitt K, Pohl SP, et al. Symptom codes and opioids: disconcerting headache practice patterns in academic primary care. Presented on April 30, 2014 at the Annual Meeting of the American Academy of Neurology, 2014.

Baden EY, et al. Intravenous dexamethasone to prevent the recurrence of benign headache after discharge from the emergency department: a randomized, double-blind, placebo-controlled clinical trial *Can J Emerg Med* 2006;8(6):393–400

Migraine Headache Author: Jasvinder Chawla, MD, MBA; Chief Editor: Helmi L Lutsep, MD emedicine.medscape.com/article/1142556

Loder E, Weizenbaum E, Frishberg B, Silberstein S; the American Headache Society Choosing Wisely Task Force. Choosing Wisely in Headache Medicine: The American Headache Society's List of Five Things Physicians and Patients Should Question. Headache. Available at onlinelibrary.wiley.com/doi/10.1111/head.12233/

Top Magn Reson Imaging, 2015;24:291

J Res Med Sci. 2014 Apr; 19(4): 331–335

Ann of EM, Vol.655:622

JEM, epub, 3/14/19

DIZZINESS PROTOCOL

When using any protocol, always follow the Guidelines of Proper Use (page 18).

Definitions

- Sensation of being off balance or of movement of body or surrounding environment

Differential Diagnosis

- Vestibular disorder of inner ear
- Cardiac arrhythmia
- Pulmonary embolism
- TIA
- CVA
- Seizures
- Dehydration
- Aortic stenosis
- Hypoglycemia
- Subarachnoid hemorrhage
- Hemorrhage
    - GI bleeding
    - Ectopic pregnancy
- Adrenal insufficiency
- Sepsis
- Hypotension

Considerations

- Vertigo: peripheral ("inner ear") or central
- Disequilibrium: suggests CNS disorder
- Increasingly common in presenting to acute care settings
- Antiemetics and vestibular suppressants should be withdrawn after a few days if possible to hasten vestibular compensation

Can be:

- Near syncope
- Generalized weakness
- Cardiopulmonary

- Metabolic
- Emotional disorder

Peripheral Vertigo

- Sensation of movement worsened with head movement or position change
- Horizontal nystagmus; rotary nystagmus
- Nausea and vomiting
- No vital sign abnormalities
- No focal neurologic deficits, neurologic complaints or other significant comorbidities
- No further testing may be needed

Central vertigo

- Not worse usually on movement
- Vertical nystagmus
- Infrequent nausea and vomiting
- Central nervous system findings present

Evaluation

- Complete history and physical examination
    - Check for nystagmus, gait abnormalities
    - Hallpike maneuver prn
- For benign peripheral vertigo no further testing may be needed
- Consider CT brain scan for
    - Ataxia
    - Vertical nystagmus
    - Neurologic deficits or complaints
    - Headache
    - Consult physician
- CBC, BMP, EKG, CXR as indicated for patients that may have a disorder besides peripheral vertigo causing symptoms
- Toxicology screen and medication levels as indicated
- Follow Chest Pain, Dyspnea, TIA, Syncope/Near syncope or other Protocols as indicated

Treatment Options

- Benign Paroxysmal Positional Vertigo: Epley maneuver

- Peripheral benign vertigo: meclizine 25 mg tid prn, or Phenergan (promethazine), or benzodiazepines can be considered
- Consider steroids and/or acyclovir (or valacyclovir — Valtrex) — or other herpes medication for vestibular neuronitis or labyrinthitis
- Avoid antihistamines if not peripheral vertigo

Discharge Criteria

- Peripheral vertigo with normal vital signs and O_2 saturation
- Not ataxic
- Acute central nervous system or metabolic disorder not suspected

Discharge instructions

- Provide dizziness aftercare instructions
- Follow up with primary care provider, neurologist or ENT within 10 days as needed

Consult Criteria

- Neurologic abnormalities or complaints
- Visual complaints or findings
- If CT brain scan needed or performed
- Cardiogenic, pulmonary, toxicology cause of dizziness
- Age ≥ 70
- Uncertain or unknown cause of dizziness
- Syncope or near syncope unless vasovagal episode in healthy nonelderly patient
- Refer to General Patient Criteria Protocol (page 22)

Lab and x-ray consult criteria

- New onset renal insufficiency or worsening renal insufficiency
- WBC ≥ 15,000 or < 3,000; Neutrophil count < 1,000
- Bandemia ≥ 15%
- Acute thrombocytopenia
- Increased anion gap
- Metabolic acidosis
- Significant electrolyte abnormally
- Glucose ≥ 400 mg/dL in diabetic patient

- Glucose ≥ 300 mg/dL in non-diabetic patient
- Pleural effusion
- New chest x–ray infiltrate(s) or increased interstitial changes
- New onset renal insufficiency or worsening renal insufficiency

Notes

References:

emedicine.medscape.com/article/2149881

Dizziness presentations in U.S. emergency departments, 1995–2004. Acad Emerg Med. 2008; 15(8):744–50

Treatment of vestibular neuritis. Curr Treat Options Neurol. 2009; 11(1):41–5

CVA/TIA PROTOCOL

When using any protocol, always follow the Guidelines of Proper Use (page 18).

Definition

- TIA — An acute and temporary neurologic dysfunction caused by a focal decrease in blood flow to the central nervous system
- CVA — A neurologic dysfunction caused by a focal decrease in blood flow to the central nervous system that causes neuronal death in the affected area

Differential Diagnosis

- CVA
- Bell's palsy
- Migraine
- Subarachnoid hemorrhage
- Brain tumor
- Multiple sclerosis
- Intracerebral hemorrhage
- Seizure disorder
- Transient global amnesia (TGA)
- Hypoglycemia

Considerations

- TIA always lasts less than 24 hours
    - They usually last 15 minutes to 1 hour in duration
- Up to 40% of patients with TIA have actually had small infarctions by MRI criteria
    - 10.5% of TIA's will have a CVA within 90 days
        - Half of these will occur within 2 days
    - Up to 21 % of CVA's will die or have a major cardiac event
- Up to 16% of TIA patients will have a headache
- Most TIA patients should be hospitalized; especially with a cardiogenic etiology and crescendo TIA's
- Syncope is seldom caused by a TIA

- Acute CVA goal is to complete evaluation and initiate thrombolytics, if indicated, within 60 minutes of patient arrival and within 3 hours of stroke onset
  - Unless intra-arterial t-PA is to be used then the 3 hour time window may be expanded in consultation with neurologist and interventional radiologist

Symptoms

- Acute in onset
- Focal
- Reaching intensity within seconds
- Begin at the same time
- Most common symptoms and signs are
  - Motor and/or sensory deficit on one side of the body
  - Loss of speech or comprehension
  - Loss of vision in one eye or one hemifield
- Vertebrobasilar CVA/TIA presenting as syncope is typically associated with other brainstem signs:
  - Diplopia
  - Ataxia

Most common symptoms and signs

- Hemiparesis
- Hemiataxia
- Hemisensory loss
- Speech difficulty
- Visual difficulty — diplopia or visual loss

High risk factors to develop CVA following TIA

- Age > 60
- Diabetes
- TIA lasting > 10 minutes
- Motor weakness
- Speech impairment

TIA mimics

Migraines

- Migraines symptoms usually migrate and grow, without the abrupt symptom onset of TIA

Syncope

- Hypoperfusion usually produces loss of consciousness, but focal deficits can occasionally be seen, especially after an episode of true syncope

Vertigo

- True vertigo without other findings is seldom central. Look especially for other brainstem signs

Epilepsy

- Focal paralysis without motor activity occurs rarely

TGA

- Transient global amnesia without any other neurologic deficit

Intracerebral hemorrhage

- Symptoms rarely are transient

Multiple sclerosis

- Onset is typically much slower than TIA

Hypoglycemia

- Some alteration in consciousness usually present

Nondescript complaints

- Acute onset of focal symptoms is occasionally a conversion reaction, but be aware of the possibility of embellishment of a real deficit

Evaluation Options

- CBC
- CMP
- EKG
- CT brain scan at time of initial presentation
- Chest x-ray
- C-RP
- ESR
- PT/INR
- Assess for focal neurologic deficits in addition to cardiac and general exam
- Check gait as needed

Assess for other causes

- Migraines
- Seizures
- Vertigo
- TGA
- Medication side effect/toxins
- Multiple sclerosis
- Intracerebral hemorrhage
- Lumbar puncture if subarachnoid hemorrhage is suspected
- Blood cultures if infected emboli are suspected (e.g., SBE)

Acute CVA presentations less than 4.5 hours from onset (notify physician)

- Rapidly perform NIHSS (NIH Stroke Scale) and examine patient
- Order stat CT brain without contrast
- Consult physician and neurologist immediately after ordering CT brain scan
    - If available and appropriate to the specific institution and the patient's clinical situation, order contrast/or perfusion CT brain to be performed after plain CT brain completed per physician (renal patients discuss with physician or radiologist prior to iodinated contrast)
- Determine patient eligibility for t-PA with physician and a course of action if possible
- Repeat NIHSS immediately when patient returns from CT brain scan and discuss with physician
    - To give thrombolysis treatment, blood pressure targets initially are:
        - SBP $\leq$ 185 mm Hg
        - DBP $\leq$ 110 mm Hg
- Follow established specific institution's acute stroke policies if present instead of this section
- Oxygen — avoid high flow oxygen
    - Hyperoxia can cause vasoconstriction of the carotid and downstream cerebral arteries
        - Avoid high O_2 saturations caused by supplemental oxygen

Current inclusion guidelines for the administration of t-PA are:

- Diagnosis of ischemic stroke causing measurable neurologic deficit
- Neurologic signs should not be clearing
- Neurologic signs not be minor and isolated
- Caution should be exercised in treating patients with major deficits (higher risk of hemorrhagic conversion)
- Symptoms not be suggestive of subarachnoid hemorrhage
- Onset of symptoms < 4.5 hours before beginning treatment
- No head trauma or prior stroke in past 3 months
- No MI in prior 3 months
- No GI/GU hemorrhage in previous 21 days
- No arterial puncture in noncompressible site during prior 7 days
- No major surgery in prior 14 days
- No history of prior intracranial bleed
- SBP < 185 mm Hg and DBP < 110 mm Hg
- No evidence of acute trauma or bleeding
- Not taking an oral anticoagulant, or if so INR < 1.7
- If taking heparin within 48 hours must have a normal activated partial thromboplastin time (aPTT)
- Platelet count > 100,000 μL
- Blood glucose level greater than 50 mg/dL (2.7 mmol)
- No seizure with residual postictal impairments
- CT scan does not show evidence of multilobar infarction (hypodensity > 1/3 hemisphere) — increased risk of hemorrhagic conversion
- Pregnancy
- The patient and family understand the potential risks and benefits of therapy

Exclusion criteria for t-PA for CVA symptoms 3–4.5 hours of duration (any 1 of the following)

- Patients older than 80 years

- All patients taking oral anticoagulants are excluded regardless of the international normalized ratio (INR)
- Patients with baseline NIHSS score > 25
- Patients with a history of stroke and diabetes
- Patients with imaging evidence of ischemic damage to more than one third of the middle cerebral artery (MCA) territory

AHA/ASA Guidelines 2018 Update

- Studies showed a clear benefit of "extended window" mechanical thrombectomy for certain patients with large vessel occlusion who could be treated out to 16-24 hours
- The benefits of intravenous (IV) tissue plasminogen activator (tPA) are time-dependent, and treatment for eligible patients should be initiated as quickly as possible (even for patients who may also be candidates for mechanical thrombectomy)
- IV tPA should be administered to all eligible acute stroke patients within 3 hours of last known normal and to a more selective group of eligible acute stroke patients (based on ECASS III exclusion criteria) within 4.5 hours of last known normal
- Centers should attempt to achieve door-to-needle times of <60 minutes in ≥50% of stroke patients treated with IV tPA
- **Prior to initiation of IV tPA in most patients, a noncontrast head computed tomography (CT) and glucose are the only required tests**
    - An INR PTT, and platelet count do not need to have resulted prior to IV tPA initiation if there is no suspicion for underlying coagulopathy
- Centers should attempt to obtain a noncontrast head CT within 20 minutes of arrival in ≥50% of stroke patients who may be candidates for IV tPA or mechanical thrombectomy
- For patients who may be candidates for mechanical thrombectomy, an urgent CT angiogram or magnetic resonance (MR) angiogram (to look for large vessel occlusion) is recommended

    - This study should not delay treatment with IV tPA if indicated
- Patients ≥18 years should undergo mechanical thrombectomy with a stent retriever
    - If they have minimal prestroke disability
    - Have a causative occlusion of the internal carotid artery or proximal middle cerebral artery
    - Have a NIHSS of ≥6
    - Have a reassuring noncontrast head CT
    - Can be treated within 6 hours of last known normal
    - No perfusion imaging (CT-P or MR-P) is required in these patients.
- In selected acute stroke patients within 6-24 hours of last known normal who have evidence of a large vessel occlusion in the anterior circulation, obtaining perfusion imaging (CT-P or MR-P) or an MRI with diffusion-weighted imaging (DWI) sequence is recommended to help determine whether the patient is a candidate for mechanical thrombectomy
- As with IV tPA, treatment with mechanical thrombectomy should be initiated as quickly as possible
- Administration of aspirin is recommended in acute stroke patients within 24-48 hours after stroke onset
    - For patients treated with IV tPA, aspirin administration is generally delayed for 24 hours. Urgent anticoagulation (e.g., heparin drip) for most stroke patients is not indicated

Time targets for t-PA candidates

- Door to Provider: 10 min
- Access to neurologic expertise: 15 min
- Door to CT scan completion: 20 min
- Door to CT scan interpretation: 45 min
- Door to treatment: 60 min
- Admission to monitored bed: 6 hr.
- Preferred thrombolytic treatment window within 3 hours of stroke onset — may be extended if CT

perfusion scan indicates potentially salvageable brain

TIA Treatment Options

- Aspirin 325 mg per day (if no cerebral hemorrhage)
- Consider Plavix (clopidogrel) for ASA failure or ASA allergy (if no cerebral hemorrhage)
- Aggrenox can be used instead of aspirin or Plavix (clopidogrel)
- Coumadin (warfarin) is more effective than above medications if atrial fibrillation present (or can use newer thrombin inhibitor agents)
  - See Stroke Prevention or atrial fibrillation sections
- Lower head of bed to flat position to improve cerebral circulation (unless intracranial hemorrhage is present)
- Avoid hypotonic IV fluids

Hypertension treatment for TIA and CVA nonthrombolysis candidates

- Consult physician for treatment preferred
  - Treat SBP ≥ 220 mm Hg or MAP ≥ 130 mm Hg carefully (avoid rapid or large decreases in BP > 15%)
    - Labetalol 10–20 mg IV over 1–2 minutes — may repeat q10min and double as needed to maximum dose of 150 mg (now controversial)

      OR
    - Nicardipine 5mg/hr. IV and titrate as needed

      OR
    - Nitroprusside 0.3–10 mcg/kg/min (NMT 10 mcg/kg/min.)—start low
  - Avoid treating SBP < 220 mm Hg or MAP < 130 mm Hg
    - Unless AMI, severe CHF, aortic dissection or hypertensive encephalopathy or ICH (intracranial hemorrhage) is present
  - Notify physician promptly if intracranial hemorrhage present
    - SBP > 180 mm Hg is treated

Admission Criteria

- Acute CVA
- Most TIA's
  - High risk criteria
  - Crescendo/recurrent TIA's
  - Cardiogenic etiology of TIA
  - Recent single TIA's are often offered admission because of the high risk of subsequent stroke and to facilitate rapid work-up
  - Septic emboli diagnosis is a possibility
  - Likelihood that patient would not return for outpatient work-up

Discharge Criteria

- Not surgical or anticoagulation candidate
- Patient declines admission for evaluation
- Fully worked up in recent past
- Neurologically stable

Discharge instructions

- TIA aftercare instructions
- Discharge instructions should include early follow-up along with what signs and symptoms to watch for, and to return immediately for further symptoms

Consult Criteria

- All TIA or CVA patients
- CT brain scan with acute findings
- Unclear diagnosis
- Refer to General Patient Criteria Protocol (page 22)

NIH stroke scale

Do not augment or interpret patient's responses on what you think the patient can do. Only record what the patient exactly does.

1a – Level of consciousness (LOC)

- 0 = **Alert;** keenly responsive

- 1 = **Not alert;** arousable by minor stimulation to obey, answer, or respond
- 2 = **Not alert;** requires repeated stimulation to attend, or is obtunded and requires strong or painful stimulation to make movements (not stereotyped)
- 3 = **Responds only** with reflex motor or autonomic effects or is totally unresponsive, flaccid, and areflexic

1b – LOC questions – asked month and age (must be exact)

- 0 = **Answers** both questions correctly
- 1 = **Answers** one question correctly
- 2 = **Answers** neither question correctly

1c – LOC commands – asked to open and close eyes and then to grip and release non-paretic hand

- 0 = **Performs** both tasks correctly
- 1 = **Performs** one task correctly
- 2 = **Performs** neither task correctly

2 – Best gaze

- 0 = Normal
- 1 = Partial gaze palsy; gaze is abnormal in one or both eyes, but forced deviation or total gaze paresis is not present
- 2 = Forced deviation, or total gaze paresis not overcome by the oculocephalic (doll's eyes) maneuver

3 – Visual

- 0 = No visual loss
- 1 = Partial hemianopsia (quadrantanopsia)
- 2 = Complete hemianopsia
- 3 = Bilateral hemianopsia (blind including cortical blindness)

4 – Facial palsy

- 0 = Normal symmetrical movements
- 1 = Minor paralysis (flattened nasolabial fold, asymmetry on smiling)
- 2 = Partial paralysis (total or near-total paralysis of lower face)

- 3 = Complete paralysis of one or both sides (absence of facial movement in the upper and lower face)

5 – Motor arm (score for each arm)

- 0 = **No drift;** limb holds 90 (or 45) degrees for full 10 seconds
- 1 = **Drift;** limb hold 90 (or 45) degrees, but drifts down before full 10 seconds; does not hit bed or other support
- 2 = **Some effort against gravity;** limb cannot get to or maintain (if cued) 90 (or 45) degrees, drifts down to bed, but has some effort against gravity
- 3 = **No effort against gravity;** limb falls
- 4 = **No movement**
- UN = **Amputation** or joint fusion, explain: ________________________________

6 – Motor leg (score for each leg)

- 0 = **No drift;** leg holds 30-degree position for full 5 seconds
- 1 = **Drift;** leg falls by the end of the 5-second period but does not hit bed
- 2 = **Some effort against gravity;** leg falls to bed by 5 seconds, but has some effort against gravity
- 3 = **No effort against gravity;** leg falls to bed immediately
- 4 = **No movement**
- UN = **Amputation** or joint fusion, explain: ________________________________

7 – Limb ataxia

- 0 = Absent
- 1 = Present in one limb
- 2 = Present in two limbs
- UN = **Amputation** or joint fusion, explain: ________________________________

8 – Sensory

- 0 = **Normal;** no sensory loss
- 1 = **Mild-to-moderate sensory loss;** patient feels pinprick is less sharp or is dull on the

affected side; or there is a loss of superficial pain with pinprick, but patient is aware of being touched.

- 2 = **Severe to total sensory loss;** patient is not aware of being touched in the face, arm, and leg

9 – Best Language

- 0 = No aphasia; normal
- 1 = Mild-to-moderate aphasia; some obvious loss of fluency or facility of comprehension, without significant limitation on ideas expressed or form of expression. Reduction of speech and/or comprehension; however, makes conversation about provided materials difficult or impossible. For example, in conversation about provided materials, examiner can identify picture or naming card content from patient's response.
- 2 = Severe aphasia; all communication is through fragmentary expression; great need for inference, questioning, and guessing by the listener. Range of information that can be exchanged is limited; listener carries burden of communication. Examiner cannot identify materials provided from patient response.
- 3 = Mute, global aphasia; no usable speech or auditory comprehension

10 – Dysarthria

- 0 = Normal
- 1 = Mild-to-moderate dysarthria; patient slurs at least some words and, at worst, can be understood with some difficulty.
- 2 = Severe dysarthria; patient's speech is so slurred as to be unintelligible in the absence of or out of proportion to any dysphasia, or is mute.
- UN = Intubated or other physical barrier, explain:______________________________

11 – Extinction and Inattention (Neglect)

- 0 = No abnormality
- 1 = Visual, tactile, auditory, spatial, or personal inattention or extinction to bilateral simultaneous stimulation in one of the sensory modalities.

- 2 = Profound hemi-inattention or extinction to more than one modality; does not recognize own hand or orients to only one side of space.

NOTE: If the patient in 1a has a score of 3, then the rest of the exams usually are scored a 3 for each category

Notes

References:

www.ninds.nih.gov/doctors/NIH_Stroke_Scale.pdf

Stroke. May 2007;38(5):1655–711

Stroke. 2010;41;2108

Cornet AD, et al. *Crit Care* 2013 Apr 18;17:313

Ischemic Stroke Workup Author: Edward C Jauch, MD, MS, FAHA, FACEP; Chief Editor: Helmi L Lutsep, MD

stroke.ahajournals.org/content/suppl/2013/01/29/STR.0b013e318284056a.DC1/Executive_Summary.pdf

emedicine.medscape.com/article/1160840
Thrombolytic Therapy in Stroke Author: Jeffrey L Saver, MD, FAHA, FAAN; Chief Editor: Helmi L Lutsep, MD

N Engl J Med 2018; 378:11-21 January 4, 2018

N Engl J Med 2018; 378:708-718 February 22, 2018

BELL'S PALSY PROTOCOL

When using any protocol, always follow the Guidelines of Proper Use (page 18).

Definition

- Dysfunction or paralysis of the 7th cranial nerve unilaterally of acute onset and usually idiopathic etiology

Differential Diagnosis

- Vascular
  - TIA
  - CVA
  - Aneurysm
- Infectious
  - Lyme disease
  - Herpes zoster
  - Mononucleosis
- Neoplastic
  - Tumor of pons or cerebellopontine angle or acoustic nerve
  - Lymphoma
  - Skull based tumor, cholesteatoma
- Multiple sclerosis

Considerations

- 7th cranial nerve dysfunction
- Affects 1 in 65 persons in a lifetime
- Complete recovery in 65% of patients at 3 months and 85% at 9 months
- Studies have shown the benefit of high-dose corticosteroids for acute cases
- Steroids and Valtrex (valacyclovir) or acyclovir recommended only in the initial 72 hours of symptoms in age 16 years or older, with complete or nearly complete paralysis — not useful otherwise
- Slowly progressive facial paralysis suggestive of cancer

- Recurrent paralysis or bilateral presentation warrants additional workup
- Bilateral 7th nerve weakness excludes Bell's palsy and is suggestive of infectious causes such as Lyme disease or VZV (varicella zoster virus)
- Forehead sparing of motor function usually indicates upper motor neuron lesion (CVA)
- Lyme disease should be considered as a cause in endemic areas
- Bell's palsy can be mimicked by pontine brainstem lesion
- Other associated signs and symptoms:
    - Vestibular signs
    - Diabetes and hypertension higher risk for pontine lesions

Signs and Symptoms

- Typical presentation is subacute weakness of one side of the face
- Often associated with pain near the ear
- No sensory loss although patient may complain of vague sensation disturbance on the face
- Hyperacusis due to paralysis of the stapedius sometimes occurs
- Distortion of taste sometimes occurs although this is seldom a presenting complaint
- Weakness of eye closure is helpful to differentiate Bell's palsy from stroke where eye opening may be impaired
- Asymmetry of mouth movement is most obvious with grimacing and smiling
- Maximal defect is 5 days from onset
- Forehead and lower facial muscles both weak
    - If forehead spared of weakness, suspect central lesion (CVA, tumor)
- Increased tear flow
- Dry eyes
- Rash or vesicles around ear on affected side suggests herpes zoster (Ramsey-Hunt syndrome). Usually significant pain near the ear

Causes

- Idiopathic usually
- Infectious causes
    - Most infectious cases of Bell's palsy are thought to be due to virus infections
        - HSV 1 or 2
        - VZV
    - EBV
    - Lyme disease is a rare cause of Bell's palsy
- Sarcoidosis can present with facial palsy, occasionally can present with bilateral facial weakness.
- Other infections such as osteomyelitis, primary ear infections, and meningitis are less likely
- Neoplasm of local tissues near the ear and skull base or neoplastic meningitis
- Pontine (brainstem) lesion, including cerebellopontine angle lesion
- Aneurysm of the basilar artery or branch with resultant neural compression
- Parotid gland mass lesions

Evaluation Options

- Usually no testing except history and physical exam
- Testing driven by suspected processes or recurrent/bilateral presentations
    - CBC
    - ESR or C-reactive protein
    - Lyme titer
    - HIV test
    - Serum glucose
    - CT brain if suspected central lesion (usually not needed)
    - Lumbar puncture if intracranial or spinal infectious process suspected

Goals of treatment

- Improve facial nerve (seventh cranial nerve) function
- Reduce neuronal damage
- Prevent complications from corneal exposure

Treatment Options

- Artificial tears
- Tape eyelids closed on affected side at night only
- Eye protection if eyelid closure is impaired
- Steroids are commonly used unless specifically contraindicated
  - Prednisone 1 mg/kg/day up to 60 mg/day × 7 days without taper (or may taper to 5 mg/day over 10 days)—use only if symptoms ≤ 3 days
- Antiviral agents (e.g., acyclovir, valacyclovir) may be considered if a herpes viral etiology is suspected, but only in combination with corticosteroids (i.e. herpes zoster rash present, etc.) within the first 72 hours of symptom onset.
  - Valtrex (valacyclovir) 1000 mg PO tid × 5 days
    - Valtrex > age 2 years: 20 mg/kg PO q8hr for 5 days; not to exceed 1 g PO q8hr

    OR

  - Acyclovir 400 mg PO 5 ×/day × 7–10 days

    OR

  - Famciclovir 500 mg tid × 5–10 days
- Physical therapy may be used for patients with moderate to severe deficits

Discharge Criteria

- Isolated 7th nerve palsy

Discharge instructions

- Bell's palsy aftercare instructions
- Follow up with primary care provider or neurologist within 7 to 10 days
- Discharge precautions noted:
  - Return if additional symptoms occur or significant worsening
  - Complete the course of medications prescribed
- Ensure follow-up after discharge

Consult Criteria

- Suspected other causes of nerve palsy

- Central nervous system findings or complaints
- Refer to General Patient Criteria Protocol (page 22) as needed

Notes

References:

Baugh RF, Basura GJ, Ishii LE, Schwartz SR, Drumheller CM, Burkholder R, et al. Clinical Practice Guideline: Bell's Palsy Executive Summary. *Otolaryngol Head Neck Surg*. Nov 2013;149(5):656–63.

Sullivan FM, Swan IR, Donnan PT, Morrison JM, Smith BH, McKinstry B, et al. Early treatment with prednisolone or acyclovir in Bell's palsy. *N Engl J Med*. Oct 18 2007;357(16):1598–607.

Engström M, Berg T, Stjernquist-Desatnik A, et al. Prednisolone and valaciclovir in Bell's palsy: a randomised, double-blind, placebo-controlled, multicentre trial. *Lancet Neurol*. Nov 2008;7(11):993–1000

Reconciling the clinical practice guidelines on Bell palsy from the AAO-HNSF and the AAN; Seth R. Schwartz, Stephanie L. Jones, Thomas S.D. Getchius, et. Al. Neurology 2014;1927–1929 May 2, 2014

ADULT SEIZURE PROTOCOL

When using any protocol, always follow the Guidelines of Proper Use (page 18).

Definition

- Focal or generalized electrical depolarizations of the brain resulting in focal or generalized neurologic and motor findings with or without loss of consciousness

Differential Diagnosis

- Pseudoseizures
- Migraines
- Encephalitis
- Meningitis
- Transient global amnesia (TGA)
- Psychogenic unresponsiveness
- TIA (rare TIA's can present with focal motor activity or unresponsiveness)
- Syncope
- Hypoglycemia
- Conversion reaction

Considerations

Generalized seizures (most common)

Classic tonic-clonic (grand mal)

- Sustained generalized muscle contractions followed by loss of consciousness

Absence seizures (petit mal)

- Brief episodes of sudden immobility and blank stares

Partial seizures

Simple

- Brief sensory or motor symptoms without loss of consciousness
  - Focal motor seizures is an example

Complex

- Mental or psychiatric symptoms
- Affect changes

- Confusion
- Automatisms
- Hallucinations
- Impaired consciousness

Status epilepticus (SE)

- Newly defined as seizure > 5 minutes or 2 or more seizures in which patient does not recover consciousness
- Older definition > 30 minutes or 2 or more seizures in which patient does not recover consciousness (controversy exists about definition)
- Mortality of 10–12%
- Failure to recognize nonconvulsive SE increases poor outcomes
- Prolonged SE leads to electromechanical dissociation
    - Exhibit minor movements: twitching of eyes, face, hands, feet; coma

Prolactin level

- Helpful if drawn within 10–20 minutes of seizure and elevated 2 times normal
    - Syncope can also elevate prolactin levels
- Normal prolactin level favors pseudoseizure but cannot differentiate seizure from syncope
- Normal prolactin does not rule out seizure however

Pseudoseizures

- Closed eyes during seizure: 96% sensitive; 98% specific in indicating pseudoseizure
- Open eyes during seizure: 98% sensitive; 96% specific in indicating true seizure

First time seizure has 25% recurrence in 2 years

Epilepsy defined as 2 or more seizures not provoked by other illness or causations

Causes

- Idiopathic
- Genetic
- Hypoglycemia or hyperglycemia
- Hypernatremia and hyponatremia
- CVA

- Cerebral mass
- Intracranial hemorrhage — especially subarachnoid or intraparenchymal
- Traumatic brain injury
- Cocaine
- Meningitis
- Encephalitis
- Eclampsia
- Fever
- Prescribed drugs (lowered seizure threshold especially with some antibiotics and analgesics)
- Withdrawal syndromes (drugs and alcohol)

Evaluation

- Assess airway and breathing
- Cardiac and O_2 saturation monitoring
- Complete history and physical
- Obtain seizure history and treatment
- Obtain history of associated symptoms
- Drug abuse history

Patients with chronic seizures and no change in typical seizure pattern, without comorbid findings or symptoms

- BMP
- U/A
- Seizure drug levels if acutely measurable

All other seizures with comorbid considerations and new onset seizures

- CMP, Mg^{++}, prolactin level in select patients
- Pregnancy test in childbearing age fertile women
- Consider lumbar puncture (LP) in immunocompromised patient or with meningitis signs
- Consider LP in patients with seizure and fever
- CBC; U/A; chest x-ray as indicated by associated symptoms or findings
- Blood alcohol and drug screen as indicated
- Serum anticonvulsant levels for anticonvulsant therapy that are acutely measurable
- CT brain scan on first time seizures if available
- CT brain scan on elderly or patients taking Coumadin or newer anticoagulants
- CT brain scan for head trauma

- Consider stat EEG for suspected nonconvulsive SE

Treatment Options

- Notify physician promptly of seizures occurring in the department or clinic
- Intubation if airway not secure
- IV NS KVO
- Nasal oxygen

Initial treatment

- Lorazepam 2–6 mg IV if actively seizing
    - May repeat q10–15 minutes for recurrent seizures prn (NMT 10 mg)

Adjunctive treatments as needed

- Thiamine 100 mg IM/IV for alcoholism history (or if not known)
- Glucose D50W 1 amp if hypoglycemic
- Prophylactic lorazepam can be given in the first 12 hours of alcoholic withdrawal
- Magnesium sulfate 4 gms IV over 5—10 minutes for eclampsia

Status epilepticus (beware of "too slow and too low" treatment)

- Lorazepam 0.1 mg/kg IV (NMT 10 mg)
- Cerebyx (fosphenytoin) 18–20 PE mg/kg IV at 100–150 mg/minute if no response in 3–5 minutes to lorazepam

Drugs that can be used if lorazepam and Cerebyx (fosphenytoin) fail

- Valproic acid 20–30 mg/kg at max rate up to 10mg/kg/minute; (NMT 40 mg/kg) — loading dose
    - 5 mg/kg/hr. drip
- Levetiracetam (Keppra) 30–50 mg/kg at 100 mg/minute (loading dose)
- Phenobarbital 10 mg/kg IV at 100 mg/hr. per physician (seldom used in adults)
- Lidocaine 1 mg/kg up to 100 mg; may be repeated (NMT 3 mg/kg)
- Propofol per physician (intubate patient)
    - 2 mg/kg; may repeat if needed in 3–5 minutes
    - Maintenance 5 mg/kg/hr.

Management of refractory status epilepticus (consult physician immediately)

- Referral to an intensive care unit
- Anesthetic agents such as midazolam, propofol, barbiturates (thiopental, pentobarbital) or ketamine for generalized convulsive status epilepticus
    - Intermittent ketamine superior to continuous infusion
- Non-anesthetic anticonvulsants such as phenobarbital or valproic acid for nonconvulsive status epilepticus

ACEP Clinical Policy: Critical Issues in the Evaluation and Management of Adult Patients Presenting to the Emergency Department with seizures (January 2014)

- Intended for emergency departments
- Adult patients ≥ 18 years with generalized convulsive seizure
- Not intended for pediatric patients, complex partial seizures, acute head or multisystem trauma, or brain tumor, immunocompromised or eclamptic patients

Level A recommendations

- Emergency providers should administer an additional antiepileptic medication in emergency department patients with refractory status epilepticus who have failed treatment with benzodiazepines

Level B recommendations

- Emergency providers may administer intravenous phenytoin, fosphenytoin, or valproate in emergency department patients with refractory status epilepticus who have failed treatment with benzodiazepines.

Level C recommendations

- Emergency providers need not initiate antiepileptic medication in the emergency department for patients who have had a first provoked seizure
- Precipitating medical conditions should be identified and treated

- Emergency providers need not initiate antiepileptic medication in the emergency department for patients who have had a first unprovoked seizure without evidence of brain disease or injury
- Emergency providers may initiate antiepileptic medication in the emergency department, or defer in coordination with other providers, for patients who experienced a first unprovoked seizure with a remote history of brain disease or injury

Level C recommendations

- Emergency providers need not admit patients with a first unprovoked seizure who have returned to their clinical baseline in the emergency department

Level C recommendations

- Emergency providers may administer intravenous levetiracetam, propofol, or barbiturates in emergency department patients with refractory status epilepticus who have failed treatment with benzodiazepines

Level C recommendations

- When resuming antiseizure medication in the emergency department is advisable, IV or oral route is acceptable at the providers discretion

Discharge Criteria

- Patient with normal neurologic exam and no concerning comorbidities
- No known structural brain disease
- Patients usually do not need to be started on seizure outpatient treatment at that time if patient had single brief seizure without previous seizure history, and has a normal exam, normal imaging and no further seizures
- With treatment, after oral or parenteral load with anticonvulsant
- Without treatment if risk of recurrent seizure is judged to be low

Discharge instructions

- Seizure aftercare instructions
- Advise of seizure precautions/safety issues prior to discharge (for example – no driving, swimming, bathtubs, climbing etc.)

Consult Criteria

- Notify physician promptly on all actively seizing patients
- Discuss all seizure patients with prior to discharge
- Notify physician of any other neurologic abnormalities
- Abnormal imaging studies
- Significant abnormal lab tests
- Abnormal vital signs and O_2 saturation < 95% on room air (<92% O_2 saturation in COPD patients)

Notes

References:

Seizure Assessment in the Emergency Department

Author: M Tyson Pillow, MD, MEd; Chief Editor: Rick Kulkarni, MD

emedicine.medscape.com/article/1609294

American College of Emergency Physicians Clinical Policy: Critical Issues in the Evaluation and Management of Adult Patients Presenting to the Emergency Department With Seizures (January 2014)

American Epilepsy Society (AES) 69th Annual Meeting. Abstracts 3.177 and 1.123

PEDIATRIC SEIZURE PROTOCOL

When using any protocol, always follow the Guidelines of Proper Use (page 18).

Definition

- Focal or generalized electrical depolarizations of the brain resulting in focal or generalized neurologic and motor findings with or without loss of consciousness

Differential Diagnosis

- Pseudoseizures
- Migraines
- Encephalitis
- Meningitis
- Cat scratch disease
- Amphetamine toxicity
- Cocaine toxicity
- Dystonic reactions
- Heavy metal toxicity
- Syncope
- Brain cancer

Considerations

Generalized seizures (most common)

Classic tonic-clonic (grand mal)

- Sustained generalized muscle contractions followed by loss of consciousness

Absence seizures (petit mal)

- Brief episodes of sudden immobility and blank stares

Partial seizures

Simple

- Brief sensory or motor symptoms without loss of consciousness
    - Focal motor seizures is an example

Complex

- Mental or psychiatric symptoms
- Affect changes
- Confusion
- Automatisms
- Hallucinations
- Impaired consciousness

Status epilepticus (SE)

- Newly defined as seizure > 5 minutes or 2 or more seizures in which patient does not recover consciousness
- Older definition > 30 minutes or 2 or more seizures in which patient does not recover consciousness (controversy exists about definition)
- Mortality of 10–12%
- Failure to recognize nonconvulsive SE increases poor outcomes
- EEG, CBC, BMP, calcium level, toxicology screen, ABG, anticonvulsant levels, LFT's
- Intubate as needed
- Prolonged SE leads to electromechanical dissociation
    - Exhibit minor movements: twitching of eyes, face, hands, feet; coma

Prolactin level

- Helpful if drawn within 10–20 minutes of seizure and elevated 2 times normal
    - Syncope can also elevate prolactin levels
- Normal prolactin level favors pseudoseizure but cannot differentiate seizure from syncope
- Normal prolactin does not rule out seizure however

Pseudoseizures

- Closed eyes during seizure: 96% sensitive; 98% specific in indicating pseudoseizure
- Open eyes during seizure: 98% sensitive; 96% specific in indicating true seizure

First time seizure has 25% recurrence in 2 years

Epilepsy defined as 2 or more seizures not provoked by other illness or causations

Causes of Seizures Amenable to Treatment

- Hypoglycemia
- Hyponatremia
- Hypocalcemia
- Hypomagnesemia
- Isoniazid ingestion treated with pyridoxine
- Hypertension

Evaluation

- Assess airway and breathing
- Cardiac and O_2 saturation monitoring
- Complete history and physical
- Obtain seizure history and treatment
- Obtain associated symptoms
- Drug abuse history

Patients with chronic seizures and no change in typical seizure pattern, without comorbid findings or symptoms

- BMP
- Seizure drug levels if acutely measurable

All other seizures with comorbid considerations and new onset seizures

- CMP, prolactin level in select patients
- Pregnancy test in childbearing age females
- Consider lumbar puncture on the immunocompromised patient or patient that has meningitis signs
- Consider LP in patients with seizure and fever unless it is a benign febrile seizure
- CBC; U/A; chest x-ray as indicated by associated symptoms or findings
- Blood alcohol and drug screen as indicated
- Serum anticonvulsant levels for anticonvulsant therapy that are acutely measurable
- CT brain scan on first time seizures if available

- CT brain scan for head trauma
- Consider stat EEG if no resolution of post-ictal lethargy and for suspected nonconvulsive SE

Treatment Options

- Intubation if airway not secure
- IV NS KVO or INT
- Nasal oxygen

Initial treatment options

- Lorazepam 0.05–0.1 mg/kg IV; may repeat q10–15 minutes prn or valium 0.2 mg/kg IV
- Diastat (diazepam rectal gel) if no IV available
  - Age up to 5 years: 0.5 mg/kg
  - Age 6–11 years: 0.3 mg/kg
  - Age > 12 years: 0.2 mg/kg
  - Round up to available dose: 2.5, 5, 7.5, 10, 12.5, 15, 17.5, 20 mg/dose
- Midazolam IV/IM/PR/ET/intranasal 0.1–0.2 mg/kg/dose; not to exceed a cumulative dose of 10 mg

Adjunctive treatments as needed

- Dextrose: 0.25–0.5 g/kg/dose (1–2 cc of 25% dextrose) intravenously for hypoglycemia; not to exceed 25 gm/dose
- Naloxone (Narcan): 0.1 mg/kg/dose intravenously preferable (if needed may administer intramuscularly or subcutaneously) for narcotic overdose (do not exceed 2 mg initially)
- Thiamine: 100 mg intramuscularly for possible deficiency
- Pyridoxine (vitamin B6): 50–100 mg intravenously/intramuscularly for possible deficiency
- Rocephin (ceftriaxone) 50–100 mg/kg IV or IM not to exceed 2 grams if meningitis suspected (may use Sanford Guide or databases), initiate treatment with antibiotics prior to cerebrospinal fluid (CSF) analysis or brain imaging
  - Give Decadron (dexamethasone) 15 minutes before antibiotics or with antibiotics

Status epilepticus (beware of "too slow and too low" treatment)

- Lorazepam 0.1 mg/kg IV (NMT 10 mg) or diazepam 0.2 mg/kg IV
- Cerebyx (fosphenytoin) 15–20 mg/kg PE IV at 100–150 mg/minute if no response in 5 minutes to lorazepam or midazolam (Versed)
    - May repeat in 20 minutes is seizure activity continues at 10 mg/kg PE IV
- Keppra (Levetiracetam) 30-40 mg/kg IV
    - 2-5 mg/kg/minute
    - NMT 2000 mg

Drugs that can be used if above medications fail

- Pentobarbital 1 mg/kg boluses IV to maximum 5 mg/kg per physician
- Valproic acid 15 mg/kg over 1–5 minutes (NMT 40 mg/kg)
    - 5 mg/kg/hr. drip
- Phenobarbital 20 mg/kg IV at 100 mg/hr. per physician
- Propofol 2 mg/kg IV bolus (patient intubated), may repeat if needed and start 5 mg/kg/hr. infusion if necessary
- Ketamine

Management of refractory status epilepticus (consult physician immediately)

- Referral to an intensive care unit
- Anesthetic agents such as midazolam, propofol, ketamine or barbiturates (thiopental, pentobarbital) for generalized convulsive status epilepticus
    - Intermittent ketamine superior to continuous infusion
- Non-anesthetic anticonvulsants such as phenobarbital or valproic acid for nonconvulsive status epilepticus

Discharge Criteria

- Patient with normal neurologic exam and no concerning comorbidities
- No known structural brain disease

- Most patients usually do not need to be started on seizure outpatient treatment at time of discharge
- No further seizures
- With treatment, after oral or parenteral load with anticonvulsant
- Without treatment if risk of recurrent seizure is judged to be low

Discharge instructions

- Seizure aftercare instructions
- Advise of seizure precautions/safety issues prior to discharge (for example – no driving)
- Contact primary care physician or provider to alert of ED visit and arrange follow up if seen in acute care setting

Consult Criteria

- Notify physician promptly on all actively seizing patients
- Discuss all seizure patients with prior to discharge
- Notify physician of any neurologic abnormalities
- Abnormal imaging studies
- Significant abnormal lab tests
- Abnormal vital signs and O_2 saturation < 95% on room air

Notes

References:

emedicine.medscape.com/article/1179097

Chamberlain JM, Okada P, Holsti M, et al. Lorazepam vs diazepam for pediatric status epilepticus: a randomized clinical trial. *JAMA*. Apr 23–30 2014;311(16):1652–60

emedicine.medscape.com/article/908394

Neuology 2012 Dec 11;79(24):2355-8. doi: 10.1212/WNL.0b013e318278b685. Epub 2012 Nov 28.

Efficacy and safety of ketamine in refractory status epilepticus in children. Rosati A, L'Erario M, Ilvento L, Cecchi C, Pisano T, Mirabile L, Guerrini R

Delirium (Altered Mental Status) Protocol

When using any protocol, always follow the Guidelines of Proper Use (page 18).

Definition

- Acute organic brain syndrome manifested by impaired thinking, confusion, deficits in attention, hallucinations, tremor, fluctuating course, impaired speech and other symptoms and signs of impaired cognition

Causes of delirium

Medications and substances

- Ethanol
- Anticholinergics
- Antihistamines
- Sedatives
- Narcotics
- Antidepressants
- Lithium
- Neuroleptics
- Tagamet (cimetidine)

Withdrawal

- Ethanol
- Benzodiazepines
- Narcotics

Metabolic

- Electrolyte abnormalities (Na and Ca)
- Hypoglycemia and hyperglycemia
- Acid-base disturbance
- Dehydration
- Hypoxia
- End organ insufficiency – liver, kidney and lungs
- Vitamin deficiency – thiamine, folate
- Fever or hypothermia

Infectious

- Urinary tract infection – especially in elderly
- Encephalitis or meningitis
- Pneumonia
- Sepsis
- Influenza

Neurologic

- Brain tumor
- Subdural hematoma
- Intracerebral hemorrhage
- Seizure disorder
- CVA
- Dementia is a risk factor

Endocrine

- Hyperthyroidism
- Hypothyroidism
- Parathyroid – hyper and hypoparathyroidism

Cardiovascular

- Congestive heart failure
- Arrhythmia
- Acute myocardial infarction

Conditions that mimic delirium

- Dementia
- Depression
- Schizophrenia
- Mania
- Wernicke's aphasia

Evaluation of delirium

Mental status examination

OMI HAT (OMI = organic disease; HAT = psychiatric or functional)

- O – Orientation
- M – Memory
- I – Intellect
- H – Hallucinations
- A – Affect disorder
- T – Thought disorder

Functional Disorder

- Age 15–40 years old
- Onset gradual
- Not confused
- Appears depressed

Organic disorder

- Middle age or elderly
- Non-adolescent children
- Labile course
- Confused
- Visual hallucinations
- Vital signs frequently abnormal

Testing Options

- CBC
- BMP
- LFT's
- U/A
- Chest x-ray
- EKG

Tested as indicated

- Drug levels
- Thyroid studies
- Urine drug screen
- Blood alcohol
- Blood cultures
- CT brain
- Lumbar puncture for CSF analysis
- Urine culture

Treatment of delirium

- Treat underlying illness
- Restore any fluid or electrolyte imbalances
- Haloperidol 0.5 mg–5 mg PO, 2–5 mg IM, or 2–10 mg IV depending on severity of symptoms
    - **Do not** use newer atypical antipsychotic medication in **dementia-related psychosis**
- Lorazepam
- Restraints avoided if possible
- Discontinue any unnecessary medication that is contributing to delirium (discuss with physician)

Consult criteria for delirium

- Discuss all cases with physician
- Physician should examine all delirium or acute altered mental status patients unless from ethanol or drug abuse

Notes

References:

Delirium Author: Kannayiram Alagiakrishnan, MD, MBBS, MHA, MPH; Chief Editor: Iqbal Ahmed, MBBS, FRCPsych (UK) emedicine.medscape.com/article/288890

American Psychiatric Association. Diagnostic and Statistical Manual of Mental Disorders, Fifth Edition. 5th ed. Washington, DC: American Psychiatric Association; 2013

Back

Section Contents

When using any protocol, always follow the Guidelines of Proper Use (page 18).

BACK PAIN PROTOCOL

When using any protocol, always follow the Guidelines of Proper Use (page 18).

Differential Diagnosis

- Muscular pain
- Aortic aneurysm
- Vertebral infection
- Epidural hematoma
- Epidural abscess
- Herniated nucleus pulposus (HNP)
- Spinal stenosis
- Renal colic
- Pyelonephritis
- Cancer
- Prostatitis
- Perirectal abscess

Considerations

- Most back pain is benign
- Usually is without acute neurologic signs
- Radiculopathy is frequently an associated complaint or finding
- Fever may be harbinger of spinal or vertebral infection in patients with IV drug abuse or recent instrumentation
- Elderly have increased risk of vertebral fractures with or without injury
- Second most common complaint in ambulatory care and third most expensive disorder behind cancer and heart disease

Spinal cord compression signs

- Urinary retention with overflow incontinence or voiding
- Fecal incontinence
- Decreased rectal tone
- Decreased perineal sensation

Cauda equina syndrome

- Urinary retention is most common finding in cauda equina syndrome
- Patients without urinary retention have an approximately 1/10,000 chance of having cauda equina syndrome
- Normal rectal tone usually excludes cauda equina syndrome
- Saddle numbness
- Extreme weakness

Warning flags in back pain

- Cancer history (Pain not relieved by rest)
- Chronic infections or fever history
- Night pain
- Prolonged pain
- Depression
- HIV history
- Unexplained weight loss
- IV substance abuse
- Disability pursuit
- Urinary retention
- Failure to improve after 6 weeks of conservative therapy

Evaluation

- Complete history and physical examination
- Check reflexes, SLR (straight leg raise), and neurovascular exam
- Check rectal tone; perineal sensation; urinary bladder retention in suspected cauda equina syndrome
- Healthy non-elderly patients without direct blunt trauma usually need no tests
- Elderly frequently need plain spine films (or CT) due to higher incidence of vertebral fractures
- Plain back/pelvic films may be needed in falls, MVC's, direct blunt trauma, depending on severity of injury mechanism
- U/A if renal disease suspected or significant injury mechanism
- D-dimer if aortic dissection considered

- CBC, C-RP (or ESR) for fever with vertebral back pain as only other symptom or finding

CT spine

- Acute neurologic complaints or findings
- Compression fracture > 30%
- Burst fracture (goes through entire vertebral body — unstable)
- Posterior vertebral involvement
- Traumatic back pain out of proportion to clinical expectation

MRI for spinal cord findings or symptoms

Treatment Options

- NSAID's more effective long term than opiates
    - Ibuprofen+acetaminophen more effective than hydrocodone 5 mg
- Short narcotic course prn for severe pain
- Preferably no prolonged bed rest unless fracture present
- Limit bed rest to no more than 2–3 days if possible (unless compression fracture)
- Return to work with restricted activities or light duty results in better long term outcomes
- Muscle relaxants of questionable usefulness
- Salmon calcitonin for compression fractures that can be discharged

Discharge Criteria

- Uncomplicated presentation and findings
- Ability to control pain and ambulate
- Orthopedic referral for fractures

Discharge instructions

- Follow up within 10 days as needed
- If HNP suspected refer to neurosurgeon or orthopedic surgeon within 10 days
- Back pain aftercare instructions

Consult Criteria

- Severe pain with inability to ambulate

- Progressive neurologic deficits
- Signs of cauda equina syndrome
- Signs of spinal cord compression or injury
- Evidence of infectious, vascular, or neoplastic etiologies
- Nontraumatic pediatric back pain
- Fracture
- Suspected aortic disease as cause of pain

Lab and x-ray consult criteria

- New onset renal insufficiency or worsening renal insufficiency
- WBC > 15,000 or < 3,000; Neutrophil count < 1,000
- Bandemia ≥ 15%
- Acute thrombocytopenia
- Metabolic acidosis
- Significant electrolyte abnormally
- Glucose ≥ 450 mg/dL in diabetic patient
- Glucose ≥ 400 mg/dL in non-diabetic patient
- Hyperglycemia with metabolic acidosis (decreased serum CO_2 or elevated anion gap)
- New pleural effusion
- New chest x–ray infiltrate(s) or increased interstitial changes
- New onset renal insufficiency or worsening renal insufficiency
- Refer to General Patient Criteria Protocol as needed

Notes

References:
emedicine.medscape.com/article/822462

Chaparro LE, Furlan AD, Deshpande A, Mailis-Gagnon A, Atlas S, Turk DC. Opioids compared to placebo or other treatments for chronic low-back pain. *Cochrane Database Syst Rev*. Aug 27 2013;8:CD004959

Kinkade S. Evaluation and treatment of acute low back pain. Am Fam Physician. Apr 15, 2007;74(8):1181–8

FLANK PAIN PROTOCOL

When using any protocol, always follow the Guidelines of Proper Use (page 18).

Differential Diagnosis

- Renal colic
- Renal infarction
- Biliary colic
- Aortic aneurysm
- Mechanical back pain
- Herpes zoster
- Pyelonephritis
- Renal vein thrombosis
- Retroperitoneal bleeding
- Appendicitis
- Splenic infarction or injury

Considerations

- Renal colic is most common misdiagnosis of ruptured abdominal aortic aneurysm
- Aortic disease cause more frequent in elderly
- No hematuria on U/A with 10–15% of kidney stones
- Flank ecchymosis indicative of intra-abdominal bleeding

Evaluation

- Detailed abdomen, back, flank, and neurovascular exam

Musculoskeletal suspected as cause

- No tests unless blunt injury occurred
- Blunt trauma consider imaging
- CBC and U/A as indicated

Kidney stone suspected

- KUB
- UA
- Noncontrast CT abdominal/pelvis may be considered

CT abdominal/pelvis scan considered

- In elderly
- Unclear diagnosis
- Aortic cause suspected
- Inadequate response to pain medications

D-dimer

- Can be used as screening test to rule out aortic disease if negative (98% specific)
- Coumadin (warfarin) can cause false negative D-dimer
- Elderly have a positive D-dimer > 50% of the time without acute process
    - D-dimer increases 10 mcg/L for every year over 50 years of age if the upper cutoff is 500 mcg/L (for example an 80 year old with d-dimer 700 mcg/L would be in the normal range)
    - If another assay used, then 2% increase/year over age 50 may be used to adjust upper limit for age

U/A

- UTI symptoms
- Obtain urine C&S if pyelonephritis suspected or a diabetic with UTI

Treatment Options

- Toradol (ketorolac) 30 mg IV with or without Dilaudid (hydromorphone) 0.5–1 mg IV (or other equipotent narcotic) and Phenergan (promethazine) 6.25 mg or Zofran (ondansetron) 4 mg IV for suspected renal colic
    - Do not use Toradol (ketorolac) if creatinine is elevated
- Musculoskeletal can be treated with Tylenol, OTC medication, NSAID or short narcotic course
- Narcotic short course prn on discharge for renal colic pain, with or without Toradol (ketorolac)
- Phenergan (promethazine) prn
- Flomax (tamsulosin) 0.4 mg PO every day for 2–4 weeks for ureteral calculus

- Simple UTI: Septra DS, cephalosporin or nitrofurantoin for 3–5 days — consider single dose therapy for appropriate agents
- Pyridium: 200 mg TID prn urinary symptoms — do not dispense more than 6 for acute cystitis (avoid in renal insufficiency)
- Pyelonephritis: 10–14 days of simple UTI antibiotic regimen
- IV Rocephin (ceftriaxone) or Invanz (ertapenem) × 1 can be given initially
- Herpes zoster Rx as indicated

Discharge Criteria

- Renal colic controlled
- Simple cystitis
- Pyelonephritis in nontoxic patient and able to hold down medication at home
- Benign musculoskeletal disorder

Discharge instructions

- Flank pain aftercare instructions
- Refer to primary care provider or urologist as indicated within 1–7 days

Consult Criteria

- Unknown cause of moderate to severe flank pain
- Unable to hold oral fluids down at home
- Heart rate ≥ 110, hypotension or relative hypotension (SBP < 105 with history of hypertension)
- Suspected vascular cause of flank pain
- Toxic UTI patient
- Unable to hold down medications at home
- WBC ≥ 14,000
- New onset anemia
- Inadequate renal colic relief
- Age ≥ 60 without firm diagnosis
- New onset renal insufficiency or worsening renal insufficiency
- Solitary kidney with ureteral calculus
- Pyelonephritis with ureteral calculus

Notes

Reference:

emedicine.medscape.com/article/1958746–overview
Causes of Flank Pain Author: J Stuart Wolf Jr, MD, FACS; Chief Editor: Bradley Fields Schwartz, DO, FACS

Age-Adjusted D-Dimer Cutoff Levels to Rule Out Pulmonary Embolism: The ADJUST-PE Study *JAMA.* 2014;311(11):1117-1124. doi:10.1001/jama.2014.2135

Gastrointestinal

Section Contents

When using any protocol, always follow the Guidelines of Proper Use (page 18).

ABDOMINAL PAIN PROTOCOL

When using any protocol, always follow the Guidelines of Proper Use (page 18).

Differential Diagnosis

- See below locations of pain

Considerations

- Appendicitis may have normal WBC
  - WBC ≥ 10,000 with left shift in 80–90% of patients
- WBC is a poor predictor of surgical disease
- Consider EKG in epigastric pain with CAD risk factors and a benign exam
- Constitutional history important

Diagnostic pitfall

- Diagnosing UTI with mildly elevated WBC's in the general range of 7–15 WBC's on U/A as the cause of moderate to severe abdominal pain and/or tenderness, especially in females and those without infectious urinary complaints

Locations of pain

RUQ

- Gallbladder disease
- Liver disease
- Peptic ulcer disease

Epigastric

- Peptic ulcer
- Cardiac ischemia
- Gallbladder disease
- Pancreatitis
- Aortic aneurysm
- Mesenteric ischemia
- Small bowel disorder

LUQ

- Colon disorder

- Spleen disorder
- Liver disease
- Constipation

Right and left flanks

- Renal colic
- Pyelonephritis
- Aortic aneurysm

Periumbilical

- Pancreatitis
- Peptic ulcer
- Mesenteric ischemia
- Aortic aneurysm
- Intussusception

RLQ

- Appendicitis
- Mesenteric adenitis
- Diverticulitis
- Renal colic
- Ectopic pregnancy
- Ovarian cyst rupture
- Colitis
- Constipation
- Intussusception

LLQ

- Diverticulitis (most common area)
- Renal colic
- Ectopic pregnancy
- Ovarian cyst rupture
- Colitis
- Intussusception
- Constipation

Suprapubic

- Cystitis
- Prostatitis
- Proctitis
- Perirectal abscess
- Constipation/fecal impaction

Groin

- Inguinal hernia
- Femoral hernia
- Inguinal ligament strain
- Femoral pseudoaneursym post cardiac catheterization

Appendicitis

- See Appendicitis Protocol

Diverticulitis

- Prevalence increases with age
- Usually pain and tenderness in LLQ of abdomen
- Fever may occur
- WBC may not be elevated in 60% of patients
- CT abdominal/pelvis imaging study of choice
    - Children start with abdominal ultrasound for radiation considerations
        - Ultrasound used to rule in appendicitis; do not use to rule out appendicitis (if negative and appendicitis a consideration, then CT abdomen/pelvis)
- Patients with mild to moderate diverticulitis without systemic signs of infection or peritoneal signs may be discharged home on antibiotics and a clear liquid diet for 2–3 days and advanced as tolerated
    - Flagyl (metronidazole) 500 mg PO qid for 10 days
    - Cipro (ciprofloxacin) 500 mg PO bid or Levaquin (levofloxacin) 500–750 mg PO qday with Flagyl (metronidazole) for 10 days
    - Septra DS PO bid can be used instead of Cipro (ciprofloxacin) or Levofloxacin if needed
    - May use Sanford guide or antibiotic database also

Biliary colic and cholecystitis

- See Gallbladder Disease Protocol

Pancreatitis

- Major causes are gallstones lodged in pancreas and ethanol consumption

- Severe pain usually in central abdomen and vomiting very common
- Chronic pancreatitis may develop (alcoholics)
  - Lipase may remain elevated with a normal amylase
- Lipase may remain elevated up to 12 days whereas amylase will return to normal after acute pancreatitis has resolved
- Level of lipase and amylase do not indicate severity of disease
- Fever may occur
- Obtain CBC, amylase, lipase, LFT's, LDH and U/A
  - Amylase may be normal early
  - Lipase and amylase elevated more than 3 times normal is diagnostic of acute pancreatitis
- Ultrasound if cholecystitis or choledocholithiasis suspected
- Treatment options
  - IV NS or LR 250–500 cc/hour for adults as clinically indicated
    - Lactated ringers (LR) may be preferred over NS
    - Caution in heart failure and renal failure patients, etc.
  - If patient hypotensive then more aggressive fluid resuscitation needed
  - Phenergan (promethazine) 6.25 mg IV or 25–50 mg IM

    OR
  - Zofran (ondansetron) 4–8 mg IM or IV
  - Stadol (butorphanol) 0.25–1 mg IV or 2 mg IM

    OR
  - Dilaudid (hydromorphone) 0.25–1 mg IV or 1–2 mg IM
  - Small narcotic doses for very elderly

Mesenteric ischemia

- Mortality high – 70–90%, especially with low flow circulatory states such as CHF
- Causes are arterial embolism, arterial thrombosis, non-occlusive mesenteric ischemia and venous

thrombosis which all lead to ischemia/reperfusion syndrome of the bowel

- Order CBC, BMP, lactate level, amylase, lipase and CT abdomen/pelvis
- Severe pain with less than expected tenderness on exam (may only have mild tenderness)
- Vomiting and diarrhea frequently present
- Risk factors are CHF, atrial fibrillation, and atherosclerotic disease
- May have metabolic acidosis secondary to bowel infarction (elevated lactic acid)
- Intestinal angina may occur after a meal

Small bowel obstruction (SBO)

- Usually from postsurgical adhesions
- Pain is usually severe if obstruction is complete
- Vomiting is very common
- Hyperactive bowels sounds seen early in process
- Abdominal distension common
- Check for hernias
- Order CBC, amylase, lipase and BMP
- Obtain flat and upright plain abdominal films — may be negative in 30%
    - Consider CT abdomen/pelvis if SBO suspected and plain films nondiagnostic
    - May need N-G tube to low suction though can be managed frequently without suction.
        - Latest data suggest may not be as effective as was thought in the past

Large bowel obstruction

- 60% from malignancy, 20% from diverticulitis and 5% from cecal volvulus
- Abdominal distension is significant
- Abdomen is hyperresonant on percussion
- Fever, rebound tenderness and rigidity suggest perforation
- Order CBC, BMP, lactate level if acidotic, and flat and upright abdominal films
- Ogilvie syndrome is acute colonic pseudoobstruction
    - Needs to be decompressed to avoid perforation

Hernia

Differential diagnosis

- Epididymitis
- Hydrocele
- Lymphogranuloma Venereum
- Testicular torsion
- Pseudoaneurym of femoral artery
- Varicocele
- Groin abscess

Considerations

- Reducible hernia can have contents returned to abdominal cavity
- Incarcerated hernia cannot be reduced
    - Not strangulated
    - Bowel obstruction not uncommon
    - Painful
- Strangulated hernia
    - Blood flow compromised with possible necrosis of bowel
    - Significant pain and tenderness
    - If reduced, pain and tenderness persists

Types of hernia

- Umbilical
    - Through umbilical ring
    - Common in childhood
    - Usually resolves by age 2 years
- Inguinal
    - Indirect inguinal hernia
        - Through inguinal ring into the inguinal canal following spermatic cord to scrotum
    - Direct inguinal hernia
        - Through Hasselbach's triangle (above inguinal ligament
- Femoral
    - Through femoral canal
    - Frequently become incarcerated or strangulated
- Ventral or incisional hernia

- Post-surgical complication
- Usually without pain or incarceration

Gastroenteritis

- See Gastroenteritis Protocols for adults and pediatrics

Flank pain or kidney stone pain (renal colic) see respective protocols

Elderly abdominal pain

- Pain perception and abdominal exam altered in elderly
- Admissions and surgery rates are higher in elderly
- Consider mesenteric and cardiac ischemia in elderly
- Elderly may have normal WBC with serious disease
- Appendicitis missed 50% of the time
- CT abdominal/pelvis commonly ordered as serious organic disease is more prevalent
- Diverticulitis: WBC is normal 50% of the time
- Consider ruptured aortic aneurysm especially with flank pain thought to be renal colic
- Polypharmacy and medication side effects can be a cause of abdominal complaints

Pediatric abdominal pain

- Peritonitis patient is immobile
- Colic patient is writhing
- Absence of fever does not rule out serious illness
- Discuss with physician prior to ordering CT abdomen/pelvis in children
- Children start with abdominal ultrasound for radiation exposure considerations
    - Ultrasound used to rule-in appendicitis; do not use to rule-out appendicitis (if negative and appendicitis a consideration, then CT abdomen/pelvis)

Pediatric appendicitis

- Frequently missed in age < 2 years
- With abdominal pain, fever is most useful sign in appendicitis

- CBC may be normal
- Absolute neutrophil count < 6750 significantly decreases the likelihood of appendicitis
- Less than 50% have classic presentation
- Missed appendicitis is second most common reason for pediatric malpractice suits in the emergency department
- Perforation occurs in majority of patients < 4 years of age with appendicitis
- Treatment delayed > 36 hours increases rate of perforations up to 65% of appendicitis cases
- C-reactive protein is nonspecific and not helpful if positive in determining cause of inflammation or abdominal pain
- U/A can have pyuria, bacteriuria or hematuria in 20–40% of patients
- MRI has a high accuracy for the diagnosis of acute appendicitis, with a sensitivity and specificity of 96% and 96% in children
- Ultrasound preferred initially over CT scan due to radiation issues
    - Can rule in appendicitis, but not rule it out

General Evaluation

History

- Pain onset and duration
- Location and migration
- Appetite
- Exacerbating factors
- Prior surgical, medical and medication history
- Vomiting and fever history
- Bowel and urinary history
- Constitutional history
- Melena or bleeding
- Last normal menstrual cycle
- Menstrual abnormalities

Physical examination

- Observe for distension
- Auscultation for bowel sounds and arterial bruits

- Gently palpate entire abdomen
- Percuss for liver size; and for ascites if present
- Perform rectal exam for masses; tenderness; prostate disease; gross blood; occult blood when indicated
- Palpation of entire abdomen and document any findings of:
    - Tenderness location and severity
    - Rebound tenderness
    - Voluntary and involuntary guarding
    - Pulsatile masses
    - Abdominal masses

Objective testing

Benign findings and complaints in nonelderly healthy patient

- Consider no tests

Moderate complaints and findings, or if diabetic

- CBC and CMP

Urine or renal disease

- U/A
- CBC and BMP if pyelonephritis suspected
- Urine culture as indicated (complicated UTI)

Pancreatitis

- Amylase and lipase
- CBC and CMP

Gallbladder disease

- Gallbladder ultrasound as needed
- CBC and BMP
- Amylase, lipase and LFT's

Hepatic or metastatic malignant disease

- Liver function tests
- CBC and BMP

Fertile female

- UCG

Constipation or obstruction

- KUB or flat/upright films

Consider CT scan in adults for

- Suspected appendicitis or diverticulitis
- Flank pain of unknown etiology
- Rebound tenderness in adults
- Suspected bowel obstruction not seen on plain flat and upright abdominal films
- Elderly with moderate to severe pain

Caution in ordering pediatric CT scans. Consult physician prior to ordering — ultrasound can be used for appendicitis evaluation instead to rule-in appendicitis (not rule-out), depending on the institution

Outpatient Treatment Considerations

- OTC medications
- Hydrocodone or synthetic codeine derivatives as needed
- Avoid Demerol (meperidine)
- Phenergan (promethazine) or Zofran (ondansetron) prn nausea or vomiting

Parenteral Treatment Considerations

- IV NS 100–1,000 cc/hour for adults as clinically indicated
- IV NS 1–2 times maintenance in children if stable, otherwise discuss with physician
- Nausea or vomiting (adjust for children)
    - Phenergan (promethazine) 6.25 mg IV (adult or pediatrics) or 25–50 mg IM adult or 0.5 mg/kg IM for children

      OR
    - Zofran (ondansetron) 4 mg IM or IV (adults and pediatrics)
- Pain control (adjust for children)
    - Stadol (butorphanol) 0.25–1 mg IV or 1–2 mg IM for adults

      OR
    - Dilaudid (hydromorphone) 0.25–1 mg IV or 1–2 mg IM for adult or 0.015 mg/Kg IV or IM for pediatrics
    - Small narcotic and Phenergan (promethazine) doses for the very elderly

Discharge Criteria

- Mild pain and tenderness in nonelderly healthy patient with normal vital signs consider symptomatic treatment if benign disease process suspected
- Biliary colic with normal vital signs and exam that resolves with treatment may not require labs and may be discharged
- Acute and self-limited process suspected such as gastroenteritis in stable nontoxic patient
- Reducible hernia with resolution of pain

Discharge instructions

- To primary care provider or surgeon for follow-up in 1 day if pain is moderate to severe, otherwise in 5–7 days
- To primary care provider for abnormal lab within 1 week unless chronic in nature
- Abdominal pain aftercare instructions

Consult Criteria

- Moderate pain in age ≥ 60 years
- Abdominal pain that develops hypotension or relative hypotension (SBP < 105 with history of hypertension)
- Toxic appearance
- Dehydration
- Significant GI blood loss or melena
- Acute surgical abdomen or rebound tenderness
- Moderate to severe pain of uncertain cause
- Severe pain with any diagnosis
- Intractable vomiting
- Return ED visit within 14 days for same acute abdominal pain complaint

Discuss with physician if following suspected or diagnosed

- Appendicitis
- Cholecystitis
- Pancreatitis
- Diverticulitis
- Aortic aneurysm

- Bowel obstruction
- Ectopic pregnancy
- Intra-abdominal abscess
- Mesenteric ischemia
- Incarcerated or strangulated hernia

Lab consult criteria (if checked)

- Hemoglobin decrease > 1 gm or creatinine increase> 0.5 from baseline
- Hemoglobin < 10 gms
- Elevated LFT's
- Elevated amylase or lipase
- WBC ≥ 14,000
- Bandemia
- Increased anion gap
- Metabolic acidosis
- Significant electrolyte abnormally
- Glucose ≥ 400 mg/dL in diabetic patient
- Glucose ≥ 300 mg/dL in non-diabetic patient
- Hyperglycemia with metabolic acidosis (decreased serum CO_2 or elevated anion gap)
- Acute thrombocytopenia

Vital sign and age consult criteria

- Any abdominal pain age ≥ 70 years
- Adult heart rate ≥ 110
- Pediatric heart rate
    - 0–4 months ≥ 180
    - 5–7 months ≥ 175
    - 8–12 months ≥ 170
    - 1–3 years ≥ 160
    - 4–5 years ≥ 145
    - 6–8 years ≥ 130
    - 9–11 years ≥ 125
    - 12–15 years ≥ 120
    - 16 years or older ≥ 115

Notes

References:

Tenner S, Baillie J, Dewitt J, et al. American College of Gastroenterology Guidelines: Management of Acute Pancreatitis. *Am J Gastroenterol*. Jul 30 201

Wu BU , et al. Â *Clin Gastroenterol Hepatol* 2011; 9:710
emedicine.medscape.com/article/181364

JICS;15(3):226-230

CT Abdominal Scan Issues

When using any protocol, always follow the Guidelines of Proper Use (page 18).

Cancer Risk from One CT Depending on Type

- Adults: 1/500–2000
- Children under 1 year of age: 1/500
- Decreasing risk with increasing age

Oral contrast considerations

- Adds little if anything to interpretation
  - Oral contrast located immediately adjacent to the bowel wall can make assessment of the degree of IV contrast enhancement difficult
  - IV contrast extravasating into bowel lumen can be masked by dense positive oral contrast
- Some radiologists uncomfortable without it
- Appendicitis diagnosed without and with contrast
  - Sensitivity 95% vs. 92%
  - Specificity 97% vs. 94%
  - Accuracy 97% vs. 89%
- Message: Non-oral contrast CT is better in diagnosing appendicitis

IV contrast considerations

- Does not improve accuracy of noncontrast studies
- In very thin patients without much body fat IV contrast is needed

There is no connection between seafood and/or shellfish allergy and IV contrast allergy

Treatment of Allergy to IV Contrast

- Benadryl (diphenhydramine) 50 mg in adult or weight based in children
- Decadron (dexamethasone) 10 mg IV in adult or 0.6 mg/kg IV in children (not to exceed 10 mg)

- May not be effective since steroid dosing should be done 12 hours before IV contrast

Prior History of Asthma

- 1/1000 chance of severe reaction to IV contrast
- No reason to withhold contrast study

Creatinine Considerations

- Majority of patients do not need a creatinine measurement
- Needed with history of risk factors
  - Renal insufficiency
  - Elderly
  - Diabetes
  - Multiple myeloma
  - Volume depletion
  - Diuretic therapy
  - NSAID's use
  - ACE inhibitor use
  - CHF
  - Anemia

Prevention of Contrast-induced Nephropathy (CIN)

- There is a lack of good data
- Dialysis is required in less than 1% of contrast nephropathy
- IV hydration NS 1–1.5 ml/kg/hr. 3 hours before contrast and continued 6–24 hours after reduces nephropathy
- Considerations for 0 or 1 risk factor above
  - Before procedure: 1 liter of D5W mixed with 3 amps of $NaHCO_3$ IV at 3 cc/kg for 1 hour
  - During procedure: low volume iso-osmolar contrast
  - After procedure: 1 liter of D5W mixed with 3 amps $NaHCO_3$ IV at 1 cc/kg for 6 hours
- Considerations for 2 or more risk factors — do above

Plus

- N-acetylcysteine 150 mg/kg IV 30 minutes before procedure and 600–1200 mg PO bid × 2 doses after procedure

OR

- Vitamin C 3 gms PO 2 hours before procedure and bid PO after procedure for 1 day

Metformin and IV contrast

- No increase in lactic acidosis if creatinine normal

Notes

References:

xrayrisk.com/calculator/calculator.php

Ionizing Radiation Exposure with Medical Imaging Author: Edward B Holmes, MD, MPH, MSc; Chief Editor: Caroline R Taylor, MD emedicine.medscape.com/article/1464228

Friedewald VE, Goldfarb S, Laskey WK, et al. The editor's roundtable: contrast-induced nephropathy. *Am J Cardiol*. Aug 1 2007;100(3):544–51

Emerg Radiol, epub 5/11/16

ADULT GASTROENTERITIS PROTOCOL

When using any protocol, always follow the Guidelines of Proper Use (page 18).

Definition

- Acute inflammatory or infectious process of the stomach and intestines

Differential Diagnosis

- Rheumatoid Colitis
- Appendicitis
- Cholecystitis
- Pancreatitis
- Mesenteric ischemia
- Aortic aneurysm
- Peptic ulcer disease
- GERD
- Biliary colic
- Renal colic
- Bowel obstruction
- Inflammatory bowel disease

Definitions

- Diarrhea > 3 loose bowel movements (BM's) per day
- Dysentery
    - Disorders with intestinal inflammation (usually colon)
    - Abdominal pain
    - Tenesmus
    - Frequent BM's with blood and mucus in stool
- Enteritis — small bowel inflammation
- Gastritis — stomach inflammation
- Gastroenteritis symptoms
    - Acute inflammation of stomach and intestines with abdominal pain
    - Weakness

- Nausea
- Diarrhea
- Anorexia
- Fever

Considerations

- Diarrhea most common manifestation (virus most common cause — norovirus)
- Enteritis — often with bloating, periumbilical pain, nausea/vomiting (viral most common cause)
- Colitis — can have localized left sided pain, rectal bleeding
- Antibiotics can cause diarrhea — C. difficile (antibiotic-associated or "pseudomembranous" colitis)
- Association between antibiotic use, enterohemorrhagic Escherichia coli and hemolytic-uremic syndrome remains unproven

Diarrhea Red Flags

- Bloody stools or pus in stool
- Infant refuses to drink anything for more than 3 to 4 hours
- Signs of dehydration and/or acute weight loss
- Abdominal pain that comes and goes or is severe
- Any fever >102°F (39°C) or a fever >101°F (38.4°C) that persists for more than 3 days
- Decreased responsiveness or lethargy
- Chronic diarrhea
- Recent antibiotic use
- Weight loss over past 1–2 months

Invasive bacteria — frequently with occult or gross blood

- Campylobacter
- Salmonella
- Shigella
- Vibrio
- Yersinia

Food-borne disease

- Staph aureus most common: 1–6 hours post food ingestion
- Bacillus cereus: 1–36 hours post food ingestion

- Cholera: profuse rice water stools
- Ciguatera: Fish — 5 minutes–30 hours post food ingestion
- Traveler's diarrhea: E. coli usually
- Camping: Giardia, water ingestion, beavers

Evaluation

- Travel, food and antibiotic history
- Healthy patient without toxicity and with acute onset of symptoms and mild to no tenderness and normal vital signs may not require further testing
- Consider CBC, CMP if vital signs abnormal or with significant tenderness
- Consider stool WBC, RBC, cultures for fever; blood in stool
- Consider rectal exam
- Imaging usually not necessary unless
    - Obstruction suspected
        - Abdominal flat and upright films
        - Consider CT abdomen/pelvis if bowel obstruction suspected and plain films negative
    - Consider CT abdomen/pelvis for elderly with abnormal vital signs and significant tenderness or pain

Treatment Options

Dehydration

Oral Rehydration Therapy (ORT) for mild to moderate dehydration

- Oral rehydration formula (WHO, Rehydralyte or Pedialyte) for mild to moderate dehydration or serum CO_2 13–18 mEq/L or Na+ 146–152 mEq/L — if able to take PO fluids
    - Zofran (ondansetron) 8 mg chewable tablet if vomiting or 4–8 mg IM
    - 15–30 cc every 1–2 minutes for 1–4 hours for age > 12 — start 20 minutes after Zofran (ondansetron) given
    - Hold ORT 10 minutes if vomiting occurs then resume

    - Re-assess for urine production, improved heart rate, and absence of severe vomiting
    - Recheck serum CO_2 if initially < 17 mEq/L or anion gap > 21
    - Mild dehydration give 20 cc/kg in < 4 hours
    - Moderate dehydration give 20–40 cc/kg in 1–4 hours
  - Severe dehydration give IV NS 200–500 cc/hour over 2–4 hours or 1000 cc/hour for 1 hour (notify physician)
    - Hypotension or signs of poor organ perfusion (lactic acid > 2) give NS at 500–1,000 cc/hour up to 2 liters or IV 500–1,000 cc bolus (consult physician promptly)

Diarrhea

- Nontoxic, non-dehydrated healthy patients with mild abdominal tenderness, benign vital signs and diarrhea may be discharged without further testing
- Pepto-Bismol — good for traveler's diarrhea
- Quinolone 1, 3 or 5 day course, especially with traveler's diarrhea
- Septra DS 1 PO bid for 5 days (DOC for age < 18 years or for shigella)
  - Septra (trimethoprim/sulfamethoxazole) 8-12 mg TMP/kg/dose or 0.5 cc/LB BID PO for PO q12hr for 5-10 days for children
  - Contraindicated in ages < 2 months
- Rifaximin (Rx) – Xifaxan 200 mg PO q8hr.
- If C. difficile colitis suspected from recent antibiotic use:
  - Mild to moderate symptoms
    - Flagyl (metronidazole) 500 mg PO tid × 10 days
    - Florastor PO bid × 10 days (OTC)

Antibiotic therapy

- World Health Organization currently recommends empiric antimicrobial therapy in the setting of febrile acute bloody diarrhea in young children
  - Infections by enteropathogenic *E coli*, when running a prolonged course — septra or ceftriaxone
  - Enteroinvasive *E coli*, based on the serologic, genetic, and pathogenic similarities with *Shigella* — septra or ceftriaxone
  - *Yersinia* infections in subjects with sickle cell disease — septra or cipro or ceftriaxone or doxycycline (avoid doxycycline in age <8 years)
  - *Salmonella* infections in very young infants, if febrile or with positive blood culture findings — ceftriaxone
    - Most salmonella infections do not require antibiotics and they may prolong the illness
- Clostridium difficile proven or clinically suspected — metronidazole (30 mg/kg/d divided qid for 7 d) can be used as a first-line agent, with oral vancomycin reserved for resistant infections
  - Severe symptoms consult physician
  - Stop offending antibiotic
  - See primary care provider within 1–2 days for follow-up

Antimotility agents

- Loperamide (most preferred due to safety profile)
- Diphenoxylate (heme negative stools only)

Vomiting

- Phenergan (promethazine) PO/PR/IM (if IV give no more than 6.25 mg/dose as single dose)
- Zofran (ondansetron) 4–8 mg PO/IM/IV

Abdominal pain treatment outpatient considerations

- OTC medications
- Hydrocodone or synthetic codeine derivatives as needed
- Avoid Demerol (meperidine)

Abdominal pain parenteral treatment considerations

- Stadol (butorphanol), Nubain (nalbuphine) or Dilaudid (hydromorphone): IV or IM
  - Stadol and Nubain may cause acute opiate withdrawal in opiate addicted patients
- Give Phenergan (promethazine) 6.25 mg (if IV) or Zofran (ondansetron) as needed for nausea
- Adjust doses for weight in pediatrics

Discharge Criteria

- Healthy nontoxic patient with stable vital signs

Discharge instructions

- Gastroenteritis aftercare instructions
- Resume regular diet as soon as possible
- Follow-up in 1–2 days if symptoms are moderate to severe if discharged, otherwise within 5–7 days if symptoms persist
- Follow up for abnormal lab within 1 week unless chronic in nature
- Return within 3 days if symptoms not improving

Consult Criteria

- Toxic appearance
- Dehydration > 5%
- Significant blood loss or melena
- Suspected or diagnosed appendicitis, cholecystitis, pancreatitis, diverticulitis, aortic aneurysm, bowel obstruction or admittable diagnosis
- Acute surgical abdomen
- Moderate pain of uncertain cause
- Severe pain
- Narcotic IM/IV dosing that is given acutely
- Intractable vomiting
- Return visit within 14 days for same acute abdominal pain complaint

Lab consult criteria (if checked)

- Metabolic acidosis (increased anion gap)
- Hemoglobin decrease > 1 gm or creatinine increase> 0.5 from baseline

- Elevated LFT's
- Elevated amylase or lipase
- WBC ≥ 15,000
- Bandemia
- Significant electrolyte abnormally
- Glucose ≥ 400 mg/dL in diabetic patient
- Glucose ≥ 300 mg/dL in non-diabetic patient
- Hyperglycemia with metabolic acidosis (decreased serum CO_2 or elevated anion gap)
- Acute thrombocytopenia

Vital sign and age consult criteria

- Age ≥ 70
- Adult heart rate > 100 post-treatment
- Hypotension or relative hypotension (SBP < 105 with history of hypertension)
- Orthostatic vital signs

Notes

References:

Payne DC, Vinjé J, Szilagyi PG, Edwards KM, Staat MA, Weinberg GA. Norovirus and medically attended gastroenteritis in U.S. children. *N Engl J Med*. Mar 21 2013;368(12):1121–30

Emergent Treatment of Gastroenteritis
Author: Arthur Diskin, MD; Chief Editor: Steven C Dronen, MD, FAAEM emedicine.medscape.com/article/775277

IRRITABLE BOWEL SYNDROME PROTOCOL

When using any protocol, always follow the Guidelines of Proper Use (page 18).

Definition

- A functional bowel disorder without specific pathology of abdominal pain and altered bowel habits

Differential Diagnosis

- Anxiety disorder
- Biliary colic
- Inflammatory bowel disease
- Ischemic colitis
- Antibiotic-associated colitis
- Endometriosis
- Gastroenteritis
- Food allergies
- Malabsorption
- Porphyria
- Colon carcinoma
- Thyroid disease

Considerations

- Is a disorder of exclusion of other disease processes
- Hypersensitivity to pain and symptoms
- Association with psychopathology is common
- Is a chronic relapsing disorder
- Females 2–3 times more likely to have the disorder than males

Common Symptoms and Findings

- Abdominal pain
- Diarrhea
- Constipation
- Mucus in stool
- Abdominal distension

- Stress related commonly
- Fibromyalgia is frequently present
- Postprandial bowel movement urgency

Symptoms not consistent with IBS

- Middle age or later onset
- New symptom presentations
- Fever
- Weight loss
- Nocturnal symptoms
- Progressive symptoms
- Rectal bleeding
- Painless diarrhea

Patterns of IBS

- IBS-D (diarrhea predominant)
- IBS-C (constipation predominant)
- IBS-M (mixed diarrhea and constipation)
- IBS-A (alternating diarrhea and constipation)

Evaluation

- History and physical examination
    - Rectal examination for occult blood as indicated
    - Testing not recommended in age < 50 years with typical IBS symptoms and no weight loss, or family history of serious bowel diseases (colon cancer, inflammatory bowel disease, etc.)

Lab test options

- CBC
- BMP
- LFT's
- Thyroid panel as indicated
- Plain flat and upright x-rays as indicated
- Amylase and lipase as indicated
- CT abdominal and pelvis scan as indicated (usually not needed)

Treatment Options

- Add fiber to diet
- Reassurance regarding symptoms and diagnosis

- Stress management suggestions
- Consider psychiatric referral

Antispasmodic agents

- Bentyl (dicyclomine) 10–40 mg PO qid ac (before meals) or with pain onset
- Levsin (hyoscyamine) 0.125– 0.25 mg q4hr and or prn (NMT 1.5 pills/day) for adults
- Levsin (hyoscyamine) 1/2–1 pill qid PO q4hr or prn (NMT 6 tabs/day) for age 2–12 years

Antidiarrheal agents

Lomotil (diphenoxylate/atropine)

- Age > 12 years: 1–2 tabs PO qid ac prn
- Age 8–12 years: 2 mg PO 5 times qday prn
- Age 5–7 years: 2 mg PO qid prn
- Age 2–4 years: 2 mg PO tid prn

Imodium (loperamide)

- Adult: 4 mg PO after 1st loose stool, then 2 mg PO after each following loose stool prn (NMT 16 mg/day)
- Pediatric: 0.1 mg/kg PO after each loose stool not to exceed adult total daily dose

Other agents

- SSRI's
- Elavil 10–100 mg PO qday prn (start with low dose)
- Rifaximin – Xifaxan 550 mg PO q8hr for 14 days (nonabsorbed antibiotic) — read drug information
- Lubiprostone – Amitiza 8 mcg PO q12hr in women ≥ 18 years with IBS–C (constipation type) — read drug information
- Linaclotide – Linzess 290 mcg PO qday at least 30 minutes before first meal of the day for adults for the treatment of irritable bowel syndrome with constipation
- Eluxadoline – Viberzi 100 mg bid PO with food for diarrhea-predominant irritable bowel syndrome (IBS-D) in adult men and women
    - Stop if constipation > 4 days
    - 75 mg bid for cholecystectomy patients or hepatic impairment

Discharge Criteria

- No other concerning disease process diagnosed

Discharge instructions

- Irritable bowel syndrome aftercare instructions
- Follow up within 10 days or as needed

Consult Criteria

- WBC ≥ 12,000
- Severe pain
- Age ≥ 60 years
- Heart rate > 100
- Dehydration
- Patient appears toxic
- Fever
- Weight loss
- Progressive symptoms
- Rectal bleeding
- See General Patient Criteria Protocol (page 22) for items not covered in this protocol

Notes

References:

Brandt LJ, Chey WD, Foxx-Orenstein AE, Schiller LR, Schoenfeld PS, Spiegel BM, et al. An evidence-based position statement on the management of irritable bowel syndrome. *Am J Gastroenterol*. Jan 2009;104 Suppl 1:S1–35

Irritable Bowel Syndrome Author: Jenifer K Lehrer, MD; Chief Editor: Julian Katz, MD
emedicine.medscape.com/article/180389–overview

APPENDICITIS PROTOCOL

When using any protocol, always follow the Guidelines of Proper Use (page 18).

Definition

- Inflammation of the appendix secondary to luminal obstruction

Differential Diagnosis

- Pelvic inflammatory disease
- Ruptured ovarian cyst
- Endometriosis
- Mesenteric adenitis
- Inflammatory bowel disease
- Colon carcinoma
- Mesenteric ischemia
- Ureteral colic
- Pyelonephritis
- Biliary colic
- Abdominal abscess
- Diverticulitis
- Ectopic pregnancy
- Ovarian torsion
- Constipation

Considerations

- Appendicitis is missed 50% of the time in elderly
- In patients with suspected acute appendicitis, use clinical findings (signs and symptoms) to risk-stratify patients and guide decisions about further testing and management
- In adult patients undergoing a CT scan for suspected appendicitis, perform abdominal and pelvic CT scan with or without contrast IV, oral, or rectal
    - Patients with little body fat may need IV contrast

    - In children, use ultrasound to confirm acute appendicitis but not to definitively exclude acute appendicitis
        - In children, use an abdominal and pelvic CT to confirm or exclude acute appendicitis if ultrasound does not rule-in appendicitis
- The duration of symptoms is less than 48 hours in approximately 80% of adults
    - Frequently longer in elderly persons and in those with perforation
- Approximately 2% of patients report duration of pain in excess of 2 weeks
- A history of similar pain is reported in as many as 23% of cases, and this history of similar pain should not be used to rule out the possibility of appendicitis
- If mesenteric adenitis is diagnosed, it can be treated with supportive care or in more severe cases antibiotics
    - Metronidazole, clindamycin, or unasyn

Presentations

- Abdominal pain is most common symptom
- Migration of pain from periumbilical area to RLQ has sensitivity and specificity of 80%
- Nausea present in 61–92% of patients
    - Vomiting that precedes pain suggests intestinal obstruction instead
- Anorexia present in 74–78% of patients
- Diarrhea or constipation noted in around 18% of patients
- Common to have low-grade fever or no fever
- High fever develops with abscess formation secondary to appendiceal rupture
- Fecaliths and lymphoid hyperplasia most common causes secondary to luminal obstruction

Physical findings

- 96% of patients with RLQ tenderness — most specific sign
- The most specific exam findings are guarding, percussion tenderness, rebound tenderness and rigidity

- Rosving, Obturator, Psoas signs present in minority of patients and their absence should not be used to rule out appendicitis

Lab findings

- Normal C-reactive protein after abdominal pain for 24 hours has a high negative predictive value ruling out appendicitis
- U/A showing WBC's and urinary complaints not uncommon in appendicitis

Pregnancy and appendicitis

- First trimester pain in RLQ
- Second trimester pain at level of umbilicus
- Third trimester pain in RUQ
- Anorexia in one-third to two-thirds of patients
- Nausea usually present
- MRI has a high accuracy for the diagnosis of acute appendicitis, with a sensitivity and specificity of 94% and 97%, respectively, in pregnant patients

Pediatric appendicitis

- Frequently missed in age < 2 years
- With abdominal pain, fever is most useful sign in appendicitis
- CBC may be normal
    - WBC >10,500 in 80–85% of adults with appendicitis
    - Less than 4% of patients with appendicitis have a WBC count less than 10,500 and neutrophilia less than 75% of WBC's
- Absolute neutrophil count < 6750 significantly decreases the likelihood of appendicitis
- Less than 50% have classic presentation
- Missed appendicitis is second most common reason for pediatric malpractice suits in the emergency department
- Perforation occurs in majority of patients < 4 years of age with appendicitis
- Treatment delayed > 36 hours increases rate of perforations up to 65% of appendicitis cases
- C-reactive protein is nonspecific and not helpful if positive in determining cause of inflammation or abdominal pain

  - Very high levels of CRP in patients with appendicitis indicate gangrenous appendix, especially if it is associated with elevated WBC and neutrophils
- Appendicitis: U/A can have pyuria, bacteriuria or hematuria in 20–40%
- MRI has a high accuracy for the diagnosis of acute appendicitis, with a sensitivity and specificity of 96% and 96% in children

Evaluation

- History and physical examination
  - Specific attention to onset and progression of symptoms

Testing

- No testing if signs and symptoms not consistent with possible appendicitis
- CBC
- BMP
- U/A
- UCG in fertile females (includes those with history of bilateral tubal ligation)
- LFT's as indicated
- Amylase and lipase as indicated
- Plain flat and upright if obstruction suspected
- CT abdominal and pelvic scan in adults as needed
- CT abdominal and pelvic scans in pediatrics need serious consideration of the risk potential for later cancer development — discuss with physician before ordering
  - Ultrasound has usefulness in pediatric appendicitis depending on radiologist experience

Discharge Criteria

- None

Consult Criteria

- All appendicitis or suspected appendicitis patients

Notes

References:

Howell JM, Eddy OL, Lukens TW, Thiessen ME, Weingart SD, Decker WW, American College of Emergency Physicians. Clinical policy: critical issues in the evaluation and management of emergency department patients with suspected appendicitis. Ann Emerg Med. 2010 Jan;55(1):71–116

Appendicitis Clinical Presentation

Author: Sandy Craig, MD; Chief Editor: Barry E Brenner, MD, PhD, FACEP emedicine.medscape.com/article/773895

AJR,2016;206:508

ANTIBIOTIC-ASSOCIATED COLITIS PROTOCOL

When using any protocol, always follow the Guidelines of Proper Use (page 18).

Definition

- Inflammation of the bowel secondary to Clostridium difficile and usually recent antibiotic use or hospitalization

Differential Diagnosis

- Crohn's disease
- Ulcerative colitis
- Irritable bowel syndrome
- Gastroenteritis
- Toxic megacolon
- Diverticulitis

Considerations

- 20% of hospitalized patients acquire the infection
  - Diarrhea develop in 30% of these
- Colitis is caused by a toxin produced by C. difficile
- Should be considered with antibiotic use past 2 months or hospitalization in past 3 days
- Asymptomatic colonization occurs in 1–3% of the healthy population
- Do not routinely test for Clostridium difficile in age < 12 months where rates can exceed 40% in asymptomatic patients
  - By age 2–3 years carrier rate of Clostridium difficile are 1–3%
  - Test in symptomatic patients with evidence of pseudomembranous colitis, toxic megacolon or clinically significant diarrhea
- A brief exposure to an antibiotic can cause C. difficile colitis
  - Symptoms usually start 3–9 days after antibiotic initiation

- Age ≥ 60 years is a risk factor
- Relapse after treatment is common
    - Recurs in 15 – 35% of patients with one previous episode and 33 – 65% of patients with more than two episodes
- Elevated WBC is found in 50–60% of patients

Symptoms and Findings

- Mild to moderate watery diarrhea
    - Usually not bloody
- Crampy abdominal pain
- Loss of appetite
- Fever usually in severe cases
- Lower abdominal tenderness
    - Rebound tenderness suggests bowel perforation

Evaluation

- History and physical examination
- Lab test options
    - CBC
    - BMP
    - U/A
    - Stool cultures for C. difficile and other pathogens
    - PCR testing
    - Enzyme immunoassay for C. difficile A and B toxins
        - Available in 2.5 hours
        - Sensitivity 75–80%
- Imaging options
    - Plain upright and flat x-rays if toxic megacolon suspected
    - CT abdominal and pelvis scan may be needed

Treatment Options

- Stop antibiotics (consult physician if antibiotic treatment crucial in treating previous condition)
    - May be all that is needed in mild cases without fever, abdominal pain and elevated WBC
- No treatment of asymptomatic carriers of C. difficile
- Mild to moderate diarrhea or colitis

    - First episode of non–severe clostridium difficile diarrhea may be treated with vancomycin 125 mg PO qid for 10 days
    - Flagyl (metronidazole) 500 mg PO tid for 10–14 days — IV can be used if needed but not as effective as PO
    - Florastor PO bid for 10–14 days (over the counter)
- More severe cases
    - Vancomycin 125 mg PO qid for 10 days
    - Florastor PO bid for 10–14 days (over the counter)
- Antidiarrheal agents should be avoided
- Analgesics
- Symptoms improve usually in 3 days on above antibiotics
- Recurrent C difficile infection can be treated with fecal-microbiota transplant

Discharge Criteria

- Mild to moderate C. difficile or antibiotic-associated colitis
- See General Patient Criteria Protocol (page 22)

Discharge instructions

- Antibiotic-associated colitis aftercare instructions
- Stop current antibiotics
- Follow up with primary care provider within 3–5 days
- Return if symptoms worsen or do not improve
- Wash hands frequently with soap and water

Consult Criteria

- Fever
- WBC ≥ 13,000
- Severe pain
- Rebound tenderness
- CT scan shows colitis
- Dehydration
- See General Patient Criteria Protocol (page 22)

Notes

References:

Clostridium Difficile Colitis

Author: Faten N Aberra, MD, MSCE; Chief Editor: Julian Katz,

emedicine.medscape.com/article/186458-overview

Sloan LM, Duresko BJ, Gustafson DR, Rosenblatt JE. Comparison of real-time PCR for detection of the tcdC gene with four toxin immunoassays and culture in diagnosis of Clostridium difficile infection. *J Clin Microbiol*. Jun 2008;46(6):1996–2001

Debast SB, Bauer MP, Kuijper EJ. European Society of Clinical Microbiology and Infectious Diseases (ESCMID): update of the treatment guidance document for Clostridium difficile infection (CDI). *Clin Microbiol Infect*. Oct 5 2013

AHQR Comparative Effectiveness Review, 172, March 2016

McDonald LC, et al. *Clin Infect Dis*. 2018 Feb 15

Fecal-Microbiota Transplant Beats Antibiotics for Recurrent C Diff - Medscape - Jan 15, 2019

INFLAMMATORY BOWEL DISEASE PROTOCOL

When using any protocol, always follow the Guidelines of Proper Use (page 18).

Definition

- Inflammatory disorder of unknown cause — ulcerative colitis or Crohn's disease

Differential Diagnosis

- Appendicitis
- Diverticulitis
- Endometriosis
- Pelvic inflammatory disease
- Colon carcinoma
- Antibiotic-associated colitis
- Irritable bowel syndrome
- Ischemic colitis

Considerations

- Ulcerative colitis is limited to the large intestine
- Crohn's disease can be anywhere in the gastrointestinal tract
- Kidney stone incidence is increased in Crohn's disease
- Smoking increases the risk Crohn's flares and severity of disease

Ulcerative colitis presentations and findings

- Bloody diarrhea
- Abdominal pain and cramping
- Fever in more severe cases
- Rectal tenesmus or urgency
- Nausea and vomiting
- Dehydration
- Anemia
- Total colectomy is curative
- Test for C. difficile infection

Crohn's disease

- Insidious onset
- Usually nonbloody diarrhea
- Half of cases have perianal fistulas or abscesses
- Weight loss
- Skip regions of intestinal involvement
- Fever
- Arthritis
- Uveitis
- Hepatitis
- Anemia

Evaluation

- History and physical examination
- Lab test options
  - CBC
  - BMP
  - LFT's
  - Amylase and lipase
  - U/A
- Imaging options
  - Plain upright and flat x-rays if toxic megacolon suspected or obstruction suspected
  - CT abdominal and pelvis scan
    - Also perform if obstruction suspected
    - No CT scan if ESR+5 x CRP ≤ 10 in crohn's disease
      - Negative predictive value of 98.1% for missing serious complications

Treatment

Step therapy

- Step 1 –aminosalicylates
- Step 2 – corticosteroids
- Step 2 – immunomodulators

Crohn's disease

Mild disease

- Sulfasalazine 0.5−1.5 gms PO 2–4 times a day for mild to moderate disease in colon
    - Caution with sulfasalazine hypersensitivity, renal insufficiency, coagulation abnormalities, pyloric stenosis, PUD, and liver disease
    - Read drug information in database
- Mesalamine (Asacol HD) 1.6 g three times daily for small bowel for remission induction of active mild to moderate – read PDR or databases
- Antidiarrheal medications qid for diarrhea without active colitis (avoid if possible)
    - Imodium (loperamide) 2 mg PO qid prn
    - Lomotil (diphenoxylate/atropine) 5 mg PO qid prn

Moderate disease

- Prednisone 30–60 mg PO qday 7−10 days
- Flagyl (metronidazole) 250−500 mg PO qid for fistula complications for 1 month

Disease not responsive to usual treatment

- Vedolizumab (Entyvio) 300 mg IV at 0, 2 and 6 weeks, then 300 mg IV q8weeks — read drug information
- Biologics (TNF inhibitors) read drug information and discuss with physician
    - Infliximab (Remicade)
    - Adalimumab – Humira

Ulcerative colitis

Mild disease

- Sulfasalazine 0.5−1.5 gms PO 2–4 times a day for mild to moderate disease in colon
    - Contraindications
        - Hypersensitivity to mesalamine or salicylates
        - Breastfeeding
        - Rectal suspension: Patients with history of sulfite hypersensitivity

- Children with chickenpox or flulike symptoms

  Caution with sulfasalazine hypersensitivity, renal insufficiency, coagulation abnormalities, pyloric stenosis, PUD, and liver disease

- Disease confined to the rectum, topical mesalazine (Asacol) given by suppository is the preferred therapy
- Antidiarrheal medications qid for diarrhea without active colitis (avoid if possible)
  - Imodium (loperamide) 2 mg PO qid prn
  - Lomotil (diphenoxylate/atropine) 5 mg PO qid prn
- Mesalamine (Asacol HD) for mild to moderate disease with differing doses depending on disease activity – read PDR or databases

Moderate disease

- Prednisone 30–60 mg PO for 7–14 days followed by taper of 5 mg/week (should see PCP within 1–3 days after discharge)

Disease not responsive to usual treatment

- Vedolizumab (Entyvio) 300 mg IV at 0, 2 and 6 weeks, then 300 mg IV q8weeks — read drug information
- Biologics (TNF inhibitors) read drug information and discuss with physician
  - Infliximab (Remicade)
  - Adalimumab – Humira

Discharge Criteria

- Mild to moderate disease
- Prior history of Crohn's disease or ulcerative colitis
- Heart rate ≤ 100 for age ≥ 14 years

Discharge instructions

- Crohn's disease or ulcerative colitis aftercare instructions
- Smoking cessation for Crohn's disease patients
- Follow up within 1–3 days as needed
- Refer perianal disease to surgeon within 7–10 days

Consult Criteria

- Severe pain
- Fever
- Heart rate > 110/minute for age ≥ 14 years
- WBC ≥ 13,000
- Dehydration
- Hypotension
- Appears toxic
- Toxic megacolon
- Unable to self–hydrate
- Vomiting
- Progressive anemia
- Hemoglobin < 10 gms
- See General Patient Criteria Protocol (page 22) for items not in this protocol

Notes

References:

Mayo Clin Proc, June 2011, pg. 557

Inflammatory Bowel Disease
Author: William A Rowe, MD; Chief Editor: Julian Katz, MD
emedicine.medscape.com/article/179037–overview

Ford AC, Bernstein CN, Khan KJ, et al. Glucocorticosteroid therapy in inflammatory bowel disease: systematic review and meta-analysis. *Am J Gastroenterol*. Apr 2011;106(4):590–9

Ulcerative Colitis Treatment & Management
Author: Marc D Basson, MD, PhD, MBA, FACS; Chief Editor: Julian Katz, MD emedicine.medscape.com/article/183084

Govani SM, Guentner AS, Waljee AK, Higgins PD. Risk stratification of emergency department patients with

Crohn's disease could reduce computed tomography use by nearly half. Clin Gastroenterol Hepatol. 2014 Oct. 12(10):1702-1707.e3

ACG Clinical Guideline: Ulcerative Colitis in Adults

David T. Rubin, MD, FACG1, Ashwin N. Ananthakrishnan, MD, MPH2, Corey A. Siegel, MD, MS3, Bryan G. Sauer, MD, MSc (Clin Res), FACG (GRADE Methodologist)4 and Millie D. Long, MD, MPH, FACG

Gastroesophageal Reflux Disease (GERD) Protocol

When using any protocol, always follow the Guidelines of Proper Use (page 18).

Definition

- When the amount of gastric juice that refluxes into the esophagus exceeds the normal limit, causing symptoms with or without associated esophageal mucosal injury

Differential Diagnosis

- Acute coronary syndrome
- Biliary colic
- Peptic ulcer disease
- Esophagitis
- Esophageal spasm
- Achalasia
- Irritable bowel syndrome
- Asthma from aspiration

Considerations

- 40% of the population experience GERD monthly
- Most patients with hiatal hernias do not experience clinically significant reflux
- Acid secretion is the same with or without GERD

Causes and effects

- Obesity
- Smoking
- Decrease in lower esophageal sphincter (LES) tone or function (most common cause)
- Erosive gastritis
- Esophageal stricture
- UGI bleeding
- Recurrent pneumonia
- Asthma

Medications that can cause GERD:

- Calcium channel blockers
- Nitrates
- Beta–blockers
- Theophylline

Foods and beverages that can cause GERD:

- Coffee
- Chocolate
- Tea
- Alcohol
- Tomato products
- Citrus products

Signs and Symptoms

- Heartburn (burning from epigastrium up into chest and throat at times)
- Dysphagia
- Odynophagia
- Regurgitation
- Belching
- Worse bending over or lying down
- Usually transiently relieved with antacids

Evaluation

- Consider high risk differential diagnoses and test as indicated

Treatment Options

- Weight loss if obese
- Antacids
- Analgesics (excluding NSAID's or aspirin)
- Avoid late night or heavy meals
- Eat last meal ≥ 3 hours before laying down
- Stop smoking and alcohol intake
- Avoid drugs and foods/beverages that decrease LES
- Reglan (metoclopramide) — caution with long term usage — tardive dyskinesia)
- H2 blockers prn
- Proton pump inhibitors prn

- Elevate head of bed 6–8 inches
- Fundoplication (refer to surgery as outpatient)

Discharge Criteria

- Uncomplicated GERD
- Follow up with primary care provider or gastroenterologist within 1–3 weeks as needed

Discharge instructions

- GERD aftercare instructions

Consult Criteria

- UGI bleeding
- Esophageal obstruction
- Dehydration
- Toxic appearing patients
- Uncertain diagnosis as cause of patient complaints
- Refer to General Patient Criteria Protocol (page 22) as needed

Notes

References:

Gastroesophageal Reflux Disease
Author: Marco G Patti, MD; Chief Editor: Julian Katz, MD
emedicine.medscape.com/article/176595

DeVault KR, Castell DO. Updated guidelines for the diagnosis and treatment of gastroesophageal reflux disease.*Am J Gastroenterol*. Jan 2005;100(1):190–200

Agency for Healthcare Research and Quality. Comparative Effectiveness of Management Strategies for Gastroesophageal Reflux Disease - Executive Summary. AHRQ pub. no. 06–EHC003–1. December 2005

PEPTIC ULCER DISEASE AND GASTRITIS PROTOCOL

When using any protocol, always follow the Guidelines of Proper Use (page 18).

Definition

- Inflammatory changes in the gastric mucosa or a discrete mucosal defect in the stomach or duodenum

Differential Diagnosis

- GERD
- Gastroenteritis
- Acute coronary syndrome
- Biliary colic
- Peptic ulcer disease
- Esophagitis
- Esophageal spasm
- Irritable bowel syndrome
- Abdominal aortic aneurysm
- Mesenteric ischemia
- Hepatitis
- Inflammatory bowel disease
- Pancreatitis
- Pulmonary embolism

Considerations

- Consider high risk differential diagnoses and test as indicated

Causes

- H. pylori responsible for 90–95% of duodenal ulcers and 80% of gastric ulcers with NSAID use
- NSAID's interfere with prostaglandin synthesis and lead to breakdown in mucosa
- Smoking
- Alcohol intake
- Aspirin
- Steroids

Signs and Symptoms

- Epigastric pain and burning 80–90%
- Epigastric tenderness
- Gastric ulcer pain worsened by food
- Duodenal ulcer pain improved by food
- Nausea
- Vomiting
- UGI bleeding
- Hematemesis
- Melena
- Peritonitis with perforation
- Anemia

Evaluation Options

- Mild symptoms and findings with normal vital signs treat symptomatically
- H. pylori testing if available
- Moderate or severe symptoms or tenderness
    - CBC
    - BMP
    - Amylase
    - Lipase
    - Consider LFT's
- Peritonitis findings
    - Upright chest x-ray and abdominal films to evaluate for free air
    - CT abdominal and pelvis if diagnosis is uncertain or age ≥ 65 years
- EKG
    - Age ≥ 60 years with unimpressive abdominal exam and no cardiac risk factors
    - Age < 60 years with cardiac risk factors for coronary artery disease with unimpressive abdominal exam
    - Consider CT abdominal/pelvis scan with age ≥ 70 if diagnosis not reasonably certain

Treatment Options

- Unstable patient notify physician immediately
- Stable nonacute patient

- Antacids prn
- H2 blockers
- Proton pump inhibitors × 1–2 months

Antibiotics with PPI only if H. pylori documented with testing

- Biaxin (clarithromycin) 500 mg PO × 14 days
- Flagyl (metronidazole) 500 mg PO × 14 days

    OR

- Biaxin (clarithromycin) 500 mg PO bid × 14 days
- Amoxicillin 1,000 mg bid × 14 days

2017 American College of Gastroenterology (ACG) guidelines for the treatment of H. pylori infection

- 10-14 days of bismuth quadruple therapy (bismuth, proton pump inhibitor [PPI], tetracycline, and metronidazole), particularly in those with previous macrolide exposure or are penicillin allergic
- Recommended option — 10-14 days of concomitant PPI, clarithromycin, amoxicillin, and metronidazole
- 14 days of clarithromycin triple therapy (clarithromycin, a PPI, and amoxicillin or metronidazole) should be reserved for patients with no previous history of macrolide exposure who live in regions where clarithromycin resistance among *H pylori* isolates is known to be low (< 15%)
- Suggested option — 5-7 days of sequential therapy with a PPI and amoxicillin, followed by 5-7 days with clarithromycin, a PPI, and metronidazole
- Suggested option — 7 days of a hybrid therapy with a PPI and amoxicillin, followed by 7 days with a PPI, amoxicillin, clarithromycin, and metronidazole
- Suggested option — 10-14 days of levofloxacin triple therapy (levofloxacin, a PPI, and amoxicillin)
- Suggested option — 5-7 days of fluoroquinolone sequential therapy (a PPI and amoxicillin), followed by 5-7 days of a PPI, fluoroquinolone,

and nitroimidazole (metronidazole or others of this class)

Discharge Criteria

- Uncomplicated exam and findings consistent with gastritis or peptic ulcer disease

Discharge instructions

- Peptic ulcer or gastritis aftercare instructions
- Follow up with primary care provider in 1 day if pain is moderate to severe, otherwise in 5–7 days
- Follow up with primary care provider for abnormal lab within 1 week unless chronic in nature
- Return within 3 days if not improving

Consult Criteria

- GI bleeding
- Moderate pain with age ≥ 65 years
- Abdominal pain that develops hypotension or relative hypotension (SBP < 105 with history of hypertension)
- Toxic appearance
- Dehydration
- Significant blood loss or melena
    - Melena can occur with as little as 50 ml of upper GI blood loss
- Suspected or diagnosed appendicitis, cholecystitis, pancreatitis, diverticulitis, aortic aneurysm, bowel obstruction
- Acute surgical abdomen or rebound tenderness
- Moderate to severe pain of uncertain cause
- Severe pain with any diagnosis
- Intractable vomiting
- Return visit within 14 days for same acute abdominal pain complaint

Lab consult criteria (if checked)

- Hemoglobin decrease > 1 gm or creatinine increase> 0.5 from baseline
- Elevated LFT's
- Elevated amylase or lipase

- WBC ≥ 15,000
- Bandemia
- Increased anion gap
- Significant electrolyte abnormally
- Glucose ≥ 450 mg/dL in diabetic patient
- Glucose ≥ 300 mg/dL in non-diabetic patient
- Hyperglycemia with metabolic acidosis (decreased serum CO_2 or elevated anion gap)
- Acute thrombocytopenia

Vital sign and age consult criteria

- Age ≥ 70 years
- Adult heart rate ≥ 110
- Pediatric heart rate
    - 0–4 months ≥ 180
    - 5–7 months ≥ 175
    - 8–12 months ≥ 170
    - 1–3 years ≥ 160
    - 4–5 years ≥ 145
    - 6–8 years ≥ 130
    - 9–11 years ≥ 125
    - 12–15 years ≥ 115
    - 16 years or older ≥ 110

Notes

References:

Peptic Ulcer Disease

Author: BS Anand, MD; Chief Editor: Julian Katz, MD

emedicine.medscape.com/article/181753

Chey WD, Wong BC. American College of Gastroenterology guideline on the management of Helicobacter pylori infection. *Am J Gastroenterol*. Aug 2007;102(8):1808–25

Chey WD, Leontiadis GI, Howden CW, Moss SF. ACG Clinical Guideline: Treatment of Helicobacter pylori infection. *Am J Gastroenterol*. 2017 Feb. 112(2):212-39

GALLBLADDER DISEASE PROTOCOL

When using any protocol, always follow the Guidelines of Proper Use (page 18).

Definition

- Disease of gallbladder from gallstone obstruction of cystic duct or infection and inflammation of the gallbladder without gallstones

Differential Diagnosis

- Peptic ulcer disease
- Acute myocardial infarction
- Angina
- Right-sided pulmonary embolism
- Right-sided pneumonia
- Right renal colic
- Hepatitis
- Mesenteric ischemia
- Cholangitis
- Right pyelonephritis
- Gastroenteritis
- Abdominal aortic aneurysm
- Pancreatitis

Considerations

- Common in females age ≥ 40 years
- 90% of cholecystitis is from gallstones
- Moderate to severe pain and tenderness RUQ of abdomen
- Nausea and vomiting very common
- Charcot's triad: (1) Jaundice, (2) Fever, (3) RUQ abdominal pain
- Fever occurs with advanced disease
- Increased morbidity and mortality in diabetes
- Ascending cholangitis is a life threatening infection of common bile duct

- May increase LFT's, amylase, lipase and bilirubin with common duct gallstones
- Acalculus cholecystitis has a higher mortality than cholecystitis with gallstones
    - Seen more in elderly and diabetic patients
- Elderly may present with vague and diminished symptoms
- Emphysematous cholecystitis more common with diabetes

Evaluation

- History for
    - Onset
    - Severity
    - Duration
    - Associated symptoms
    - Previous episodes
- Abdominal exam for
    - Tenderness
    - Guarding
    - Rebound tenderness
    - Distension

Testing options

- CBC
- U/A
- UCG if fertile female
- LFT's
- Amylase
- Lipase
- Gallbladder ultrasound may be needed with elevated WBC and if amylase or lipase elevated
- If pain, tenderness and vomiting resolve with treatment, testing may not be needed

Treatment Options

- IV NS or LR 1 liter bolus if hypotensive (notify physician promptly)
- Pain and vomiting treatment
- Dilaudid (hydromorphone) prn
- Stadol (butorphanol) prn

- Nubain (nalbuphine) prn
- Phenergan (promethazine) or Zofran (ondansetron) prn

Discharge Criteria

- Resolution of pain, tenderness, vomiting
- Gallbladder ultrasound without findings of cholecystitis or choledocholithiasis (if performed)
- No fever or chills
- Diagnosis reasonable certain for biliary colic

Discharge instructions

- Gallbladder disease aftercare instructions
- Return within 1 day if pain persists or worsens
- Refer to general surgeon or primary care provider within 7 days

Consult Criteria

- WBC ≥ 13,000
- Bandemia ≥ 15%
- Rebound tenderness
- Intractable nausea or vomiting
- Pain not resolved with treatment
- Cholecystitis
- Choledocholithiasis
- Cholangitis

Lab consult criteria

- Hemoglobin decrease > 1 gm or creatinine increase> 0.5 from baseline
- Elevated LFT's
- Elevated amylase or lipase
- Increased anion gap
- Acute thrombocytopenia
- Significant electrolyte abnormally
- Glucose ≥ 300 mg/dL in diabetic patient
- Glucose ≥ 200 mg/dL in non-diabetic patient
- Hyperglycemia with metabolic acidosis (decreased serum CO_2 or elevated anion gap)
- Lactic acidosis

Vital sign and age consult criteria

- Age ≥ 60
- Adult HR ≥ 110 post treatment
- Hypotension or orthostatic vital signs

Notes

References:

Cholecystitis Author: Alan A Bloom, MD; Chief Editor: Julian Katz, MD emedicine.medscape.com/article/171886

Huffman JL, Schenker S. Acute acalculous cholecystitis - a review. *Clin Gastroenterol Hepatol*. Sep 9 2009

ACUTE HEPATITIS PROTOCOL

When using any protocol, always follow the Guidelines of Proper Use (page 18).

Definition

- Inflammation of the liver

Differential Diagnosis

- Biliary colic
- Cholecystitis
- Cholangitis
- Peptic ulcer disease
- Gastritis
- Gastroenteritis
- Aortic aneurysm
- Pancreatitis

Considerations

- Frequently asymptomatic
- Ranges from asymptomatic to fulminate hepatitis and liver failure
- Misdiagnosed frequently as nonspecific viral syndrome
- Viral causes are most frequent: hepatitis A – 40%, hepatitis B – 30%, hepatitis C – 20%
    - Hepatitis A: fecal-oral transmission most common cause
    - Hepatitis B: exposure to infected blood or body fluids most common cause
    - Hepatitis C: percutaneous exposures most common cause
- Screening for hepatitis B and HCV recommended in high risk patients
- Chronic hepatitis develops in 75% of acute hepatitis C patients
    - Contacted largely from IV drug abuse or contaminated needles. Less often from tattoos, sharing razors, acupuncture or blood transfusions
- Autoimmune disorders can cause hepatitis
- Toxic causes

- Acetaminophen is a frequent worldwide cause (can cause liver failure)
- Ethanol (causes 50% of end-stage liver disease in U.S.)
- Isoniazid
- Ecstasy (MDMA)
- Industrial solvents and cleaning solutions
- Iron

Viral hepatitis

Risk factors

- Male homosexuality
- Hemodialysis
- IV drug abuse
- Raw seafood
- Blood product transfusion
- Tattoos or body piercing
- Foreign travel
- Sexual exposure to hepatitis B carrier

Preicteric phase

- Flu-like illness with fever, chills and malaise
- Nausea, vomiting, anorexia

Icteric phase

- Dark urine
- Light stools
- Pruritus
- Right upper quadrant tenderness
- Tender hepatomegaly

Nonalcoholic fatty liver most common cause of elevated LFT's in U.S. (ALT > AST frequently)

- Associated with obesity, Type-II DM, and/or hyperlipidemia
- Most patients asymptomatic
- Bilirubin rarely elevated
- Can lead to hepatic cirrhosis
- Treatment is weight loss
- Usually a benign course

Evaluation

- Complete history and physical exam
- Alcohol and drug history
- Special attention to acetaminophen or acetaminophen containing medicines
- Check acetaminophen level if ALT elevated with possible history of acetaminophen containing medication usage
- CBC
- BMP
- LFT's (SGOT/AST is commonly 2 times > SGPT/ALT in alcoholic hepatitis)
  - ALT > AST in fatty liver usually
- PT/PTT/INR
- Ammonia level if encephalopathic
- Rectal exam if encephalopathic for stool blood or if BUN elevated out of proportion to creatinine level
- U/A
- Consider viral serology
- Monospot if pharyngitis present
- Acetaminophen level if suspected usage

Treatment Options

- IV D50W 1 amp if hypoglycemic
- Hypotension give 250–500 cc NS bolus and notify physician
- Treat ongoing hypoglycemia with D5 1/2NS drip of 100–150 cc/hour
- Usually supportive
- Acetadote for acetaminophen toxicity as indicated
  - May need treatment if ALT elevated with history of recent acetaminophen containing medication usage, even if acetaminophen level is 0
- Cessation of ethanol use
- No acetaminophen

Discharge Criteria

- Stable patient
- PT < 3 seconds elevation
- INR < 1.5

- See General Patient Criteria Protocol (page 22)

Discharge instructions

- Hepatitis aftercare instructions
- Primary care provider within 1–2 days
- Gastroenterology within 1–2 days unless chronic liver disease without acute exacerbation

Consult Criteria

- Toxic acetaminophen level on nomogram or elevated ALT regardless of level if acetaminophen containing medication usage is suspected
- Hypoglycemia
- Altered mental status
- PT prolonged > 3 seconds
- INR > 1.5
- Bilirubin > 5
- Intractable vomiting
- Significant comorbid conditions
- Significant electrolyte or fluid disturbances
- Age ≥ 70
- Ascites
- GI bleeding
- Immunosuppression
- Fever
- LFT's > 5 times normal

Notes

Hepatitis B Author: Nikolaos T Pyrsopoulos, MD, PhD, MBA, FACP, AGAF; Chief Editor: Julian Katz, MD
emedicine.medscape.com/article/177632

Centers for Disease Control and Prevention. Hepatitis B information for health professionals: hepatitis B FAQs for health professionals
cdc.gov/hepatitis/HBV/index.htm

[Guideline] Ghany MG, Strader DB, Thomas DL, Seeff LB. Diagnosis, management, and treatment of hepatitis C: an update. *Hepatology*. Apr 2009;49(4):1335–74

Gastrointestinal Bleeding Protocol

When using any protocol, always follow the Guidelines of Proper Use (page 18).

Differential Diagnosis

- Peptic ulcer disease
- Esophagitis
- Mallory-Weiss tear
- Esophageal varices
- Diverticular disease
- Colon cancer
- Colon polyps
- Arteriovenous malformation
- Aortoenteric fistula
- Hemorrhoids

Considerations

- Upper gastrointestinal (UGI) bleeding as little as 50 ml can cause melena
    - Melena may be produced from proximal large intestine also
- UGI bleeding
    - Rapid transit can cause gross blood per rectum
    - Elevates BUN out of proportion to creatinine
    - Can lead to hepatic encephalopathy in hepatic cirrhosis patients
    - FFP should not be used in esophageal variceal bleeding in hepatic cirrhosis patients with high INR
        - Actually cirrhotic patients can be hypercoagulable due to imbalance of thrombotic and antithrombotic factors
- Lower gastrointestinal (LGI) bleeding
    - Bright or dark red gross blood
    - Frequently painless
    - Frequently from a colon diverticular source in elderly
- Hemorrhoidal bleeding usually bright red and not mixed with stools

- Can present with dyspnea, chest pain; syncope, altered mental status

Lower GI Bleeding and Risk of Severe Bleeding

- Heart rate 100 beats per minute or more (1 point)
- SBP ≤ 115 mmHg (1 point)
- Patient had associated syncope (1 point)
- Blood per rectum during first 4 hours of evaluation (1 point)
- Patient on aspirin (1 point)
- 3 or more comorbid conditions present (1 point)

0 points = 9% risk

1–3 points = 43% risk

4–6 points = 84% risk

Evaluation

- Complete history and physical exam (including rectal exam for hemoccult testing or gross bleeding)
- Medication history
- Prior GI history
- CBC
- BMP
- PT/INR
- PTT if on heparin
- Ammonia and LFT's if mental status altered
- Type and screen for history of significant bleeding
- Type and cross if
  - Hypotensive
  - Adult heart rate ≥ 120
  - Orthostatic vital signs
- Hemorrhoidal bleeding with benign bleeding history and normal vital signs may not need lab tests

Treatment Options

- IV NS 500cc bolus if hypotensive adult (notify physician promptly) — see Bleeding Protocol
- Avoid > 1 liter of isotonic fluids for acute blood loss before blood products transfusion started if possible
- Avoid hypertension
- Target systolic blood pressure of 80-90 mm Hg until major bleeding has been stopped
- Target Hgb of 7-9 g/dl after termination of major bleeding

- Pediatric: 20 cc/kg IV NS bolus, start blood and plasma for continued hypotension and bleeding (notify physician promptly)
- Proton pump inhibitors (PPI) for upper GI bleeding or peptic ulcer disease/gastritis/esophagitis
- Transfusion with PRBC's/FFP/platelets 1:1:1 ratio if hypotension persists or significant acute anemia
  - Recommendations range from 4:1:1 to 1:1:1 (consult physician promptly first)
- Consider N-G tube for UGI bleeding (consult physician)
- Somatostatin IV for UGI bleeding as needed
- <u>45 - 66% cirrhotic patients with upper GI bleeding develop bacterial infection within the first 5-7 days of the bleeding episode</u>
  - Ceftriaxone IV or other broad spectrum antibiotics decrease infection, improves bleeding, prevents rebleeding and improves survival

Hemorrhoids

External hemorrhoids

Medical treatment for mild to moderate painful thrombosed hemorrhoids

- Warm soaks (sitz baths) or hot towel applied in lateral decubitus position
- Stool softeners
- Anusol, Anusol HC or Protofoam HC topical preparations
- Tuck's pads prn (witch hazel)
- Analgesics
- Avoid exacerbating activities

Excisional treatment for severe painful acute thrombosed hemorrhoids (usually within 72 hours of symptoms)

- Prep area with betadine
- Spread buttocks with assistant's help or use tape
- Infiltrate base of hemorrhoid with 2–5 cc of 1% lidocaine with epinephrine (use plain lidocaine in coronary artery disease patients)
- Infiltrate into the hemorrhoid with 1–2 cc of lidocaine with epinephrine (use plain lidocaine in coronary artery disease patients)

- Elliptical incision (preferred) in roof/top of hemorrhoid 2–3 mm wide radially in line from anus
    - Avoid deeper anal verge and sphincter
- Remove clots(s) by expressing or with forceps
- May be packed with 0.25 gauze (removed in 6 hours) or have gelfoam applied as needed
- Analgesics

Internal hemorrhoids

Medical treatment similar to external hemorrhoid treatment

Discharge Criteria

- Healthy patient
- Normal vital signs
- Stable CBC if checked
- Normal coagulation studies if checked
- Good follow up
- Negative or insignificant blood on rectal exam

Discharge instructions

- GI bleeding or hemorrhoid aftercare instructions
- Refer to primary care provider or GI physician within 5–7 days

Consult Criteria

- Significant blood loss or melena present
- Hematemesis
- Suspected or diagnosed aortic aneurysm
- Acute surgical abdomen
- Moderate to severe pain of uncertain cause
- Severe pain with any diagnosis
- Return ED visit within 14 days for same complaint

Vital signs and age consult criteria

- Age ≥ 70
- SBP < 90 or relative hypotension (SBP < 110 with history of hypertension)
- Adult heart rate > 100
- Orthostatic vital signs
- Pediatric heart
    - 0–4 months ≥ 180

- 5–7 months ≥ 175
- 6–12 months ≥ 170

Lab consult criteria

- Hemoglobin < 12 gms unless chronic
- Hemoglobin decrease > 1 gm
- Bandemia ≥ 15%
- Metabolic acidosis
- Significant electrolyte abnormally
- Glucose ≥ 400 mg/dL in diabetic patient or > 300 mg/dL in non-diabetic patient
- Hyperglycemia with metabolic acidosis (decreased serum CO_2 or elevated anion gap)
- Acute thrombocytopenia (common in alcoholics)
- Elevated coagulation studies
- Creatinine increase > 0.5 from baseline
- Elevated LFT's

Notes

References:

JAMA, Vol.307:1072–1079

Strate LL, Orav EJ, Syngal S. Early predictors of severity in acute lower intestinal tract bleeding. *Arch Intern Med*. 2003; 163: 838–43

Scottish Intercollegiate Guidelines Network (SIGN). *Management of acute upper and lower gastrointestinal bleeding. A national clinical guideline*. (SIGN publication; no. 105). Edinburgh (Scotland): Scottish Intercollegiate Guidelines Network (SIGN); Sep 2008

Hemorrhoids Treatment & Management
Author: Scott C Thornton, MD; Chief Editor: John Geibel, MD, DSc, MA emedicine.medscape.com/article/775407

Imperiale TF, Birgisson S. Somatostatin or octreotide compared with H2 antagonists and placebo in the

management of acute nonvariceal upper gastrointestinal hemorrhage: a meta-analysis
Ann Intern Med 1997 Dec 15;127(12):1062–1071

Tripodi A, et al. *N Engl J Med* 2011;365:147-156

Nadim. Management of the critically ill patient with cirrhosis: A multidisciplinary perspective. *Journal of Hepatology* 2016;64(3):717-735

Jalan R, et al. *J Hepatol* 2014;60(6):1310-24

Chavez-Tapia, N.C., et al. *Cochrane Database Syst Rev* 2010; 9: CD002907

Rossaint R, Bouillon B, Cerny V, Coats TJ, Duranteau J, Fernández-Mondéjar E, et al. The European guideline on management of major bleeding and coagulopathy following trauma: fourth edition. *Crit Care.* 2016 Apr 12. 20 (1):100

Gastrointestinal Foreign Body Protocol

When using any protocol, always follow the Guidelines of Proper Use (page 18).

Definition

- Ingestion of a foreign body that may or may not be impacted

Considerations

- Most pass without assistance or danger once past the pylorus
- Sharp objects > 5 cm or multiple in number may need endoscopic removal

Esophageal foreign body

Symptoms

- Foreign body sensation
- Dysphagia

Areas of narrowing

- Cricopharyngeus muscle (most common)
    - C6
- Aortic arch and tracheal carina
    - T4
    - T6
- Lower esophageal sphincter (GE junction)
    - T11

Evaluation options

Chest x-ray findings

- Coins
    - Tracheal foreign body
        - Oriented anterior–posterior
    - Esophageal foreign body
        - Oriented transversely
- Bones may be seen on chest x-ray

Gastrograffin or barium swallow

- For nonopaque foreign bodies

CT scan

- For nonopaque foreign bodies
- Superior to gastrograffin or barium swallow

Button battery

- Must be removed immediately if lodged in esophagus
    - If passed esophagus does not need immediate removal
    - If passed pylorus in 48 hours does not need removal
- Rapid burns occur within 6 hours if impacted
- Lithium batteries have worse outcomes
- Consult physician immediately for retained esophageal button battery
    - **Intranasal button batteries need immediate removal**

Esophageal food impaction

- Esophageal disease present usually
    - Esophageal stricture from GERD common
- Complete obstruction patient cannot hold saliva down

Treatment options

- Endoscopic removal
- Glucagon (not too successful)
    - Adult 1–2 mg IV may repeat in 10–20 minutes if needed
    - Pediatric 0.02–0.03 mg/kg IV (NMT 0.5 mg)
- Foley catheter removal
    - Performed by physician if available
    - Do not use
        - If esophageal disease present
        - Foreign body present more than 72 hours

Discharge Criteria

- Resolved foreign body impaction
- Benign foreign body that will likely pass
- Button battery
    - If passed esophagus

- If passed pylorus in 48 hours

Discharge instructions

- Esophageal or gastrointestinal foreign body aftercare instructions
- Refer to GI or PCP within 48 hours to assess foreign body evacuation

Consult Criteria

- Retained esophageal foreign bodies
- Sharp foreign bodies
- Button battery in esophagus
- Unresolved esophageal food impaction
- Continued symptoms of foreign body
- Continued dysphagia
- Foreign bodies unlikely to spontaneously pass

Notes

References:

Gastrointestinal Foreign Bodies Workup

Author: David W Munter, MD, MBA; Chief Editor: Steven C Dronen, MD, FAAEM
emedicine.medscape.com/article/776566

Disk Battery Ingestion Follow-up

Author: Daniel J Dire, MD, FACEP, FAAP, FAAEM; Chief Editor: Asim Tarabar, MD

emedicine.medscape.com/article/774838

ANORECTAL DISORDER PROTOCOL

When using any protocol, always follow the Guidelines of Proper Use (page 18).

Conditions

- Hemorrhoids
- Anal Fissure
- Perianal/perirectal abscess
- Rectal prolapse
- Pruritus ani
- Pilonidal cyst/abscess

Hemorrhoids

Definition

- Pathologic swelling of veins in the rectum

Differential diagnosis

- Rectal prolapse
- Proctitis
- Crohn's disease and ulcerative colitis
- Condyloma acuminata
- Pregnancy related vein engorgement

Considerations

- Symptoms range from none to severe pain
- External hemorrhoids develop distal to the dentate line
    - Are bluish-purplish in color
- Internal hemorrhoids are above the dentate line
    - No sensory innervation and usually painless
    - Usually cannot be felt when not prolapsed
- Bright blood that drips into toilet or as streaks on stool is commonly from internal hemorrhoids
- Commonly thought to be from constipation or straining, but this is controversial
- Blood is not mixed inside stool

Internal hemorrhoid grading

- 1st degree = projects into canal

- 2nd degree = protrudes with defection then retracts
- 3rd degree = protrudes with straining but only retracts by manual manipulation
- 4th degree = prolapsed and cannot be reduced

Evaluation options

- Usually history and physical examination with rectal exam is all that is needed
- CBC for tachycardia or history of moderate to severe bleeding
- PT/INR if on Coumadin (warfarin)

Treatment options

External hemorrhoids

Medical treatment for mild to moderately painful thrombosed hemorrhoids

- Warm soaks (sitz baths) or hot towel applied in lateral decubitus position
- Stool softeners
- Anusol, Anusol HC or Proctofoam HC topical preparations
- Tuck's pads prn (witch hazel)
- Analgesics
- Avoid exacerbating activities

Excisional treatment for severe painful acute thrombosed hemorrhoids (usually within 72 hours of symptoms)

- Prep area with betadine
- Spread buttocks with assistant's help or use tape
- Infiltrate base of hemorrhoid with 2–5 cc of 1% lidocaine with epinephrine
- Infiltrate into the hemorrhoid with 1–2 cc of lidocaine with epinephrine
- Elliptical incision (preferred) in roof/top of hemorrhoid 2–3 mm wide radially in line from anus
    - Avoid the deeper anal verge and sphincter
- Remove clots(s) by expressing or with forceps

- May be packed with 0.25 inch gauze (removed in 6 hours) or have gelfoam applied as needed
- Analgesics

Internal hemorrhoids

Medical treatment similar to external hemorrhoid treatment

Surgical referral and treatment

- Failure of conservative treatment
- Excessive and/or prolonged bleeding
- Gangrenous 4th degree hemorrhoid (emergency)
- Concurrent anal fistula or fissure
- 3rd and 4th degree internal hemorrhoids with severe symptoms
- Patient requests referral

Discharge criteria

- Uncomplicated internal and external hemorrhoids

Discharge instructions

- Warm soaks (sitz baths) or hot towel applied in lateral decubitus position
- Stool softeners and bulk laxatives (psyllium fiber)
- Anusol, Anusol HC or Proctofoam HC topical preparations
- Hemorrhoid aftercare instructions

Consult criteria

- See surgical referral above

Anal fissure

Definition

- Superficial linear tear of the anus

Differential diagnosis

- Crohn's disease
- Ulcerative colitis
- Carcinoma
- Syphilis, gonorrhea and other STD
- HIV and AIDS
- Herpes simplex

- Rectal foreign bodies (as a cause)
- Pilonidal cyst or sinus
- Proctitis

Considerations

- Most common cause of painful rectal bleeding
- Distal to the dentate line
- Usually occur in posterior anal midline (90%) or anterior anal midline (10%)
    - If not in midline consider other diseases
- Most resolve in 2–4 weeks (may last several months)
- Refractory cases may require surgery
- Causes increased anal sphincter pressures

Evaluation

- Usually only need history and rectal exam

Treatment options

- WASH regimen
    - Warm water, shower or sitz bath after bowel movement
    - Analgesics
    - Stool softener
    - High-fiber diet
- Intra-anal nitroglycerin ointment 0.4% bid topically applied for 2 weeks if failure of WASH regimen
- Botulinum toxin injection locally
- Topical application of clove oil cream for chronic anal fissure
- Topical 0.5% nitroglycin ointment

Discharge criteria

- Uncomplicated anal fissure

Discharge instructions

- Anal fissure aftercare instructions
- WASH regimen

Consult criteria

- Refractory anal fissure
- Other disease process suspected
- Anal fistula

Perianal abscess

Definition

- Infection and collection of pus just outside the anus

Differential diagnosis

- Perirectal abscess
- Squamous cell carcinoma
- Crohn's disease

Considerations

- May be associated with a fistula tract into rectum
- Peak incidence is third to fourth decade of life
- Males affected more than females
- Common in infants
- Arises from obstruction of the anal crypts
- Usually patient is afebrile

Evaluation

- Usually history and physical exam is all that is needed

Treatment

- Incision and drainage of abscess avoiding anal verge
    - Pack abscess for 1–2 days (patient removes pack or return visit for removal)
- Antibiotics usually are not necessary
- Analgesics prn

Discharge criteria

- Uncomplicated perianal abscess

Discharge instructions

- Sitz baths 3 times a day and after bowel movements for 3–4 days
- Stool softeners
- Perianal abscess aftercare instructions

Consult criteria

- Perirectal abscess suspected
- Anal fistula
- Other disease process suspected
- Fever
- Immunocompromised patient

Perirectal abscess

Definition

- Abscess in the deeper perirectal spaces

Differential diagnosis

- Perianal abscess
- Crohn's disease
- Inflammatory bowel disease
- Rectal carcinoma
- Foreign body
- Sexually transmitted disease
- Proctitis
- Hemorrhoids
- Necrotizing fasciitis

Considerations

- Caused by obstruction of the anal crypts
- Fever and leukocytosis common (WBC can be normal)
- Severe pain present
- Sepsis can occur
- Increased pain with sitting, coughing or bowel movement
- Rectal or perirectal drainage in ¼ of patients
- Severe tenderness in rectum on digital examination
- May or may not be palpable
- Results in fistula in 25–50% of patients
- Urinary retention in 5% of patients

Evaluation options

- History and physical examination including rectal exam
- CBC
- BMP if diabetic
- Blood cultures if toxic appearing or immunocompromised
- CT abdomen/pelvis scan if diagnosis is in doubt on history and physical examination
- If in doubt and CT not performed, an 18 or 20 gauge needle aspiration of the most tender and/or swollen area after sterile skin prep can be used to help diagnose abscess (not to be used for definitive treatment

Treatment

- Per physician and/or surgeon
- Analgesics parentally prn

Discharge criteria

- Do not discharge

Consult criteria

- All perirectal abscess patients

Rectal prolapse

Definition

- Mucosal or full thickness prolapse of rectal tissue through anus

Differential diagnosis

- Hemorrhoids
- Proctitis
- Intussusception

Considerations

- Fecal incontinence and constipation commonly develop after prolapse
- Ulceration of rectal tissue may occur
- May be caused by staining and constipation
- 90% of children with rectal prolapse will spontaneously resolve
- Peak incidence is the 4th and 7th decades of life
- Much more common in females (80–90% of total)
- Children peak incidence less 1 year of age
    - Cystitis fibrosis associated with prolapse

Findings

- Protruding rectal mucosa
- Thick concentric mucosal ring
- Gap noted between anal canal and rectum
- Decreased anal sphincter tone

Evaluation

- History and physical examination including rectal exam
- Barium enema (preferred) or colonoscopy
- Tests for any associated conditions as needed

Treatment

- Adults are treated surgically
- Children usually treated nonsurgically and underlying condition is treated
- Attempt gentle digital reduction of rectum
    - Granulated table sugar applied to the rectal tissue causes an osmotic shift of fluid out of the mucosa decreasing the swelling in a few minutes that facilitates reduction of the prolapse
- Stool softeners

Discharge criteria

- Reducible mucosal or rectal prolapse

Discharge instructions

- Rectal prolapse aftercare instructions if available
- Stool softeners

Consult criteria

- All patients should be referred to surgeon
- Emergency consultation if incarcerated, ischemic or perforated rectal tissue

Pruritus ani

Definition

- Chronic anal itching

Differential diagnosis

- Eczema
- Psoriasis
- Pinworm infestation
- Scabies
- Urticaria
- Contact dermatitis
- Hemorrhoids

Considerations

- Worse at night usually
- Can be caused by increased moisture around anus or fecal leakage
- May be from certain foods, clothing, poor rectal hygiene, or medications

Evaluation options

- Cellophane tape when waking up in morning for pinworms if suspected
- 10% KOH skin scraping for fungus

Treatment options

- Diphenhydramine or hydroxyzine prn for itching
- Hydrocortisone cream 1% course bid prn for 5–10 days
- Avoid offending foods, clothing or agents
- Treat underlying condition if known
- Clean anus completely post-defecation
- Corn starch powder to dry skin

Discharge criteria

- Uncomplicated cases

Discharge instructions

- Pruritus ani aftercare instructions

Consult criteria

- Refractory cases refer to gastroenterologist

Pilonidal cyst/abscess

Definition

- A cyst that develops in the skin of the sacrococcygeal region 4–5 cm posterior to the anus

Differential diagnosis

- Anal fistula
- Perirectal abscess
- Hidradenitis suppurativa

Considerations

- Thought to be an acquired condition for folliculitis from hair that gets impacted into the skin
- More common in males
- Affects 26 out of 100,000 persons in the U.S.
- Occurs most commonly in late teens and early twenties
- Painful when acutely infected

Evaluation

- History and physical examination is usually all that is needed

Treatment

- For abscess perform I&D off midline, angulating into abscess cavity
    - See Soft Tissue Abscess section in book
- Remove any hair and granulation tissue
- Pack with gauze (medicated ribbon gauze has no added benefit)
    - Remove packing in 1–2 days
- No I&D for asymptomatic patients without significant symptoms
- Phenol injection into cyst by experience Providers

Discharge criteria

- Uncomplicated pilonidal cyst or abscess after procedural I&D
- Asymptomatic patients

Discharge instructions

- Pilonidal cyst aftercare instructions
- Return if pain returns or fever develops
- Refer to surgeon for definitive treatment

Consult criteria

- Pilonidal abscess near anus
- Patient toxicity
- Fever ≥ 101°F (38.3°C)

Notes

References:

Hemorrhoids Treatment & Management

Author: Scott C Thornton, MD; Chief Editor: John Geibel, MD, DSc, MA emedicine.medscape.com/article/775407

Pilonidal Disease Treatment & Management

Author: James de Caestecker, DO; Chief Editor: John Geibel, MD, DSc, MA emedicine.medscape.com/article/192668

Anal Fissure Treatment & Management

emedicine.medscape.com/article/196297

Schiano di Visconte M, Munegato G. Glyceryl trinitrate ointment (0.25%) and anal cryothermal dilators in the treatment of chronic anal fissures. *J Gastrointest Surg*. Jul 2009;13(7):1283–91

Rectal Prolapse Author: Jan Rakinic, MD; Chief Editor: John Geibel, MD, DSc, MA
emedicine.medscape.com/article/2026460

CONSTIPATION PROTOCOL

When using any protocol, always follow the Guidelines of Proper Use (page 18).

Definition

- A gastrointestinal motility disorder resulting in 2 of the following
  - Less than 3 bowels movements per week
  - Hard lumpy stools
  - Straining
  - Incomplete defecation sensation
  - Anorectal obstruction sensation
  - Manually assisted defecation

Differential diagnosis

- Large bowel obstruction
- Abdominal hernia
- Hypothyroidism
- Irritable bowel syndrome
- Anxiety disorders
- Toxic megacolon
- Colon cancer
- Diverticulitis

Considerations

- Most common digestive complaint
- Affects 15% of the U.S. population
- Usually treated medically with improvement in symptoms
- 30% higher incidence in nonwhite population
- May be asymptomatic or have pain with above definition symptoms

Red flag symptoms

- Unexplained weight loss
- Vomiting
- Inability to pass flatus
- Abdominal pain
- Rectal bleeding

Types

Primary or idiopathic constipation

- Normal transit constipation
- Slow transit constipation
  - Infrequent stools and decreased urgency
  - Impaired phasic colon activity
- Pelvic floor dysfunction
  - Dysfunction of pelvic floor or anal sphincter

Secondary constipation

- Caused by
  - Low fiber diet
  - Decreased fluid intake
  - Lack of exercise
  - Anal fissures
  - Diabetes mellitus, hypothyroidism
  - Stroke, spinal cord injuries, multiple sclerosis
  - Parkinson's disease
  - Antidepressants
  - Anticholinergics
  - Narcotics
  - Calcium channel blockers
  - Antacids
  - NSAID's
  - Depression

Evaluation options

- Usually history and examination is all that is needed
- CBC for weight loss, fever or bleeding
- CMP for diabetes mellitus or vomiting
- Abdominal flat and upright films for vomiting
- CT abdominal/pelvic scan for vomiting, weight loss or unusually severe pain

Treatment options

Prevention

- Good fluid intake
- Exercise
- High fiber diet
- Avoid constipating medications

Acute ED or office treatment

- Fleets mineral oil enema
  - Adult 1 bottle
  - Pediatric 30–60 ml (Age 2–11 years)
- Fleet bisacodyl enema
  - Adult 30 ml (1 bottle)
  - Pediatric (2–12 years) 15 ml
- Fleet enema
  - Adult 118 ml (1 bottle)
  - Pediatric 5–12 years Pedia-Lax 1 bottle 59 ml
  - Pediatric 2–5 years Pedia-Lax ½ bottle
  - Do not use in megacolon, CHF, ascites, renal failure or intestinal obstruction
- Glycerin suppository
  - Age > 6 years 1 suppository
  - Age 2–6 years Fleet's Babylax applicator (4 ml)
- Digital disimpaction
- Milk and molasses enema in children not allergic to milk

Acute home treatment

- Dulcolax suppository or tablet
- Colace
- Fleet's enema
- Prune juice

Chronic home treatment

- High fiber diet
- Psyllium (Metamucil)
  - < 6 years 1 gm PO qday-tid in water or juice
  - Age 6–11 years 1.7 gm (powder) in water or juice PO qday-tid or 1 oral wafer, increase slowly as needed
  - > 12 years 2–6 caps qday-tid or 2 wafers PO qday increasing as needed
- Magnesium hydroxide (Milk of magnesia)
  - Age 6–11 years 15–30 ml PO qday prn
  - Age > 12 years 30–60 ml PO qday prn
- Polyethylene glycol (MiraLax)
  - Age < 17 years – 0.8 gm/kg in 8 oz. of liquid PO qday prn up to 4 days
  - Age ≥ 17 years – 1 capful in 8 oz. liquid PO qday prn up to 4 days
- Lubiprostone (Amitiza) 24 mcg PO q12hr for chronic constipation; IBS-C 8 mcg PO q12hr

- Lactulose 15–30 mL (10–20 g) PO once daily; may be increased to 60 mL (40 g) once daily
  - Children 0.7–2 g/kg/day (1–3 mL/kg/day) PO in divided doses; not to exceed 40 g/day (60 mL/day)

Constipation induced by opioids with advanced illness

- Methylnaltrexone (Relistor) weight-base dosing

Discharge criteria

- Uncomplicated findings
- Normal vital signs

Discharge instructions

- Constipation aftercare instructions
- See Gastroenterologist referral criteria

Consult criteria

- Red flag symptoms
- Fever
- Vomiting
- Tachycardia
- Metabolic acidosis
- Significant gross rectal bleeding
- Melena
- Rebound abdominal tenderness
- Moderate to severe tenderness

Referral to gastroenterologist criteria

- Recent onset
- Rectal bleeding
- Weight loss
- Recent bowel habit changes

Notes

References:

Constipation Author: Marc D Basson, MD, PhD, MBA, FACS; Chief Editor: Julian Katz, MD emedicine.medscape.com/article/184704

Noguera A, Centeno C, Librada S, Nabal M. Screening for Constipation in Palliative Care Patients. *J Palliat Med*. Sep 11 2009

[Guideline] North American Society for Pediatric Gastroenterology, Hepatology and Nutrition. Evaluation and treatment of constipation in children: summary of updated recommendations of the North American Society for Pediatric Gastroenterology, Hepatology and Nutrition. *J Pediatr Gastroenterol Nutr*. Sep 2006;43(3):405–7

Pediatric Constipation Medication

Author: Stephen Borowitz, MD; Chief Editor: Carmen Cuffari, MD emedicine.medscape.com/article/928185

Urinary and Male Genitourinary

Section Contents

When using any protocol, always follow the Guidelines of Proper Use (page 18).

KIDNEY STONE PROTOCOL

When using any protocol, always follow the Guidelines of Proper Use (page 18).

Definition

- Ureteral colic produced by passage of renal calculus from kidney into the ureter

Differential Diagnosis

- Biliary colic
- Aortic aneurysm
- Mechanical back pain
- Herpes zoster
- Pyelonephritis
- Renal vein thrombosis
- Renal infarction
- Retroperitoneal bleeding
- Appendicitis
- Pulmonary embolism
- Testicular and ovarian torsion
- Ectopic pregnancy

Considerations

- Calcium stones account for 75% of kidney stones
- Sudden severe pain onset located in the lateral mid to lower back or lower quadrant with occasional radiation to the groin
- Nausea or vomiting usually occurs
- Fever usually absent
- Groin pain felt when kidney stone at ureterovesicular junction (UVJ)
    - Most common location of impaction
- Aortic aneurysm can mimic ureteral colic
    - Renal colic is most common misdiagnosis of ruptured abdominal aortic aneurysm
- Retained kidney stones in the renal calyces rarely cause pain
- Hematuria on U/A absent 10–15% of the time

- KUB reveals approximately 30–60% of the kidney stones (calcium stones)
- Pelvic calcifications commonly are phleboliths (benign)
- Abdominal exam frequently benign
- Abdominal tenderness can occur with high grade ureteral obstruction
- Flomax (tamsulosin) 0.4 mg qday Rx outpatient allows larger kidney stones to pass frequently — up to 1 cm
    - Flomax (tamsulosin) may be given for 2–4 weeks to pass ureteral calculus
- Most kidney stones pass given time
- Stones up to 1 cm can be managed conservatively in the absence of fever, infection and renal failure if pain is controlled
    - Most large stones will need removal by urology
- CT abdomen/pelvis 97% accurate
- Thrombocytosis can occur with ureteral obstruction in pyelonephritis patients

Evaluation Options

U/A and KUB

- More useful in patients with known kidney stone disease
- May be all that is needed on healthy patients with typical presentation

Ultrasound in children and pregnant patients

- Sensitivity of 98.3% and specificity of 100% in study of 318 patients
- Failed to find stones in 40% of children

UCG in sexually active fertile females

BMP and CBC for any below

- Diabetic patient
- Fever present
- Tachycardia present
- Hypotension present
- SBP < 105 with history of hypertension

Consider CT abdomen and pelvis without contrast

- Uncertain diagnosis

- Age ≥ 60
- Abdominal pulsatile mass
- Possibility of aortic aneurysm considered
- CT has a sensitivity of 94% to 100% and specificity of 92% to 100% in evaluating urinary and non-urinary flank pain

Urine culture if fever or pyuria present

Treatment Options

Acute treatment

- Toradol (ketorolac) 30 mg IV with or without Dilaudid (hydromorphone) 0.5– 1 mg (or equipotent narcotic IV) and Phenergan (promethazine) 6.25 mg IV or Zofran (ondansetron) 4 mg IV; may repeat narcotics × 2 prn if stable vital signs and no significant altered mental status or respiratory depression
- Toradol (ketorolac) 60 mg IM with or without Dilaudid (hydromorphone) 1–2 mg IM (or equipotent narcotic) and Phenergan (promethazine) 25 mg IM or Zofran (ondansetron) 4 mg IM if IV access not readily available
    - Do not use Toradol (ketorolac) if creatinine is elevated
- Do not give increased IV fluids except as needed for dehydration or hypotension

Discharge treatments

- Flomax (tamsulosin)) 0.4 mg PO each day for 2–4 weeks if discharged home (can cause passage of larger stones)
- UTI antibiotics if lower urinary tract infection present without pyelonephritis or fever

Discharge symptom treatment options

- Toradol (ketorolac) 10 mg PO QID prn up to 7 days
    - Do not use Toradol (ketorolac) if creatinine is elevated
- Hydrocodone or oxycodone 5–10 mg PO QID prn up to 7 days

- Phenergan (promethazine) 12.5–25 mg QID PO/PR prn nausea or vomiting

Discharge Criteria

- Pain resolved or tolerable by patient and the patient is agreeable to go home
- No upper tract urinary infection
- No solitary kidney
- No acute renal dysfunction

Discharge instructions

- Kidney stone aftercare instructions
- Increase or additional oral hydration 1–2 liters per day
- Low salt, low protein diet if type of stone not known
- Follow up within 7–10 days with urologist
- Urine strainer and turn in any stone for analysis

Consult Criteria

- Ureteral stone ≥ 6 mm
- Pain and/or vomiting not controlled to clinician or patient's satisfaction
- Uncertain diagnosis
- Concurrent upper tract urinary infection (pyelonephritis)
- Solitary functioning kidney with ureteral calculus
- Pyelonephritis
- Fever

Vital sign and age consult criteria

- Age ≥ 65
- Fever
- Adult heart rate ≥ 110
- Developing hypotension or relative hypotension (SBP < 105 with history of hypertension)

Lab consult criteria

- WBC ≥ 14,000
- Bandemia
- Metabolic acidosis
- Significant electrolyte abnormality

- Glucose ≥ 400 mg/dL in diabetic patient
- Glucose ≥ 300 mg/dL in non-diabetic patient
- Hyperglycemia with metabolic acidosis (decreased serum CO_2 or elevated anion gap)
- Hemoglobin decrease > 1 gm
- Creatinine increase > 0.5 from baseline
- Renal insufficiency
- Acute thrombocytosis
- Acute thrombocytopenia

Notes

___

___

___

References:

Medical therapy for calculus disease

BJU INTERNATIONAL Volume 107, Issue 3, February 2011, Pages: 356–368, Shrawan K. Singh, Mayank Mohan Agarwal and Sumit Sharma

Talner L, Vaughn M. Nonobstructive renal causes of flank pain: findings on noncontrast helical CT (CT KUB). Abdom Imaging. 2003; 28:210–216

Tamm EP, Silverman PM, Shuman WP. Evaluation of the patient with flank pain and possible ureteral calculus. Radiology. 2003;228(2): 319–329 (Clinical radiologic review)

Park SJ, Yi BH, Lee HK, et al. Evaluation of patients with suspected ureteral calculi using sonography as an initial diagnostic tool: how can we improve diagnostic accuracy? Ultrasound Med. 2008; 27:1441–1450 (Prospective study; 318 patients

URINARY TRACT INFECTION PROTOCOL

When using any protocol, always follow the Guidelines of Proper Use (page 18).

Definition

- Bacteriuria with the presence of symptoms

Differential Diagnosis

- Cystitis
- PID
- Ovarian cyst pain
- Gonococcal urethritis
- Nonspecific urethritis (chlamydia or ureaplasma)
- Renal colic
- Bladder outlet obstruction
- Neurogenic bladder
- Pelvic pain disorder
- Endometriosis
- Vaginitis
- Orchitis
- Epididymitis

Considerations

- Female > male incidence until age 50 or in neonates
- 0–3 months of age associated with 30% incidence of sepsis (80% of time the U/A may be normal in neonates with UTI)
- E. coli most common cause
- Sexually active males frequently have prostatitis or urethritis as cause of urinary symptoms (frequently gonorrhea or chlamydia)
- Asymptomatic bacteriuria present in 20% women > 65 years of age
    - Borderline WBC counts of 6-10 cells/mL may reflect the state of hydration such as in patients with oliguria or anuria (dialysis) will usually have some degree of pyuria

    - WBCs may also be seen with moderate hematuria
- Elderly often have atypical presentation
    - Altered mental status
    - Confusion
    - Acute incontinence
    - GI symptoms
    - Urinary retention
- Fever and/or vomiting suggest upper tract urinary infection
- Gross hematuria usually present in lower tract infection
- Acute thrombocytosis with upper tract infection (pyelonephritis) may indicate obstruction from ureteral calculus

UTI facts

- Visual inspection of urine clarity is not useful in diagnosing UTI in women
- Foul-smelling urine is an unreliable indicator of infection in catheterized patients
- Asymptomatic bacteriuria is common in all ages and frequently over-treated
- Virtually 100% of patients with an indwelling Foley catheter are colonized within 2 weeks of placement with 2–5 organisms
- Younger women with true recurrent UTI, bacteriuria may be "protective" for future UTI from more pathogenic organisms
- Leukopenic patients may have artificially low urine WBC
- Noninfectious conditions may result in pyuria — for example acute renal failure, STD, or noninfectious cystitis from a catheter
- Pyuria is a nonspecific, frequent finding in older patients with or without bacteriuria and is not diagnostic of UTI or indicate a need for antibiotics
    - The absence of pyuria has a negative predictive value of > 95% to rule out UTI
- Urine nitrates should not be used alone to start antibiotics
    - Bacteriuria, as noted above, does not define a clinically significant UTI

- Occurrence of candiduria in the catheterized patient is common, and most often reflects colonization or asymptomatic infection
    - Treatment of candida in the urine should occur only in rare situations, such as clear signs and symptoms of infection and no alternative source of infection
- Attributing altered mental status to bacteriuria can result in failure to identify the true cause
    - Without clinical instability or other signs or symptoms of UTI, AMS in elderly can reasonably be observed for resolution of confusion for 24-48 hrs. without antibiotics, while searching for other causes of confusion

Children with UTI admission criteria

- Patients who are toxic or septic
- Patients with signs of urinary obstruction or significant underlying disease
- Patients who are unable to tolerate adequate oral fluids or medications
- Infants younger than 2 months with febrile UTI (presumed pyelonephritis)
- All infants younger than 1 month with suspected UTI, even if not febrile

High risk

- Diabetes
- **Pregnancy**
    - Higher incidence of premature rupture of membranes and fetal demise with UTI (even if asymptomatic)
- Renal failure
- Sickle cell anemia
- Immunocompromised

Complicated UTI

- High risk criteria listed above
- Structural abnormalities
- Mechanical (catheter, stones, stents, instrumentation)
- Functional (reflux or neurogenic bladder)
- Males
- Resistant pathogens

Acute urethral syndrome

- Dysuria without pyuria
- Empiric treatment for STD

Differential of acute urethral syndrome

- Chlamydia
- Gonorrhea
- Herpes
- Vaginitis

Evaluation

- Complete history and physical exam
- Abdominal and costovertebral exam
- Pelvic exam in females and genital exam in males if STD suspected
- U/A – clean catch; catheter specimen if contamination suspected
    - Positive nitrite highly specific (low false positives)
- CBC if vomiting, fever or tachycardia present
- BMP if diabetic or for dehydration/tachycardia if present
- Prostate and urethral meatus exam in males at risk for STI

Urine culture

- For high risk patient or complicated UTI
- Symptoms after > 2 days of treatment or relapse
- Pyelonephritis

Treatment Options

Asymptomatic bacteriurias do not treat unless

- Pregnant (obtain culture)
- Neutropenic
- Abnormal renal functions
- Transplant patient
- Undergoing urologic procedure

Uncomplicated UTI options

- 3 days of one choice below
    - Septra (trimethoprim/sulfamethoxazole)
        - Pediatric 0.5 ml/kg bid (max dose 20 ml)

    - Augmentin (amoxicillin/clavulanate)
- Macrobid (nitrofurantoin) × 7 days — do not use in renal impairment or in upper tract infections
- Cephalexin 20–50 mg/kg/day
- 3rd generation cephalosporin
- Fosfomycin 3 gm PO x 1 with 3–4 oz. of water
- Avoid quinolones if locally high resistance
- May use Sanford Guide or antibiotic database

Complicated UTI

- Cystitis same as uncomplicated UTI but for 5–7 days of antibiotics (excluding Fosfomycin and nitrofurantoin)
- Ertapenem (Invanz) 1 gm IV
- Ciprofloxacin or levofloxacin may be used if known resistance is < 10%
    - Not first line antibiotic in children due to potential complications of arthropathy
- Obtain culture

Pyelonephritis

- Obtain culture
- Antibiotics for 14 days
- Consider IM or IV antibiotic first dose if discharged — Rocephin (ceftriaxone) 1–2 gms IV/IM in adults, 50 mg/kg in children – not to exceed adult dose)
    - May give gentamicin 24 hour dose also
- Antibiotics same as for uncomplicated UTI except for parentally dosing (excluding nitrofurantoin)
- Ciprofloxacin or levofloxacin may be used if known resistance is < 10%
    - Not first line antibiotic in children due to potential complications of arthropathy
- Ertapenem (Invanz) 1 gm IV/IM — adjust for renal dosing

Sexually transmitted diseases

- See Sexually Transmitted Disease Protocol

Pain and nausea medication prn

- Narcotics short course
- OTC medications

- Pyridium (phenazopyridium) 100–200 mg TID (NMT 6 pills)
    - Avoid in renal insufficiency—can cause renal failure
- Phenergan (promethazine) — may need suppository if actively vomiting)
- Zofran (ondansetron)

Discharge Criteria

- Uncomplicated UTI without toxicity
- Able to hold PO intake and medications down
- Healthy patients with uncomplicated pyelonephritis

Discharge instructions

- UTI aftercare instructions
- Follow up primary care provider or urologist within 7 days as needed

Consult Criteria

- Complicated UTI
- Toxic appearance
- Failed outpatient treatment
- Immunocompromised
- Persistent vomiting
- Unable to hold PO meds down
- Unable to self-hydrate
- Pregnancy
- Progressive renal insufficiency
- Poor follow-up
- Male children with first UTI

Vital signs and age consult criteria

- Age ≥ 70
- Age < 24 months
- Adult heart rate ≥ 110
- Hypotension (or relative hypotension: SBP < 105 in patient with hypertension history)
- Pediatric heart rate — see General Patient Criteria Protocol (page 22)

Lab consult criteria

- WBC ≥ 15,000 or < 3,000; neutropenia < 1,000

- Bandemia ≥ 15%
- Acute thrombocytopenia
- Acute thrombocytosis
- Creatinine increase > 0.5 from baseline
- Renal insufficiency
- Increased anion gap
- Significant electrolyte abnormality
- Glucose ≥ 400 mg/dL in diabetic patient
- Glucose ≥ 300 mg/dL in non-diabetic patient
- Hyperglycemia with metabolic acidosis (decreased serum CO_2 or elevated anion gap)
- Lactic acidosis

Notes

References:

International Clinical Practice Guidelines For The Treatment Of Acute Uncomplicated Cystitis And Pyelonephritis In Women: A 2010 Update By The Infectious Diseases Society Of America And The European Society For Microbiology And Infectious Diseases. Clinical Infectious Diseases. 2011;52(5):e103–e120

Management Of Suspected Bacterial Urinary Tract Infection In Adults. A National Clinical Guideline.1 Scottish Intercollegiate Guidelines Network. 2012. www.sign.ac.uk/pdf/sign88.pdf

Cystitis in Females
Author: John L Brusch, MD, FACP; Chief Editor: Michael Stuart Bronze, MD
emedicine.medscape.com/article/233101

American College of Obstetricians and Gynecologists (ACOG). 2008. Treatment of urinary tract infections in nonpregnant women

Gupta K, Hooton TM, Naber KG, et al. International clinical practice guidelines for the treatment of acute uncomplicated cystitis and pyelonephritis in women: A 2010 update by the Infectious Diseases Society of America and the European Society for Microbiology and Infectious Diseases. Clin Infect Dis. Mar 2011;52(5):e103–20

Urinary Tract Infection in Males Medication
Author: John L Brusch, MD, FACP; Chief Editor: Michael Stuart Bronze, MD
emedicine.medscape.com/article/231574

Pediatric Urinary Tract Infection
Author: Donna J Fisher, MD; Chief Editor: Russell W Steele, MD emedicine.medscape.com/article/969643

Schulz L, et al. *Journal of Emerg Med,* April 7 2016. [Epub]

Nicolle LE, et al. *Clin Infect Dis*. 2005; 40: 643–654

Emedhome.com Clinical Pearls: 6 UTI Myths
Published April 13, 2016

JEM, 7/16:25

NEJM,2016;374:562

CHRONIC RENAL FAILURE PROTOCOL

When using any protocol, always follow the Guidelines of Proper Use (page 18).

Definition

- Decreased kidney glomerular filtration rate (GFR) of less than 60 mL/min

Differential Diagnosis

- Acute renal failure
- Acute on chronic renal failure

Considerations

- Normal glomerular filtration rate (GFR) in healthy adult is 120 cc/minute
- Uremia occurs when GFR is 10–20 cc/minute

Main causes

- Diabetes
- Hypertension
- Obstruction (usually in men)
- Polycystic kidney disease (inherited)
- NSAIDs are among the most common causes of drug-induced renal injury
  - Prostaglandin-induced renal vasodilation is critical for maintaining renal perfusion
    - Prostaglandin inhibition by NSAIDs impairs this vasodilation — magnified in hypovolemic patients or those taking ACE inhibitors

Signs, Symptoms and Associated Disorders

- Malaise; weakness; fatigue
- Anorexia; nausea; vomiting
- Gastritis and peptic ulcer disease

- Peripheral neuropathy
- Anemia
- Pruritus
- Volume overload
- CHF
- Hypocalcemia
- Increased infections
- Dialysis catheter infections
- Pericarditis
- Peritonitis in peritoneal dialysis (CAPD) patients

Dialysis disequilibrium syndrome

- Overdialysis
- Weakness
- Dizziness
- Headache
- Mental status changes in severe cases

Hyperkalemia

- EKG cannot reliably predict K+ level
- Caused frequently by medications (ACEI/ARB/spironolactone/epleronone)
- May be caused by potassium supplements

K+ level

- 5.0–6.5 mEq/L — T wave peaking; shortening QTc interval
- 6.5–8.0 mEq/L — PR interval prolongation; loss of P waves; QRS widening
- Greater than 8.0 mEq/L — IVCD; bundle branch blocks; sine wave complex

Evaluation

- Complete history and physical exam
- Last dialysis noted if currently being treated
- BMP

Testing options

- CBC
- Troponin (frequently elevated due to volume overload and CHF only)
- BNP (commonly very elevated and of questionable utility)

- U/A if producing urine and UTI suspected (cath urine sample for fever or lower abdominal pain)
- Chest x-ray if volume overload suspected
- EKG if K+ elevated
- DO NOT ORDER IV CONTRAST unless approved by physician
- Digoxin level if taking it

Treatment Options

Emergent hypertension (consult physician promptly)

- Treat with nitroglycerin SL (NTG) up to 3 doses prn
- NTG paste 1–2 inches prn
- Nitroprusside drip IV
- Dialysis if due to volume overload and patient is on dialysis. Usually an urgent treatment and other steps need to be taken first

Asymptomatic hypertension

- Per Hypertension Protocol (usually no treatment needed)

Hyperkalemia > 5.5 mEq/L (consult physician)

- EKG with peaked T waves or widened QRS complex may or may not be seen
- EKG may not reflect degree of hyperkalemia
- Emergent treatment is indicated if the ECG is abnormal even before the lab test returns
    - Emergent treatment is otherwise not indicated without the lab results
    - Frequently no treatment acutely needed with K+ < 6.0–6.5 mEq/L unless EKG changes or cardiotoxicity present

Calcium gluconate (safer peripheral IV than CaCl) or calcium chloride up to 1 amp IV over 2–3 minutes with patient on monitor

- Calcium chloride 3 three times more potent than calcium gluconate
    - Give 10 ml of calcium gluconate or 5 ml of calcium chloride initially — may repeat as needed per physician

- Duration of action 30–60 minutes
- May be repeated in 5–10 minutes if EKG not improved
- Does not lower serum potassium levels
- Stabilizes cardiac membranes from effects of high potassium
- Controversial whether dangerous or not in Digoxin (digitalis) toxic patients — give Digibind

D50W 1 amp (if patient not hyperglycemic) followed by regular insulin 5–10 units IV

- **In chronic kidney disease patients use regular insulin 5 units IV to avoid hypoglycemia**
- Starts to lower K+ by 0.5–1.5 mEq/L in 15 minutes
- Peak effect in 60 minutes
- Effect lasts 4–6 hours
- Recheck blood glucose in 60–75 minutes for hypoglycemia
- If initial blood glucose is ≥ 250, then D50W is not given
- Check K+ and glucose every 2 hours

Albuterol aerosol inhalation

- 10–20 mg of Albuterol in chamber with a few cc's of NS
- Onset of action within 20–30 minutes
- Peak effect in 90 minutes
- May cause tachycardia

Sodium bicarbonate not acutely effective in treating hyperkalemia in renal failure patients

Kayexalate

- 30–60 gms in 20% sorbitol or water PO
    - Onset of action 1–3 hours
- 60 gms without sorbitol PR
    - Longer onset of action than PO
- Recent controversy on effectiveness
- May cause colonic necrosis

Patiromer (*Veltassa*, Relypsa)

- New agent approved in 2015

- Binds medications so need at least 6 hour delay from taking other medications
- Not for emergency treatment of hyperkalemia due to delay in action

Dialysis

CHF and volume overload (consult physician prior to treatment)

- BNP usually elevated even in asymptomatic patients

Hypertension treatment options

- NTG SL
- NTG paste 1–2 inches
- NTG drip IV
- Dialysis best treatment

Hypotension

- Rule out sepsis
- IV NS 200 bolus if not in clinical fluid overload
- Notify physician promptly

Bleeding

- Direct pressure
- DDAVP (more for oozing than brisk bleeding)

CAPD peritonitis

- Consult physician

Discharge Criteria

- Chronic renal failure patient who is stable and at baseline without acute significant electrolyte abnormalities

Discharge instructions

- Chronic renal failure aftercare instructions
- Avoid potassium supplements
- See Hyperkalemia Protocol

Consult Criteria (supervising physician)

- Hyperkalemia
- Volume overload
- Heart failure

- Significant electrolyte abnormalities or active comorbidities
- Abnormal vital signs or O_2 desaturation

Notes

References:

Weisberg LS. Management of severe hyperkalemia. *Crit Care Med* 2008;36:3246–3251

Sood MM, et al. Emergency Management and Commonly Encountered Outpatient Scenarios in Patients With Hyperkalemia *Mayo Clin Proc* 2007;82:1553–1561

Annals Int Med 110(6):426, March 15, 1989

Levine M, et al. The Effects of Intravenous Calcium in Patients with Digoxin Toxicity *J Emerg Med* 2011 Jan;40(1):41–6

Dialysis Complications of Chronic Renal Failure
Author: Richard S Krause, MD; Chief Editor: Erik D Schraga, MD emedicine.medscape.com/article/1918879

Int J Nephr Renovas Dis,7:459

LaRue H, et al. *Pharmacotherapy*. 2017 Oct 4

Li T, et al. *Clin Kidney J*. 2014 Jun;7(3):239-41

Allon M, et al. *Kidney Int* 1990; 38(5): 869-872

Hyperkalemia Treatment & Management Updated: Jun 20, 2018 Author: Eleanor Lederer, MD, FASN; Chief Editor: Vecihi Batuman, MD, FASN

MALE GENITOURINARY PROTOCOL

When using any protocol, always follow the Guidelines of Proper Use (page 18).

Urethritis and Epididymoorchitis

Definition

- Infection or inflammation of the urethra, epididymis or testicle

Differential diagnosis for epididymoorchitis

- Testicular torsion
- Mumps
- Trauma
- Hernia
- Tumor — usually painless

Considerations

- Gonorrhea and chlamydia are the main causes and coexist 25–50% of the time
- Urethral discharge
- Tender and swollen epididymis and/or testicle

Gonorrhea

- Dysuria
- Thick purulent discharge from urethra
- Gram negative intracellular diplococci

Chlamydia

- Thinner discharge from urethra
- Little to no discomfort

Evaluation

- Sexual history
- Genital exam
- Smear with intracellular gram negative diplococci can be performed
- Culture
- RPR prn

Treatment options

- Follow CDC guidelines
- May use Sanford Guide or drug databases
- Analgesics prn
- Rocephin (ceftriaxone) 250 mg IM PLUS azithromycin 1 gm PO
- Second line drug is doxycycline 100 mg PO bid × 7 days to cover chlamydia instead of azithromycin only for urethral, cervical and rectal—do not use with pharyngeal gonorrheal
- If concerned about syphilis coinfection then doxycycline 100 mg bid PO for 15 days

Discharge criteria

- Nontoxic patient

Discharge instructions

- Epididymoorchitis aftercare instructions
- Return if worse
- Follow up with PCP or urologist in 3–7 days

Consult criteria

- Systemic toxicity
- Refer to General Patient Criteria Protocol prn (page 22)

Testicular Torsion

Definition

- Torsion of the testicle and spermatic cord with subsequent loss of blood flow to the testicle causing loss of testicular function and eventual testicular death and necrosis

Differential diagnosis

- Torsion of testicular or epididymal appendage (blue dot sign in light skinned patients may be present) — can be discharged home if diagnosed
- Epididymitis
- Epididymoorchitis
- Orchitis
- Hydrocele
- Testicular tumor or carcinoma
- Scrotal edema

- Inguinal hernia
- Fournier gangrene
- Testicular trauma
- Henoch-Schonlein Purpura
- Varicocele
- Appendicitis

Considerations

- True urologic emergency
- Complete torsion occurs with ≥ 360° rotation
- Partial torsion occurs with < 360° rotation
- Testicular salvage rate 90–100% with detorsion within 6 hours of pain onset
- Testicular viability 20–50% after 12 hours
- Peak age is 14 years of age, with second peak in first year of life
- Most torsions rotate inward and toward midline

Signs and symptoms

- Usually rapid onset of unilateral severe testicular pain
- Can occur from activity or trauma
- Can occur during sleep
- High-riding testicle occurs on affected side
- Scrotal swelling
- Nausea and/or vomiting
- Abdominal pain around 20–30%
- Fever not very common
- Cremasteric reflex absent on affected side

Evaluation

- Clinical diagnosis if classic history and findings
- Ultrasound color flow Doppler if unsure of diagnosis
    - 94% sensitive
    - 96% specific

Lab tests not usually very useful (used to evaluate for inflammatory processes with low suspicion of torsion)

- CBC – can be normal or elevated in torsion
- U/A – can have WBC's in 30% of torsions
- C-reactive protein – not too helpful

Treatment

- Pain control
- Manual rotation of testicles outward like opening a book
    - May need to be repeated 2–3 times to obtain relief
- Emergent surgery if unable to detorse testicle
- Urgent surgery if testicle detorsed
- All testicular torsion patients should have surgery and not be discharged

Consult criteria

- Discuss suspected testicular torsion with physician or urologist immediately

Prostatitis

Definition

- Infection or inflammation of the prostate gland

Differential diagnosis

- Prostate cancer
- Urethritis
- Mechanical back pain
- UTI

Considerations

- Gonorrhea and chlamydia are the main causes in men age < 35 years and coexist 25–50% of the time
- Prostate tender (caution with vigorous palpation if fever or toxicity present)
- Age > 35 years the usual cause is bacterial
- Nonbacterial prostatitis is an inflammatory condition without infection
- Chronic prostatitis
    - Increases risk of UTI and BPH

Acute bacterial prostatitis age > 35 years

- Fever
- Chills
- Perineal prostatic pain
- Dysuria

- Obstructive bladder symptoms
- Low back pain
- Low abdominal pain
- Spontaneous urethral discharge

Evaluation options

- U/A
- CBC

Treatment options

Age < 35 years

- Follow CDC guidelines
- May use Sanford Guide or drug databases
- Analgesics prn
- Rocephin (ceftriaxone) 250 mg IM PLUS azithromycin 1 gm PO

  \+
- Doxycycline 100 mg PO bid × 14–28 days
- Treatment for sexual partners or refer for treatment for STD
- Flomaxor similar alpha blockers to assist in urine flow and decrease recurrence

Age > 35 years

- May use Sanford Guide or other drug databases
- Septra DS 1 PO bid × 14–28 days (chronic bacterial prostatitis 4–6 weeks)
- Quinolone 14–28 days
- NSAID's and/or narcotics prn
- May given pyridium for discomfort prn

Discharge criteria

- Nontoxic patient
- Refer to General Patient Criteria Protocol prn (page 22)

Discharge instructions

- Prostatitis aftercare instructions
- Return if worse
- Follow up with PCP or urologist in 3–7 days

Consult criteria

- Systemic toxicity
- Urinary retention

Priapism

Definition

- Persistent erection unrelated to sexual desire that is usually painful

Differential considerations

- Penile implant
- Urethral foreign body
- Peyronie disease
- Erection from sexual arousal

Causes

- Idiopathic 35–50% of the time
- Sickle cell anemia
- Leukemia
- Trauma
- Spinal cord injury
- Vasoactive drugs

Low-flow priapism

- Painful
- Ischemia and impotence can occur
- From venous obstruction

High-flow priapism

- From arterial high flow state in penis
- Not usually painful
- Less common than low-flow priapism
- Trauma most frequent cause

Evaluation of priapism

- CBC
- Sickle prep or screen if suspected as a cause
- Color flow ultrasound if not sure if high or low-flow priapism

Treatment options

Low-flow priapism

- Analgesia
- Sickle cell patients may need exchange transfusion
- Terbutaline 0.25 mg SQ may help
- Pseudoephedrine 30–60 mg PO may help
- 1–2 ml of 1% lidocaine with epinephrine 1/100,000 premix injected into proximal corpora cavernosa on lateral penile shaft (one side only) post betadine and alcohol prep — use 27 gauge needle or smaller if possible
    - Aspirate some blood to ensure corpora cavernosa has been entered before injection
    - Caution with coronary artery disease history
    - Hold pressure 30–60 seconds post injection
- Phenylephrine 250–500 mcg can be used instead of 1% lidocaine with epinephrine
- Corpora cavernosa injections usually resolve priapism in 5–15 minutes

High-flow priapism

- Analgesia prn
- Ice packs

Discuss with physician and consult urology immediately

Paraphimosis

Definition

- Entrapment and inability of foreskin to be pulled back (forward) over the glans penis from the shaft in uncircumcised or partially uncircumcised males

Differential diagnosis

- Anasarca
- Balanitis
- Cellulitis
- Insect bite

- Carcinoma
- Penile fracture
- Penile hematoma
- Contact dermatitis
- Hair tourniquet

Considerations

- True emergency
- Can result in penile necrosis

Treatment

- Manual reduction after 5 minutes of ice in exam glove — pushing glans penis under foreskin while holding foreskin in place successful up to 90% of the time
- Dorsal slit of foreskin (consult physician)

Discharge criteria

- Successful reduction of paraphimosis
- No ischemic tissue damage

Discharge instructions

- Referral to urology for circumcision within 7–14 days

Consult criteria

- Inability to reduce the paraphimosis
- Penile tissue ischemic injury

Phimosis

Definition

- Inability to retract foreskin over glans penis

Considerations

- Can lead to venous congestion and eventually tissue damage
- Can lead to paraphimosis

Treatment

- Small hemostat can be passed into foreskin orifice to dilate it and deliver glans penis

Discharge criteria

- Usually can be discharged

Discharge instructions

- Refer to urology

Consult criteria

- Tissue ischemia
- Cellulitis

Hydrocele

Definition

- Collection of serous fluid in scrotum in up to 1% of males

Differential diagnosis

- Orchitis
- Testicular torsion
- Indirect inguinal hernia
- Epididymitis
- Trauma

Considerations

- Usually asymptomatic or subclinical
- Located anterior and superior to testicles
- A light shines through the hydrocele
- Most pediatric cases are congenital
- Can be from trauma, orchitis, or epididymitis

Evaluation options

- History and physical examination only may be all that is needed (transillumination)
- CBC
- U/A
- Ultrasound can be used in diagnosis uncertain

Treatment

- Usually no acute treatment needed

Discharge criteria

- Nonpainful, non-inflamed scrotal hydrocele

Discharge instructions

- Hydrocele aftercare instructions
- Refer to urology

Consult criteria

- Painful scrotum
- Scrotal cellulitis
- Fever

Notes

References:

Lewis AG, Bukoswki TP, Jarvis PD et al. Evaluation of the acute scrotum in the emergency department. J Pediatr Surg 1995;30:2:277–82

Orchitis; Author: Nataisia Terry, MD; Chief Editor: Erik D Schraga, MD; emedicine.medscape.com/article/777456

Paraphimosis Treatment & Management

Author: Jeffrey M Donohoe, MD, FAAP; Chief Editor: Bradley Fields Schwartz, DO, FACS

emedicine.medscape.com/article/442883

Roberts JR, Price C, Mazzeo T. Intracavernous epinephrine: a minimally invasive treatment for priapism in the emergency department. *J Emerg Med*. Apr 2009;36(3):285–9

Chronic Bacterial Prostatitis Medication

Author: Sunil K Ahuja, MD; Chief Editor: Edward David Kim, MD, FACS emedicine.medscape.com/article/458391

Prostatitis Author: Paul J Turek, MD; Chief Editor: Jeter (Jay) Pritchard Taylor, III, MD

emedicine.medscape.com/article/785418

ACUTE URINARY RETENTION PROTOCOL

When using any protocol, always follow the Guidelines of Proper Use (page 18).

Definition

- Acute or subacute inability to voluntarily void sufficiently causing significant retention in the urinary bladder often requiring immediate attention and intervention

Considerations

Causes (some)

- Benign prostatic hypertrophy (BPH) most common cause in men of acute urinary retention (AUR) — most common cause overall
- Bladder masses, gynecologic surgery, and pelvic prolapse most common cause in women (relatively uncommon cause of AUR)
- AUR rarely secondary to spinal cord compression
- Diabetic neuropathy may cause AUR
- Urethral stricture
- Herpes genitalis

Medications causing AUR

- Anticholinergics or antihistamines that inhibit detrusor muscle activity
- Sympathomimetic drugs that increase alpha-adrenergic tone in the prostate
- NSAIDs that may inhibit prostaglandin-mediated detrusor muscle contraction
- Chronic opioid therapy causing a reduced bladder-fullness sensation

Symptoms

- Abdominal pain and/or distension
- Back pain may be confused with renal pathology or spinal tumors
- Urinary complaints (e.g., frequency, dribbling)

- Genital pain

Evaluation

- History of medications
- Voiding history
- Associated symptoms such as fever, chills, dysuria, new onset constipation, low back pain
- Rectal and genital exam as indicated
- U/A
- CBC, BMP as needed to assess renal function and for SIRS
- Bladder scan and possibly renal ultrasound (if needed)
- CT abdomen/pelvis without contrast if ureteral calculi or other significant disease process suspected

Treatment

- Double lumen foley catheter
- Coude catheter for significant BPH and difficulty passing standard foley
- Triple lumen foley catheter if irrigation needed (16F-20F)
- Tamsulosin (Flomax) 0.4 mg PO qday with catheter
    - Improves spontaneous voiding when catheter removed
- Antibiotics not needed unless existing UTI is present
- No evidence for the need to clamp foley with rapid bladder emptying
- 70% of men had a recurrent episode of AUR within 1 week if the bladder was drained only initially on presentation
- BPH and AUR catheterized for ≤ 3 days had greater success with spontaneous voiding than those catheterized for > 3 days
- Antibiotics for lower tract UTI

Discharge criteria

- Resolution of AUR with foley
- No significant comorbidities

Discharge instructions

- Follow up with urologist ≤ 3 days
- Foley instructions
- Leg bag
- Return if fever, increased pain, vomiting or other concerning symptoms occur

Consult criteria

- Inability to pass foley
- Fever
- Pyelonephritis
- SIRS
- Significant comorbid disease processes or causes of AUR

Notes

References:

Vilke GM, Ufberg JW, Harrigan RA, et al. Evaluation and treatment of acute urinary retention. J Emerg Med. 2008;35(2):193–198. (Review)

Afonso AS, Verhamme KM, Stricker BH, et al. Inhaled anticholinergic drugs and risk of acute urinary retention. BJU Int. 2011;107(8):1265–1272

Kaplan SA. AUA guidelines and their impact on the management of BPH: an update. Rev Urol. 2004;6 Suppl 9:S46– S52

Nyman MA, Schwenk NM, Silverstein MD. Management of urinary retention: rapid versus gradual decompression and risk of complications. Mayo Clin Proc. 1997;72(10):951–956

Breum L, Klarskov P, Munck LK, et al. Significance of acute urinary retention due to intravesical obstruction. Scand J Urol Nephrol. 1982;16(1):21–24

An Evidence-Based Approach To The Emergency Department Management of Acute Urinary Retention in Men and Women January 2014 review article; EB Medicine

Electrolyte and Acid/Base Disturbances

Section Contents

When using any protocol, always follow the Guidelines of Proper Use (page 18).

HYPERKALEMIA PROTOCOL

When using any protocol, always follow the Guidelines of Proper Use (page 18).

Definition

- Elevated serum potassium levels

Differential Diagnosis

- Hypocalcemia
- Acute tubular necrosis
- Acute renal failure
- Chronic renal failure
- Metabolic acidosis
- Digoxin toxicity
- Burns
- Rhabdomyolysis
- Tumor lysis syndrome
- Head trauma

Considerations

- EKG cannot reliably predict K^+ level
    - K^+ level
        - 5.0–6.5 mEq/L — T wave peaking; shortening QTc interval
        - 6.5–8.0 mEq/L — PR interval prolongation; loss of P waves; QRS widening
        - Greater than 8.0 mEq/L — IVCD; bundle branch blocks; sine wave complex

Causes

- Renal failure
- K^+ supplementation
- Medications (ACEI/ARB/spironolactone/epleronone)
- High potassium foods
- Hemolysis from blood draw
- Hemolysis
- DIC
- Tissue injury or ischemia

Evaluation

- Complete history and physical exam
- Last dialysis noted if being currently treated
- BMP
- Chest x-ray if volume overload suspected
- EKG

Testing options

- CBC
- Troponin questionable value (frequently elevated due to volume overload and CHF only)
- BNP questionable value (commonly very elevated)
- U/A if producing urine (cath urine sample for fever or lower abdominal pain)
- DO NOT ORDER IV CONTRAST STUDIES UNLESS APPROVED BY PHYSICIAN

Treatment Options

Hyperkalemia > 5.5 mEq/L (consult physician)

- EKG with peaked T waves or widened QRS complex may or may not be seen
- EKG may not reflect degree of hyperkalemia
- Emergent treatment is indicated if the ECG is abnormal even before the lab test returns
    - Emergent treatment is otherwise not indicated without the lab results
    - Frequently no treatment acutely needed with K+ < 6.0–6.5 mEq/L unless EKG changes or cardiotoxicity present

Calcium gluconate (safer peripheral IV than CaCl) or calcium chloride up to 1 amp IV over 2–3 minutes with patient on monitor

- Calcium chloride 3 three times more potent than calcium gluconate
    - Give 10 ml of calcium gluconate or 5 ml of calcium chloride initially — may repeat as needed per physician
- Duration of action 30–60 minutes
- May be repeated in 5–10 minutes if EKG not improved

- Does not lower serum potassium levels
- Stabilizes cardiac membranes from effects of high potassium
- Controversial whether dangerous or not in Digoxin (digitalis) toxic patients — give Digibind

D50W 1 amp (if patient not hyperglycemic) followed by regular insulin 5–10 units IV

- **In chronic kidney disease patients use regular insulin 5 units IV to avoid hypoglycemia**
- Starts to lower K+ by 0.5–1.5 mEq/L in 15 minutes
- Peak effect in 60 minutes
- Effect lasts 4–6 hours
- Recheck blood glucose in 60–75 minutes for hypoglycemia
- If initial blood glucose is ≥ 250, then D50W is not given
- Check K+ and glucose every 2 hours

Albuterol aerosol inhalation

- 10–20 mg of Albuterol in chamber with a few cc's of NS
- Onset of action within 20–30 minutes
- Peak effect in 90 minutes
- May cause tachycardia

Sodium bicarbonate not acutely effective in treating hyperkalemia in renal failure patients

Kayexalate

- 30–60 gms in 20% sorbitol or water PO
    - Onset of action 1–3 hours
- 60 gms without sorbitol PR
    - Longer onset of action than PO
- Recent controversy on effectiveness
- May cause colonic necrosis
- Some controversy about effectiveness and has FDA warning about combining with sorbitol

Patiromer (*Veltassa*, Relypsa)

- New agent approved in 2015

- Binds medications so need at least 6 hour delay from taking other medications
- Not for emergency treatment of hyperkalemia due to delay in action

Dialysis

Discharge Criteria

- Mild hyperkalemia < 6.0 mEq/L
- Acceptable treatment response
- Further potassium rises not anticipated

Discharge instructions

Close follow up

- Hyperkalemia aftercare instructions
- Chronic renal failure aftercare instructions if indicated

Consult Criteria

- Discuss with supervising physician if potassium > 5.5 mEq/L
- End-stage renal disease with abnormal vital signs or O_2 desaturation
- Significant comorbidities

Notes

References:

Weisberg LS. Management of severe hyperkalemia. *Crit Care Med* 2008;36:3246–3251

Sood MM, et al. Emergency Management and Commonly Encountered Outpatient Scenarios in Patients With Hyperkalemia *Mayo Clin Proc* 2007;82:1553–1561

Annals Int Med 110(6):426, March 15, 1989

Levine M, et al. The Effects of Intravenous Calcium in Patients with Digoxin Toxicity *J Emerg Med* 2011 Jan;40(1):41–6

Dialysis Complications of Chronic Renal Failure
Author: Richard S Krause, MD; Chief Editor: Erik D Schraga, MD; emedicine.medscape.com/article/1918879

FDA Asks for Drug Interaction Studies on Kayexalate
medscape.com/viewarticle/853117

LaRue H, et al. *Pharmacotherapy*. 2017 Oct 4

Li T, et al. *Clin Kidney J*. 2014 Jun;7(3):239-41

Allon M, et al. *Kidney Int* 1990; 38(5): 869-872

Hyperkalemia Treatment & Management Updated: Jun 20, 2018 Author: Eleanor Lederer, MD, FASN; Chief Editor: Vecihi Batuman, MD, FASN

HYPOKALEMIA PROTOCOL

When using any protocol, always follow the Guidelines of Proper Use (page 18).

Definition

- Serum potassium level < 3.5 mEq/L

Differential Diagnosis

- Cushing syndrome
- Hypocalcemia
- Hypomagnesemia

Considerations

- Very common
- Increases dysrhythmias
- Increases Digoxin (digitalis) toxicity effects
- Mild 3.0–3.4 mEq/L
- Moderate 2.5–2.9 mEq/L
- Severe < 2.5 mEq/L
- Serum potassium decreases by 0.3 mEq/L for each 100 mEq of potassium reduction in total-body stores, but the response is extremely variable

Causes

- Diuretics
- Hyperventilation
- Hypomagnesemia
- Poor nutrition
- Diarrhea
- Metabolic alkalosis
- Renal tubular acidosis
- Adrenal conditions
- Hyperaldosteronism
- Gastrointestinal losses (vomiting, diarrhea, NG suction)
- Familial Periodic Hypokalemia Paralysis

Signs and Symptoms

- Severe weakness K^+ < 2.5 mEq/L

- Paralysis can occur with rapid development of K^+ < 2.0 mEq/L
- Paresthesias
- Muscle weakness
- Muscle cramps
- Constipation
- Cardiac dysrhythmias
- EKG changes
    - Low voltage T waves
    - ST segment depression
    - U waves
    - Small P waves
    - PAC's
    - PVC's

Evaluation

- BMP
- EKG if potassium < 2.5 mEq/L
- Magnesium level not needed usually

Treatment Options

- Oral replacement preferred when indicated
- Oral potassium 40–60 mEq can raise serum potassium 1–1.5 mEq/L; 135–160 mEq PO raises serum potassium 2.5–3.5 mEq/L (transient elevation since potassium taken up in cells)
- Potassium level < 2.5 mEq/L give IV replacement no faster than 10 mEq per hour
- MgSO4 (magnesium sulfate) replacement can improve potassium replacement
    - 2–4 gms IV over 30 minutes if needed
    - Mg gluconate 200–400 mg PO TID prn if hypokalemia is asymptomatic (adults)

Discharge Criteria

- Asymptomatic patient
- Able to replenish potassium orally
- Potassium level > 2.5 mEq/L

Discharge instructions

- Hypokalemia aftercare instructions

- Follow up with primary care provider within 2–3 days

Consult Criteria

- Potassium ≤ 2.5 mEq/L
- Symptomatic patient
- EKG changes

Notes

References:
Hypokalemia in Emergency Medicine
Author: David Garth, MD; Chief Editor: Erik D Schraga, MD
emedicine.medscape.com/article/767448

Agarwal A, Wingo CS. Treatment of hypokalemia *N Engl J Med* 1999;340: 154-5

Gennari FJ. Hypokalemia *N Engl J Med* 1998;339:451-458

Nicolis, GL, et al. Glucose-induced hyperkalemia in diabetic subjects *Arch Intern Med* 1981;141:49

HYPERNATREMIA PROTOCOL

When using any protocol, always follow the Guidelines of Proper Use (page 18).

Definition

- Serum Na^+ level > 145 mEq/L

Differential Diagnosis

- Hyperglycemic hyperosmolar state
- Diabetes insipidus
- Salt ingestion
- Hypertonic dehydration

Considerations

Dehydration

- Secondary to volume depletion
- Poor oral intake of fluids
- Commonly seen in nursing home patients
- PEG tube feeding patients
- Bedridden patients
- Stroke patients
- Patients unable to care for themselves
- Medication induced diuresis
- Accompanied by metabolic acidosis frequently
- High risk condition for mortality in elderly
- Usually in patients with significant comorbidities
- Na^+ 150–170 mEq/L usually indicates dehydration
- Na^+ > 170 mEq/L usually indicates diabetes insipidus
- Na^+ > 190 mEq/L usually indicates long term salt ingestion

Diabetes insipidus

Decreased urine concentration ability of kidneys

- Lithium
- Sickle cell anemia
- Post obstructive diuresis after treatment of bladder outlet obstruction

- Na^+ > 170 mEq/L usually indicates diabetes insipidus

Decreased secretion of ADH (antidiuretic hormone)

- Brain tumors
- Brain injury
- Cerebral infectious processes

Signs and symptoms

- Altered mental status
- Decreased responsiveness
- Tachycardia
- Hypotension may occur
- Tachypnea
- Poor skin turgor
- Decreased capillary refill
- Dry mucous membranes
- Decreased urine output
- Hard stools

Evaluation Options

- BMP
- CBC
- U/A
- Chest x-ray usually performed to rule out concurrent disease process
- CT brain scan if central process suspected
- Urine for spot Na and osmolarity if serum sodium > 170 mEq/L (usually indicates diabetes insipidus)

Treatment Options

- Restore plasma volume first
- Oral rehydration therapy (ORT) preferred over IV in mild to moderate dehydration if appropriate to patient's condition and ability to self-hydrate

Serum Na correction no more than 1 mEq/L per hour

- Too rapid correction may cause cerebral edema

Adult dehydration

Oral Rehydration Therapy (ORT) for mild to moderate dehydration if able to self-hydrate

- Oral rehydration formula (WHO formula, Rehydralyte or Pedialyte) for mild to moderate dehydration or serum CO_2 is 14–18 mEq/L or NA^+ 146–152 mEq/L
  - Zofran (ondansetron) 8 mg chewable tablet or 4–8 mg IM if vomiting
  - 15–30 cc every 1–2 minutes for adults (age > 12) for 1–4 hours — start 20 minutes after Zofran (ondansetron) given
  - Hold ORT 10 minutes if vomiting occurs then resume
  - Reassess for urine production, improved heart rate, and absence of severe vomiting
  - Recheck serum CO_2 if initially < 17 mEq/L
  - Mild dehydration give 50 cc/kg in < 4 hours
  - Moderate dehydration give 50–100 cc/kg in 1–4 hours

IV rehydration

- Moderate to severe dehydration (Na^+ > 152 mEq/L), give IV NS or LR 150–300 cc/hour over 2–4 hours
  - Normal saline has 154 mEq/L of sodium
  - Lactated ringers has 130 mEq/L of sodium
- Hypotension or signs of poor organ perfusion (lactic acid > 2), give NS or LR at 500–1000 cc/hour up to 2 liters (consult physician promptly) — caution if CHF history

Pediatric dehydration

Dehydration assessment

Mild ≤ 5%

- Alert
- Mucous membranes variable dry
- Skin turgor normal
- Fontanel flat
- Blood pressure normal

- Heart rate normal
- Capillary refill < 2 seconds
- Urine output decreased

Moderate 6–9%

- Irritable
- Mucous membranes dry
- Skin turgor variably reduced
- Fontanel depressed
- Blood pressure variably orthostatic
- Heart rate tachycardic
- Capillary refill 2–3 seconds
- Urine output decreased — oliguria

Severe ≥ 10%

- Lethargic
- Mucous membranes dry
- Skin turgor reduced
- Fontanel depressed
- Blood pressure orthostatic or hypotensive
- Heart rate markedly tachycardic
- Capillary refill ≥ 4 seconds
- Urine output decreased - oliguria/anuria

Oral Rehydration Therapy (ORT) for mild to moderate dehydration

- Zofran (ondansetron) oral chewable tablet in ED for frequent vomiting
  - 2 mg for 8–15 kg; 4 mg for 15–30 kg; 8 mg for > 30 kg
  - Zofran (ondansetron) 2–4 doses can be prescribed for home if indicated

Oral rehydration formula for mild to moderate dehydration; serum CO_2 14–18 mEq/L or serum Na 146–155 mEq/L

- 5 cc every 1–2 minutes for small children by caretaker for < 4 hours — start 20 minutes after Zofran (ondansetron) given
- 5–10 cc every 1–2 minutes for larger children by caretaker for 1–4 hours
- Hold ORT 10 minutes if vomiting occurs then resume

- Reassess for urine production, weight gain, improved HR and alertness, and absence of severe vomiting
- Recheck serum CO_2 if initially < 17
- Mild dehydration give 50 cc/kg in < 4 hours
- Moderate dehydration give 50–100 cc/kg over 1–4 hours

Severe dehydration give IV NS bolus 20 cc/kg; may repeat × 2

Exclusion Criteria for Oral Rehydration Therapy

- Age < 6 months of age
- Hematemesis
- Bilious vomiting
- Bloody diarrhea
- VP shunt
- Head trauma
- Focal RLQ tenderness (possible appendicitis)
- Severe dehydration
- Patient vomits 3 or more times after starting ORT

IV therapy criteria and treatment for moderate to severe dehydration

- IV NS hydration for CO_2 < 14 mEq/L or Na > 155 mEq/L
- ORT failure
- IV NS 20 cc/kg bolus, may repeat × 2
- Consult physician
- Maintenance IV with D5NS (dextrose decreases return visits)

Discharge Criteria

- Patient responds to rehydration
- Healthy without significant comorbid conditions
- Good social support systems
- Unlikely to acutely become hypernatremic post discharge

Discharge instructions

- Dehydration or hypernatremia aftercare instructions

- Follow up with primary care providers within 1–3 days

Consult Criteria

Discuss with physician

- Patients with significant comorbid conditions or findings
- Serum Na > 150 mEq/L
- Age > 60
- Age < 6 months

Vital signs consult criteria

- Adult heart rate > 100 post treatment
- Hypotension or relative hypotension (SBP < 105 with history of hypertension)
- Orthostatic vital signs
- Pediatric heart rate
    - 0–4 months ≥ 180
    - 5–7 months ≥ 175
    - 8–12 months ≥ 170
    - 1–3 years ≥ 160

Notes

References:

Hypernatremia in Emergency Medicine

Author: Zina Semenovskaya, MD; Chief Editor: Romesh Khardori, MD, PhD, FACP

emedicine.medscape.com /article/76668

HYPONATREMIA PROTOCOL

When using any protocol, always follow the Guidelines of Proper Use (page 18).

Definition

- Serum sodium level < 135 mEq/L

Differential Diagnosis

- SIADH
- Hepatitis cirrhosis
- Adrenal insufficiency
- Adrenal crisis
- CHF
- Water intoxication
- Gastroenteritis
- Renal failure
- Hypothyroidism
- Nephrotic syndrome

Considerations

- Acute hyponatremia is more symptomatic
- Chronic hyponatremia can be asymptomatic
- Central pontine myelinolysis can occur from too rapid correction of hyponatremia
    - Dysarthria
    - Dysphagia
    - Seizures
    - Altered mental status
    - Quadriplegia
    - Hypotension
- Correction of severe symptomatic hyponatremia should not raise serum sodium level more than 4 mEq/L acutely
- Chronic hyponatremia usually does not need rapid correction (can be dangerous to do so)
- Chronic hyponatremia is much more common than acute hyponatremia

- Serum Na^+ is lowered 1.6 mEq/L for every blood glucose level increase of 100 mg% over normal
  - Will correct with correction of hyperglycemia alone
- Children more prone to iatrogenic water intoxication by parents giving excessive water to replace GI fluid losses

Signs and symptoms

- Mild or none in some chronic hyponatremic patients with $Na^+ > 120$ mEq/L

Acute hyponatremia

- Serum sodium > 120 mEq/L
  - Headache
  - Nausea; vomiting
  - Muscle cramps
  - Weakness
  - Anorexia
  - Rhabdomyolysis
- Serum sodium 110–120 mEq/L
  - Hyperventilation
  - Decreased responsiveness
  - Hallucinations
  - Behavior disturbances
  - Incontinence
  - Ataxia
- Serum sodium < 110 mEq/L
  - Posturing
  - Hypertension
  - Bradycardia
  - Impaired temperature regulation
  - Seizures
  - Coma
  - Respiratory arrest

Causes

Hypovolemic

- Excess fluid losses replaced with hypotonic solutions by patient
  - Vomiting
  - Diarrhea
  - Third spacing of fluids

- Burns
- Excessive sweating
- Diuretics

Hypervolemic

- Excessive water intake (water intoxication)
- Hepatic cirrhosis
- CHF
- Nephrotic syndrome
- Renal insufficiency

Euvolemic

- Hypothyroidism
- Adrenal insufficiency
- SIADH
- Psychogenic polydipsia

Medications

- Diuretics
- NSAID's
- Oral hypoglycemic agents
- ACE inhibitors
- ARB's
- PPI's

Sodium Requirement (mEq/L)

- Na^+ deficit is total body water (Kg × 0.6) times (desired Na – Serum Na)

Hypertonic saline

- 513 mEq/L of NaCl

Normal saline

- 154 mEq/L of NaCl

Lactated ringers

- 130 mEq/L of Na^+

Evaluation

- BMP
- Urine spot Na^+ level (consider if SIADH suspected)
- Urine osmolarity (if SIADH suspected, which has inappropriately concentrated urine)
- Serum cortisol level if adrenal insufficiency suspected

- TSH and thyroid function tests if hypothyroidism suspected

Treatment Options

Chronic hyponatremia with mild to moderately severe symptoms

(Do not increase serum Na^+ by more than 10–12 mEq/L in first 24 hours)

- Hypovolemia: IV NS
- Hypervolemia: restrict free water and sodium
- Euvolemia: restrict free water — may add Lasix (furosemide) short term

Acute hyponatremia — Na^+ < 120 mEq/L with severe symptoms (or chronic hyponatremia with severe symptoms such as seizures, coma, severe altered mental status) consult physician

- 3% saline at 100 cc/hr. × 2 hours and recheck serum sodium for adults
- Pediatric calculation of TBW (kg × 0.6) × 4 mEq/L = acute Na^+ deficit to be replenished over 2 hours
- Do not raise Na^+ acutely more than 4 mEq/L

Discharge Criteria

- Asymptomatic serum sodium > 125 mEq/L without comorbid conditions

Discharge instructions

- Follow up within 1–3 days for serum sodium < 130 mEq/L with primary care provider
- Hyponatremia aftercare instructions

Consult Criteria

- Serum sodium ≤ 125 mEq/L
- Comorbid conditions or symptoms
- Refer to General Patient Criteria Protocol prn (page 22)

Notes

References:

Hyponatremia in Emergency Medicine Clinical Presentation
Author: Sandy Craig, MD; Chief Editor: Romesh Khardori, MD, PhD, FACP
emedicine.medscape.com/article/767624

Verbalis JG, Goldsmith SR, Greenberg A, Schrier RW, Sterns RH. Hyponatremia treatment guidelines 2007: expert panel recommendations. *Am J Med*. Nov 2007;120(11 Suppl 1):S1–21

METABOLIC ACIDOSIS PROTOCOL

When using any protocol, always follow the Guidelines of Proper Use (page 18).

Definition

- Disease process with an increase in plasma acidity

Differential Diagnosis

- See A CAT MUDPILES below

Considerations

- Normal pH is 7.39–7.41 (~7.35–7.45 depending on lab)
- Kidneys excrete H^+ and reabsorb HCO_{3-} normally

Metabolic acidosis

- pH lower than normal unless over-compensated by a primary metabolic or respiratory alkalosis (unusual) — can occur with aspirin overdose initially
- Elevated H^+ concentration in guise of various acids
- Low HCO_{3-}
- Goal of therapy is to raise pH to 7.2 usually by treating the process causing the acidosis
  - HCO_{3-} not used unless pH < 7.0, and not usually even then (check with physician)
- K^+ may be elevated and will decrease sometimes significantly when acidosis is treated whether initially elevated or not

Nonanion gap acidosis

- Diarrhea
- Renal tubular acidosis
- Carbonic anhydrase inhibitors — Diamox (acetazolamide)
- Hypoaldosteronism

Anion gap calculation

- Na^+ minus (HCO_{3-} – Chloride)
- Normal range 5–12 ± 3 mEq/L

Respiratory compensation

- Expected pCO_2 is $1.5[HCO_3] + 8$
- If higher, then primary respiratory acidosis exists and there is inadequate respiratory compensation
- Death can result from intubation and ventilation that does not adequately compensates enough for severe metabolic acidosis (or maintains sufficient respiratory compensation with hyperventilation if intubated)

Respiratory acidosis

- Acute: HCO3 increased by 1 mEq/L for each 10 mm Hg increase in pCO_2
- Chronic: HCO3 increased by 4 mEq/L for each mm Hg increase in pCO_2

Anion gap mnemonic — A CAT MUDPILES

A – Alcoholic ketoacidosis
C – Cyanide; carbon monoxide
A – Aspirin; other salicylates
T – Toluene
M – Methanol; metformin
U – Uremia
D – DKA
P – Paraldehyde; phenformin
I – Iron; INH
L – Lactic acidosis (dehydration or tissue ischemia commonly)
E – Ethylene glycol
S – Starvation

Osmolol gap > 10–20 suspect substance ingestion (Normal < 10)

- Gap = Osmolality measured – Osmolality calculated (calculation equation: 2(Na+K) + glucose/18 + BUN/2.8; normal 280–300 mOsm/L)
- Ethanol mg%/4.6 is added to osmolol gap equation if present
- Gap > 50 carries high specificity for toxic alcohol such as methanol, ethylene glycol, or isopropyl alcohol
- Normal gap < 10
- Refer to Toxicology Protocol

Signs and Symptoms

- Tachypnea or Kussmaul respirations
- Tachycardia
- Confusion
- Depends on the degree and type of acidosis

Evaluation

- Complete history and physical examination
- CBC
- BMP
- Serum ketones if diabetic
- Lactic acid level
- ABG for
  - Severe acidosis
  - Altered mental status
  - Significant tachycardia
- Chest x-ray if indicated
- EKG if indicated
- Toxicology tests as indicated

Treatment Options

- Treat underlying process
- pH < 7.0 can consider IV HCO3 (some controversy over degree of acidosis needing this treatment) — consult physician immediately
- See Adult and Pediatric Gastroenteritis Protocols

Discharge Criteria

- Resolving metabolic acidosis with treatable outpatient process
- HCO3 > 17
- Anion gap ≤ 19
- No significant comorbidities
- Nontoxic

Discharge instructions

- Aftercare instructions relevant to cause of acidosis
- Follow up with primary care provider within 1 day

Consult Criteria

- $HCO_3 < 18$
- Anion gap ≥ 20
- Age ≥ 60
- Condition not likely to improve as outpatient
- Respiratory acidosis
- Hypotension or relative hypotension (SBP < 105 with history of hypertension)
- Toxic appearance
- Adult heart rate ≥ 110
- Pediatric heart rate
    - 0–4 months ≥ 180
    - 5–7 months ≥ 175
    - 8–12 months ≥ 170
    - 1–3 years ≥ 160
    - 4–5 years ≥ 145
    - 6–8 years ≥ 130
    - 9–11 years ≥ 125
    - 12–15 years ≥ 115
    - 16 years or older ≥ 110

Notes

___

___

___

References:

Metabolic Acidosis Author: Christie P Thomas, MBBS, FRCP, FASN, FAHA; Chief Editor: Vecihi Batuman, MD, FACP, FASN emedicine.medscape.com/article/242975

Metabolic Acidosis in Emergency Medicine
Author: Antonia Quinn, DO; Chief Editor: Romesh Khardori, MD, PhD, FACP
emedicine.medscape.com/article/768268

Head Trauma and Neck Pain

Section Contents

When using any protocol, always follow the Guidelines of Proper Use (page 18).

Adult Minor Head Trauma Protocol

When using any protocol, always follow the Guidelines of Proper Use (page 18).

Definition

- Head trauma with Glasgow coma scale ≥ 14 and no focal neurologic deficits or complaints

Differential Diagnosis

- Subarachnoid hemorrhage
- Subdural hematoma
- Epidural hematoma
- Cerebral contusion
- Skull fracture

Considerations

- Loss of consciousness (LOC), amnesia, headache, vomiting and seizures have low sensitivity and specificity for detecting intracranial injury
- Cervical spine exam and evaluation important
- Skull films mainly replaced by CT evaluation of adult head trauma — may consider skull films for laceration > 5 cm or that extends deep to the skull
  - Violent mechanism of injury
- Significant maxillofacial injuries can coexist

Concussion Definitions

Grade 1 concussion

- Transient confusion
- No LOC
- Duration of mental status abnormalities < 15 minutes

Grade 2 concussion

- Transient confusion
- No LOC

- Duration of mental status abnormalities > 15 minutes

Grade 3 concussion

- Loss of consciousness

Postconcussion Syndrome

- Symptoms of headache, dizziness, trouble concentrating days to weeks following a concussion and can persist for months
- Can occur in up to 30% of concussions
- Anxiety and depression reported by patients
- Issues of compensation and litigation associated at times with persistent symptoms
- Disequilibrium and vertigo from vestibular concussion
- Reassurance decreases incidence and duration of symptoms
- Avoid narcotics
- Can use mild analgesics
- Can use meclizine or Phenergan (promethazine) for vestibular symptoms
- Rarely seen in young children
- Countries with low litigation have low postconcussion syndrome disability

Evaluation

- CT brain scan for concussion with loss of consciousness
- CT brain scan for patients on Coumadin (warfarin), DOAC agents (dabigatran, apixaban, or rivaroxaban) or Plavix (clopidogrel) with more than trivial injury
- Evaluate for other injuries, especially C-spine
- Retinal exam: hemorrhages present in 65–90% with abuse inflicted head injury
- Detailed neurologic exam
- INR if on Coumadin (warfarin)
- Suspected intracranial injury
- Glasgow coma scale < 15
- Evaluate for other injuries, especially C-spine
- Retinal exam: hemorrhages present in 65–90% with abuse inflicted head injury

- Detailed neurologic exam
- INR if on Coumadin (warfarin)

ENT exam

- Check for hemotympanum
- CSF rhinorrhea
- Battle's sign
- Cranial nerve palsy

CT Head Rules (your choice)

New Orleans CT brain criteria (for ordering noncontrast CT brain)

- Normal neurologic exam and one of the following
    - Abnormal GCS
    - Headache
    - Vomiting
    - Age > 60
    - Persistent anterograde amnesia
    - Drug or alcohol intoxication
    - Visible trauma above the clavicle
    - Seizure

Canadian CT Head Rule

- Any positive below then perform head CT
    - GCS < 15 at 2 hours after injury
    - Suspected or open skull fracture
    - Signs of basilar skull fracture
    - Vomiting ≥ 2 episodes
    - Age ≥ 65 years
    - Pre–impact amnesia ≥ 30 minutes
    - Dangerous mechanism

Noncontrast CT brain scan for acute brain injury

(From ACEP/CDC Clinical Policy)

Order noncontrast CT brain scan

- Loss of consciousness
- No loss of consciousness with one of the following:
    - Headache
    - Vomiting

- Age > 60 years
- Persistent anterograde amnesia
- Focal neurologic deficit
- Coagulopathy
- Drug or alcohol intoxication
- Visible trauma above the clavicle
- Posttraumatic Seizure
- GCS < 15

Consider noncontrast CT brain scan with no LOC and one of following

- Signs of basilar skull fracture
- Age > 65 years
- Dangerous mechanism of injury (includes)
    - Motor vehicle ejection
    - Pedestrian struck by motor vehicle
    - Fall from > 3 feet or 5 stairs
- Patients on warfarin
    - Minor head trauma patients on warfarin or anticoagulation with a normal initial CT brain, it is recommended that 24 hours observation and repeat CT brain scan be perfomed
    - Higher risk with INR > 3.0 for delayed intracranial bleeding

Treatment Options

- Tylenol (no ASA or NSAID's for 36 hours)
- Avoid more potent analgesics so progression of symptoms can be detected
- Head injury instruction sheet
- Return for any neurologic changes
- Follow up with primary care provider or neurologist/neurosurgeon

Discharge Criteria

- Stable condition
- Normal neurologic exam
- No other significant trauma
- No radiologic abnormalities

Discharge instructions

- Head injury aftercare instructions

Consult Criteria

- Age > 65
- Bleeding potential from medications or preexisting disease processes
- Patients on warfarin therapy
- Concussions with loss of consciousness should be discussed with physician
- Dementia
- Persistent vomiting
- Severe persistent headache
- Focal neurologic deficits
- Inadequate home observation

Notes

References:

Ann of Emergency Medicine, June 2012 (Vol. 59 | No. 6 | Pages 451–455)

ACEP Clinical Policy: Neuroimaging and Decision making in Adult Mild Traumatic Brain Injury in the Acute Setting

Head Trauma Treatment & Management
Author: David W Crippen, MD, FCCM; Chief Editor: John Geibel, MD, DSc, M
emedicine.medscape.com/article/433855

Closed Head Trauma
Author: Leonardo Rangel-Castilla, MD; Chief Editor: Allen R Wyler, MD emedicine.medscape.com/article/251834

Pediatric Minor Head Trauma Protocol

When using any protocol, always follow the Guidelines of Proper Use (page 18).

Definition

- Head trauma with Glasgow coma scale ≥ 14 and no focal neurologic deficits or complaints

Differential Diagnosis

- Subarachnoid hemorrhage
- Subdural hematoma
- Epidural hematoma
- Cerebral contusion
- Skull fracture
- Child abuse and neglect

Considerations

- Loss of consciousness (LOC), amnesia, headache, vomiting and seizures have low sensitivity and specificity for detecting intracranial injury
- Children < 2 years have a higher risk of skull fracture and intracranial injury after minor mechanisms of injury
    - Skull fracture associated with a 20–fold increase in intracranial injury
    - Most skull fractures are associated with scalp hematomas
- Scalp hematomas indicative of skull fractures is the most sensitive predictor of intracranial injury of the clinical signs of brain injury
- Infant's clinical signs of brain injury less reliable

Postconcussion Syndrome

- Symptoms of headache, dizziness, trouble concentrating days to weeks following a concussion and can persist for months
- Anxiety and depression reported by patients

- Issues of compensation and litigation associated at times with persistent symptoms
- Disequilibrium and vertigo from vestibular concussion
- Reassurance decreases incidence and duration of symptoms
- Avoid narcotics
- Can use mild analgesics
- Can use meclizine or Phenergan (promethazine) for vestibular symptoms
- Rarely seen in young children
- Countries with low litigation have low postconcussion syndrome disability

Evaluation

- Evaluate for other injuries besides head
- Retinal exam: hemorrhages present in 65–90% with abuse inflicted head injury
- ENT exam for:
    - Hemotympanum
    - CSF rhinorrhea
    - Battle's sign
    - Cranial nerve palsy
- Awake, alert and asymptomatic children without LOC usually do not require imaging

CT scan rules

Pecarn Algorithm Age < 2 years

- Order CT head if any positive
    - Abnormal GCS
    - Palpable skull fracture
    - Signs of altered mental status
    - Occipital, parietal or temporal scalp hematoma
    - History of loss of consciousness ≥ 5 seconds
    - Severe mechanism
    - Not acting normally

Pecarn Algorithm Age ≥ 2 years for pediatric head trauma

- Order CT head if any positive

- Abnormal GCS
- Palpable skull fracture
- Signs of altered mental status
- History of loss of consciousness
- History of vomiting
- Severe mechanism
- Severe headache

CT brain scan other considerations

- Anticoagulation therapy
- Preexisting CNS disease such AVM or ventriculoperitoneal shunt

Treatment Options

- Tylenol (no ASA or NSAID's for 36 hours)
- Avoid more potent analgesics so progression of symptoms can be detected
- Quiet play or activities can be resumed if no significant symptoms
- Head injury instruction sheet
- Return for any neurologic changes
- Follow up with primary care provider or neurologist

Discharge Criteria

- Stable condition
- Normal neurologic exam
- No other significant trauma
- No radiologic abnormalities

Discharge instructions

- Head injury aftercare instructions
- Refer or arrange for follow-up with primary care physician or provider for concussion

Consult Criteria

- Concussion
- Skull fracture
- CT findings of intracranial injury
- Acute neurologic abnormalities
- Intracranial bleeding potential
- Persistent vomiting

- Severe persistent headache
- Focal neurologic deficits
- Inadequate home observation
- Serial visits for head injury symptoms needed
- Patients on warfarin or other anticoagulation therapy

Concussion Definitions and Return-to-sports Recommendations

Grade 1 concussion

- Transient confusion
- No loss of consciousness (LOC)
- Duration of mental status abnormalities < 15 minutes

Grade 2 concussion

- Transient confusion
- No LOC
- Duration of mental status abnormalities > 15 minutes

Grade 3 concussion

- Loss of consciousness

Return to Sports Stages (CISG 2017)

For all concussions

- Rest no more than 24–48 hours
- Symptom limited activities that do not provoke symptoms ≥ 24 hours followed by
- Light aerobic activities ≥ 24 hours (no resistance training) followed by
- Sport–specific exercise ≥ 24 hours (i.e. running, skating but no head impact activity) followed by
- Non–contact exercises ≥ 24 hours (i.e. passing drills, resistence training) followed by
- Full contact exercises after medical clearance

If symptoms recur in any stage then go back to prior stage and try to progress again after 24 hours

Notes

References:

Kuppermann N, Holmes JF, Dayan PS, et al. Identification of children at very low risk of clinically-important brain injuries after head trauma: a prospective cohort study. *Lancet*. Oct 3 2009;374(9696):1160–70

Pediatric Head Trauma

Author: Michael J Verive, MD, FAAP; Chief Editor: Timothy E Corden, MD emedicine.medscape.com/article/907273

AMERICAN ACADEMY OF PEDIATRICS

The Management of Minor Closed Head Injury in Children Committee on Quality Improvement, American Academy of Pediatrics Commission on Clinical Policies and Research, American Academy of Family Physicians

The Use of Computed Tomography in Pediatric Patients with Minor Head Injury - Micelle J. Haydel, MD Assistant Residency Director, Section of Emergency Medicine Clinical Assistant Professor of Medicine Louisiana State University Health Science Center at New Orleans

Consensus statement on concussion in sport—the 5th international conference on concussion in sport held in Berlin, October 2016

JAMA,306(1):79-86

Pediatr Neurol. 2015 Apr 11

NEJM, Vol. 356, pg. 166

NECK PAIN PROTOCOL

When using any protocol, always follow the Guidelines of Proper Use (page 18).

Definition

- Various disorders causing neck pain

Differential Diagnosis

- Muscle strain
- "Whiplash" injury
- Cervical fracture
- HNP
- Soft tissue infection
- Retropharyngeal abscess
- Cervical lymphadenitis
- Spinal stenosis
- Rheumatoid arthritis
- Endocarditis
- Thoracic outlet syndrome

Considerations

- Common neck pain causes
    - Torticollis ("wry neck") from muscle spasm
    - Cervical disc disease
    - Soft tissue disorder
    - Cervical spine injury
    - Muscular and ligament strain
    - Ankylosing spondylitis
        - Can have cranial–cervical disassociation
        - Put in Philadelphia or rigid cervical collar
        - Exercise caution with patient's neck

Torticollis

- Discomfort caused by cervical spine motion
- May be secondary to:
    - C-spine injury
    - Muscle injury

    - Ligamentous injury
- Usually acute in children and of muscular etiology
- Infectious causes
    - URI
    - Cervical adenitis
    - Pharyngitis
    - Retropharyngeal abscess
        - Measurements of retropharyngeal space:
            - At C2: < 7 mm
            - At C6: < 22 mm in adults; < 14 mm in children
    - Epiglottitis
    - Upper lobe pneumonia
    - Meningitis
    - Dystonic reaction to medication (treat with Benadryl)

Evaluation

- Neurologic and neck exam
- If fever present order
    - CBC
    - Soft tissue neck films
    - C-reactive protein if diagnosis not evident
    - CT neck for severe pain and possible deep space infection
- No fever
    - C-spine plain films if injured
    - CT C-spine scan if
        - Significant pain and mechanism of injury
        - Neurologic deficit or complaint

Treatment options

- Benign infectious processes treat per Protocols
- Benign muscular etiology treat with NSAID's and heat or ice
- I&D superficial neck abscess

Discharge criteria

- Benign process
- Chronic stable condition
- Cervical radiculopathy controlled with analgesics

Consult criteria

- Fever
- Meningitis concerns
- Airway concerns
- Severe pain
- Epiglottitis
- Retropharyngeal abscess
- Neurologic deficit

Neck Trauma

Cervical strain

- Neck pain increases at 12–72 hours
- Perform neurologic exam
- Plain films if trauma is minor
- CT cervical scan for significant mechanism of injury, concern for fracture or dislocation

Quebec Taskforce on Whiplash-Associated Disorders classification

- Grades 0–2 no special imaging recommended
- 0: No neck pain complaints, no physical signs
- 1: Neck pain complaints, only stiffness or tenderness, no other physical signs
- 2: Neck complaints and musculoskeletal signs (decreased range of motion [ROM] and point tenderness)
- 3: Neck complaints and neurologic signs (weakness, sensory and reflex changes) — CT C–spine
- 4: Neck complaints with suspected fracture and/or dislocation — CT C–spine

Treatment options

- NSAID's +/– acetaminophen
- Ice packs first 72 hours
  - May alternate with heat if helpful after 72 hours
- Muscle relaxants
- Physical therapy
- Soft cervical collar

Penetrating neck trauma

- Consult physician unless very superficial laceration
- Do not explore Zone 2 penetrating deep neck injuries
    - Angle of mandible to cricoid cartilage
    - Consult physician/surgeon
- Stop any bleeding with pressure

Cervical spine trauma

- Leave cervical collar on until patient examined and cleared of cervical vertebra/spine injury
- Plain C-spine x-ray 3 views

Exclusionary criteria for C-spine films

- No neurologic deficit
- No distracting injuries
- No evidence of intoxication
- Normal mentation
- No posterior midline tenderness

CT C-spine indications

- Moderate to high risk of cervical fracture
- Significant mechanism of injury
- Fracture on plain C-spine films
- Neurologic deficit or complaint
- Inadequate plain C-spine films
- Whiplash-Associated Disorders classification
    - 3: Neck complaints and neurologic signs (weakness, sensory and reflex changes)
    - 4: Neck complaints with suspected <u>fracture</u> and/or dislocation
- Severe neck pain with normal plain C-spine films
- Patient will not move neck actively (on their own) without external support of patient's hands ("head in hand sign")
- Obtunded patients

Flexion-extension plain films

- Significant pain with negative plain and CT imaging after the acute trauma has subsided for subacute presentations
- Evaluates for ligamentous instability

MRI C-spine if spinal cord findings or symptoms present and CT scan unremarkable (consult physician)

Treatment options

- If C-spine cleared: analgesics and ice packs prn

Discharge criteria

- Benign neck injury
- No fracture

Discharge instructions

- Neck pain or injury aftercare instructions
- Refer to primary care provider or neurosurgeon within 3 days if not improving
- Avoid discharging with cervical collar if possible

Consult criteria

- Cervical fracture or dislocation/subluxation
- Neurologic deficit or complaint
- Significant pain
- Significant mechanism of injury

Notes

References:

Torticollis Author: Michael C Kruer, MD; Chief Editor: Selim R Benbadis, MD

emedicine.medscape.com/article/1152543

Spitzer WO, Skovron ML, Salmi LR, et al. Scientific monograph of the Quebec Task Force on Whiplash-Associated Disorders: redefining "whiplash" and its management. *Spine*. Apr 15 1995;20(8 Suppl):1S-73S

Cervical Sprain and Strain Workup
Author: Oregon K Hunter Jr, MD; Chief Editor: Consuelo T Lorenzo, MD
emedicine.medscape.com/article/306176

Cervical Spine Sprain/Strain Injuries
Author: Gerard A Malanga, MD; Chief Editor: Sherwin SW Ho, MD; emedicine.medscape.com/article/94387

HEENT

Section Contents

When using any protocol, always follow the Guidelines of Proper Use (page 18).

SORE THROAT PROTOCOL

When using any protocol, always follow the Guidelines of Proper Use (page 18).

Definition

- Pain located or perceived in the throat or anterior neck region

Differential Diagnosis

- GABHS (Group A beta-hemolytic streptococcus)
- Mononucleosis
- Gonococcal pharyngitis
- Peritonsillar abscess
- Epiglottitis
- Retropharyngeal abscess
- Diphtheria (rare)
- Cervical lymphadenitis
- Thyrotoxicosis
- Gastroesophageal reflux

Considerations

- Viral 40%
- Bacterial 30%
- Strep throat – Group A beta-hemolytic Strep (GABHS)
    - 15–30% childhood pharyngitis
    - 5–10% of adult pharyngitis
    - Peak ages 4–11 years
    - Peak months January – May
    - Associated symptoms and findings
        - Sudden onset
        - Odynophagia
        - Fever
        - Headache
        - Abdominal pain
        - Nausea and vomiting;
- Viral pharyngitis
    - Cough
    - Rhinorrhea

  - Lack of cervical adenopathy
- Lemierre syndrome — spread of pharyngitis infection (usually Fusobacterium necrophorum) to cause septic thrombophlebitis of internal jugular vein
  - Up to 50% mortality
  - Septic emboli can occur if unrecognized

Viral Pharyngitis

URI

- Treat symptomatically

Mononucleosis

Findings

- Exudative tonsillitis
- Fever
- Posterior cervical chain lymphadenopathy considered diagnostic
- Monospot
  - 90% sensitive age > 5 years
  - 75% sensitive age 2–4 years
  - Less than 30% sensitive age < 2 years
- Consider CMV and EBV IgM/IgG for age < 10 years
- CBC: 50% lymphocytes, 10% atypical lymphocytes
- Liver function tests elevated in 80–85% of patients up to 3 times normal
- Splenomegaly
- Hepatomegaly
- Encephalitis
- Meningitis

Treatment options

- Treat symptomatically
- No contact sports or gym for 4 weeks after onset of illness
  - Follow up with primary care provider before resuming sports or gym
- Ampicillin or amoxicillin rash can occur if prescribed

- Steroids may decrease symptoms and swelling but may also delay recovery and there is a concern for association with development chronic EBV syndrome
- Steroid dosing if used:
  - Adult or patients heavier than 40 kg: prednisone 40 mg PO daily for 4 days
    - May increase risk of secondary bacterial infection
  - Pediatrics: prednisone 1 mg/kg PO daily for 4 days (NMT 40 mg)

Strep throat — GABHS

- Rheumatic fever can be prevented if antibiotic treatment started within 9 days of onset—very rare now
  - Number needed to treat to prevent one case of acute rheumatic fever would be 1,430,000 on 2003 review
- Glomerulonephritis cannot be prevented with antibiotic treatment
- Self-limited resolving in 3–4 days
- Reason for antibiotic treatment is the prevention of rheumatic fever and complications such as abscess
- Pharyngitis from GABHS is often self-limited
- Without antibiotic therapy, symptoms typically resolve in 3 -5 days for most patients
- Antibiotics have been found to reduce symptoms by 12-16 hrs. when compared to placebo

Evaluation

Center criteria

- Tonsillar exudates
- Tender anterior cervical lymphadenopathy
- Fever by history
- Absence of cough
  - If 3 present: 40–60% have GABHS
  - If 3 or 4 absent: 80% negative predictive value
  - None or one criterion present: No testing or treatment needed for GABHS

Consider Rapid Strep Tests

- Sensitivity 85–95%
- Specificity 96–99%
- May be positive with carriage state and another cause of acute pharyngitis besides GABHS may exist

Treatment options

- Per Sanford Guide or drug database
- Antibiotic treatment without rapid strep testing permissible if 3 or 4 Centor criteria present
- Treatment of symptomatic household contacts if patient has positive GABHS testing for 10 days is recommended
- Pen VK or cephalexin or Augmentin or cefdinir
    - Third generation cephalosporin with improved cure rates and significantly less recurrence
- Clindamycin if penicillin allergic is usually safe
- Zithromax and erythromycin less effective due to resistance
- Steroids one dose
    - Prednisone 40–60 mg PO > 40 kg
    - Prednisone or prednisolone 1 mg/kg PO (NMT 60 mg)
    - Decadron (dexamethasone) 10 mg IM if unable to take PO
    - Decadron (dexamethasone) 0.06 mg/kg IM (NMT 10 mg) if unable to take PO

Epiglottitis or suspected epiglottitis

- Now more common in adults than children
    - Adults may not be in distress
- Constitutes an airway emergency — consult anesthesia and ENT
- Do not agitate or aggressively exam
    - If patient is in distress
    - Drooling present
    - Tripod position or sniff position present
- Pain on moving thyroid cartilage
- Lateral neck films findings — only obtain in stable patient

    - Thumb sign
    - Vallecula sign — loss of vallecula
    - False positives may occur with x-ray being rotated slightly
    - Consider CT neck if needed (may do prone if supine position not tolerated)
    - Review or listen to radiology report
- Notify physician promptly before x-ray if epiglottitis suspected or patient in distress

Peritonsillar abscess

- Sore throat 100%
- Fever 26–97%
- Voice change (hot potato)
- Dysphagia
- Drooling
- Headache
- Trismus
- Uvular deviation and peritonsillar bulge
- Asymmetric lymphadenopathy
- Peritonsillar phlegmon
- Neck CT scan may be required to delineate abscess from necrotic lymph node
- Antibiotic choices
    - Clindamycin or augmentin
    - Dexamethasone dose may be considered
- Notify physician if diagnosed or suspected

Retropharyngeal abscess

- Usually age 3–5 years

Complications

- Airway compromise
- Aspiration pneumonia
- Internal jugular vein thrombosis
- Carotid artery erosion
- Cranial nerve palsies

History and findings

- Fever
- Dysphagia
- Decreased oral intake
- Stridor or dyspnea

- Neck swelling
- Neck motion pain
- Ill appearing
- Duck-like voice

X-ray findings

- Neck CT scan much more sensitive than lateral neck plain films
- Lateral soft-tissue neck films (neck flexion may cause false positive reading)
- Retropharyngeal space anterior to C2 > 7 mm or > half the width of vertebral body
- Space anterior to C6 > 14 mm in preschool children or > 22 mm in adults

Treatment

- Supplemental oxygen (avoid patient agitation)
- Keep child calm
- Notify physician promptly

Discharge Criteria for Sore throat

- Nontoxic
- No airway obstruction concerns
- Can tolerate oral intake
- Benign diagnosis

Discharge instructions

- Sore throat or pharyngitis aftercare instructions
- Follow up with primary care provider or ENT surgeon within 5 days as needed

Consult Criteria for Sore throat

- Airway compromise
- Toxic
- Dehydration > 5%
- Suspected epiglottitis
- Peritonsillar or retropharyngeal abscess
- Unable to tolerate oral intake
- Immunosuppression

Vital signs consult criteria

- Adult heart rate ≥ 120
- Pediatric heart rate

- 0–4 months ≥ 180
- 5–7 months ≥ 175
- 8–12 months ≥ 170
- 1–3 years ≥ 160
- 4–5 years ≥ 145
- 6–8 years ≥ 130
- 9–11 years ≥ 125
- 12–15 years ≥ 120
- 16 years or older ≥ 120

* Hypotension
* O_2 saturation < 95% on room air

Lab consult criteria

- WBC ≥ 18,000 or < 3,000
- Bandemia ≥ 15%
- Acute thrombocytopenia
- Metabolic acidosis

Notes

References:

Practice Guidelines for the diagnosis and management of group A streptococcal pharyngitis
Clin Infect Dis. 2002;35(2):113–125 Guideline statement

[Guideline] Gerber MA, Baltimore RS, Eaton CB, et al. Prevention of rheumatic fever and diagnosis and treatment of acute Streptococcal pharyngitis: a scientific statement from the American Heart Association Rheumatic Fever, Endocarditis, and Kawasaki Disease Committee of the Council on Cardiovascular Disease in the Young, the Interdisciplinary Council on Functional Genomics and Translational Biology, and the Interdisciplinary Council on Quality of Care and Outcomes Research: endorsed by the American Academy of Pediatrics. *Circulation*. Mar 24 2009;119(11):1541–51

Pharyngitis Treatment & Management

Author: John R Acerra, MD; Chief Editor: Pamela L Dyne, MD; emedicine.medscape.com/article/764304

Del Mar CB, Glasziou PP, Spinks AB. Antibiotics for sore throat (Review). *The Cochrane Collaboration*. 2007;(1):1–41

Retropharyngeal Abscess
Author: Joseph H Kahn, MD; Chief Editor: Robert E O'Connor, MD, MPH medicine.medscape.com/article/764421

Epiglottitis Clinical Presentation
Author: Sandra G Gompf, MD, FACP, FIDSA; Chief Editor: Pamela L Dyne, MD
emedicine.medscape.com/article/763612

Ducic Y, Hébert PC, MacLachlan L, Neufeld K, Lamothe A. Description and evaluation of the vallecula sign: a new radiologic sign in the diagnosis of adult epiglottitis. *Ann Emerg Med*. Jul 1997;30(1):1–6

Gottlieb M, et al. *J Emerg Med*. 2018 Mar 6. [Epub ahead of print]

Pelucchi, C, et al. Clin Microbiol Infect. 2012;18: 1-28

Del Mar, CB, et al. *Cochrane Database Syst Rev*. 2006; CD000023

OTITIS EXTERNA PROTOCOL

When using any protocol, always follow the Guidelines of Proper Use (page 18).

Definition

- Inflammation of the external auditory canal

Differential Diagnosis

- Auditory canal foreign body
- Otitis media with perforation
- Cholesteatoma
- Chondroma
- Herpes zoster

Considerations

- Caused by breakdown in protective barrier of ear canal
  - Pseudomonas; staph; strep species; fungi
- Pain increased with movement of external ear or touching external ear canal
- Discharge common
- Fever uncommon

Malignant Otitis Externa

- Elderly
- Diabetes
- Immunocompromised — pseudomonas frequent concern
- Marked swelling
- Headache
- Possible cranial nerve deficit

Clinical Practice Guideline: acute otitis externa executive summary

- Distinguish diffuse acute otitis externa (AOE) from other causes of otalgia, otorrhea, and inflammation of the external ear canal
- Assess the patient with diffuse AOE for factors that modify management (non-intact tympanic membrane, tympanostomy tube,

diabetes, immunocompromised state, prior radiotherapy)

- Assess patients with AOE for pain and recommend analgesic treatment based on the severity of pain
- Do not prescribe systemic antimicrobials as initial therapy for diffuse, uncomplicated AOE unless there is extension outside the ear canal or the presence of specific host factors that would indicate a need for systemic therapy
- Use topical preparations for initial therapy of diffuse, uncomplicated AOE
- Inform patients how to administer topical drops and should enhance delivery of topical drops when the ear canal is obstructed by performing aural toilet, placing a wick, or both
- Non-intact tympanic membrane when the patient has a known or suspected perforation of the tympanic membrane, including a tympanostomy tube, the clinician should recommend a non-ototoxic topical preparation (fluoroquinolone suspension drops)
- If the patient fails to respond to the initial therapeutic option within 48–72 hours the clinician should reassess the patient to confirm the diagnosis of diffuse AOE and to exclude other causes of illness
- Avoid water in ear

Evaluation

- Usually none except otoscope and external ear exam
- Serum glucose if diabetic
- Suspected malignant otitis externa
    - CBC
    - C-reactive protein
    - Cultures

CT scan indications

- Neurologic abnormalities
- Toxic appearing patient
- Malignant otitis externa

  - Fever

Treatment Options

- Clean ear canal (most important aspect of treatment)
- Irrigate or ear loop curettage (may be difficult due to pain)
  - Use ½ peroxide and ½ water (or water only) — if TM (tympanic membrane) visible and intact (keep liquid near body temperature)
- Can use ear wick if canal markedly swollen — remove in 3 days; replace if canal still very swollen
- NSAID's or narcotics prn

Antibiotic choices

- Acetic acid 2% (Domeboro otic) 4–6 drops q4–6h for 7–10 days or until ear canal normal for 2 days
- Cortisporin otic suspension or solution (has neomycin which can cause allergy) 4 drops qid for 7–10 days or until ear canal normal for 2 days (use Ofloxin suspension if tympanic membrane (TM) perforated)
- Ofloxin 5 drops bid for 7–10 days or until ear canal normal for 2 days (drug of choice for TM perforation)
- Dexamethasone/ciprofloxacin (Ciprodex) age > 6 months: 4 drops in affected ear q12hr for 7 days
  - For acute otitis media with tympanostomy tube
  - Not for use < 6 months of age
- Oral antibiotics for facial or neck cellulitis, significant edema of ear canal, or when TM (tympanic membrane) cannot be visualized
- Diabetics may be treated also with ciprofloxacin PO for 10–14 days
- May use Sanford Guide or drug database

Discharge Criteria

- Benign otitis externa

Discharge instructions

- Otitis externa aftercare instructions
- Keep ear dry for 3 weeks (no swimming) — cotton with vasoline in ears during showers

- Prophylaxis for future OE after swimming with rubbing alcohol or acetic acid 2% if no TM (tympanic membrane) perforation
- Follow up with primary care provider or ENT surgeon within 7–10 days if needed

Consult Criteria

- Malignant external otitis (needs ENT consultation and IV antibiotics)
- Fever
- Return visit for same episode
- Glucose ≥ 400 mg/dL in diabetic patient
- Hyperglycemia with metabolic acidosis (decreased serum CO_2 or elevated anion gap)

Notes

References:

Rosenfeld RM, Schwartz SR, Cannon CR, Roland PS, Simon GR, Kumar KA, et al. Clinical practice guideline: acute otitis externa executive summary. *Otolaryngol Head Neck Surg*. Feb 2014;150(2):161–8

Wall GM, Stroman DW, Roland PS, Dohar J. Ciprofloxacin 0.3%/dexamethasone 0.1% sterile otic suspension for the topical treatment of ear infections: a review of the literature. *Pediatr Infect Dis J*. Feb 2009;28(2):141–4

Otitis Externa Medication
Author: Ariel A Waitzman, MD, FRCS(C); Chief Editor: Arlen D Meyers, MD, MBA
emedicine.medscape.com/article/994550

EYE PROTOCOLS

When using any protocol, always follow the Guidelines of Proper Use (page 18).

Considerations

- Most conjunctival infections are viral
- Allergic manifestations common
- Contact lens keratitis can be bacterial or from oxygen deficit of cornea

Evaluation

- Visual acuity if complaints of decreased vision
- Examination of
  - Conjunctiva
  - Cornea
  - Pupils
  - Extraocular motion
  - Any discharge
  - For consensual photophobia (light shined in unaffected eye causes pain in affected eye — have affected eye closed during exam)
  - Periorbital tissues
  - Anterior and posterior chambers
  - Visual fields examination as indicated
- See specific conditions below

Conjunctivitis

Allergic

- Itching and redness; watery
- Papillary hypertrophy

Treatment options

- Systemic antihistamine
- Remove offending agent if known
- Choices:
  - Naphcon-A ophthalmic 1–2 drops qid prn
  - Ketorolac ophthalmic 1 drop qid prn

- Low dose steroid eye drops prn — short course
  - Dexamethasone ophthalmic 1–2 drops tid-qid prn or similar ophthalmic steroid
  - Contraindications:
    - Herpes simplex infection (corneal dendrite)
    - Glaucoma
    - Fungal infection

Discharge criteria

- Benign presentation and findings

Consult criteria

- Photophobia
- Visual changes

Viral

- Adenovirus most common
  - Viral conjunctivitis due to adenoviruses (65% - 90% of VC cases) is highly contagious
  - Spreads through direct contact via contaminated fingers, swimming pool water, medical instruments, or personal items
- Watery mucus discharge
- Gritty or foreign body sensation
- HSV: vesicles eyelid margins or periorbital skin; corneal dendrites

Treatment options

- Usually no specific therapy
- Artificial tears prn
- HSV
  - Viroptic ophthalmic drops 1 gtt q2h not to exceed 9 gtts qday
  - Consult physician if herpes infection present
  - Ophthalmology referral within 1 day for HSV infection

Bacterial

- Purulent discharge
- Staph most common
- Gonorrhea: profuse purulent discharge

- Chlamydial: mucopurulent discharge; photophobia occasionally
- Contact lens: pseudomonas possible

Treatment options

Common drugs

- Erythromycin eye ointment
- Sulfa eye drops
- Gentamicin eye drops
- All medications given for 7 days

Contact lens complications

- Remove lens until eye normal for 2 days
- Ciloxan 1–2 drops QID × 7 days
- Consult physician

Chlamydia

- Doxycycline 100 BID × 3 weeks

  OR

- Erythromycin 500 mg QID PO × 3 weeks (erythromycin pediatric dose 50 mg/kg PO divided into 4 doses × 14 days — NMT 500 mg per dose)
- May give azithromycin 1 gm PO once instead of doxycycline or erythromycin

  Azithromycin ophthalmic solution: Instill 1 drop BID for 2 days, then 1 drop for 5 days in addition to PO medications
- Mother of children and other close contacts at risk — treat with doxycycline 100 mg BID × 7 days in age > 8 years, otherwise erythromycin treatment

Gonococcal

- Doxycycline 100 BID × 3 weeks or erythromycin 500 mg QID PO × 3 weeks
- Rocephin (ceftriaxone) 1000 mg IM (can be given daily for 3 days)
- Neonates: Rocephin (ceftriaxone) 50 mg/kg IV daily for 7 days; erythromycin eye ointment QID × 14 days

- May use Sanford Guide or other drug databases

Discharge criteria

- Benign, non-herpetic conjunctivitis

Discharge instructions

- Conjunctivitis aftercare instructions
- Follow up with primary care provider or ophthalmology within 1 day for contact lens complications, gonococcal or chlamydial infections
- Consult criteria
- Visual change
- Photophobia
- Suspected gonococcal or chlamydial infection
- Significant pain
- Contact lens complications

Infectious Keratitis

Causes

- HSV
- Staph
- Herpes zoster

Evaluation

- Direct visualization
- Fluorescein staining and wood's lamp
- Look for dendritic lesions

Treatment options

HSV

- Viroptic 1 drop q2hr while awake (NMT 9 drops qday)
- Follow up with ophthalmologist within 24 hours

Bacterial (all treatments for 7 days)

- Erythromycin eye ointment
- Sulfa eye drops
- Gentamicin eye drops

Discharge instructions

- Appropriate keratitis aftercare instructions if discharged

Consult criteria

- All infectious keratitis

Blepharitis, Hordeolum (Stye) and Chalazion

Stye

- Painful, swollen, tender and red eyelid
- Staph 90–95% of the time
- Usually will drain spontaneously

Treatment options

- Warm soaks 3–4 days a day until resolved
- Erythromycin eye ointment or sulfa eye drops or gentamicin eye drops (all for 7–10 days)
- Clean eyelid margins with baby shampoo
- Oral cephalexin or staph medications for 7–10 days if infection spread beyond hordeolum or lymph nodes are swollen
- Refer to ophthalmologist in 10–14 days if not resolved

Chalazion

- Treatment similar to Stye

Blepharitis

- Treatment similar to Stye

Discharge instructions

- Appropriate aftercare instructions

Periorbital (Preseptal) Cellulitis

- Usually from S. aureus
- More common in children
- Age < 3 years can progress to bacteremia
- Is anterior to orbital septum

Signs

- Red swollen eyelid
- No vision changes
- Ocular mobility normal
- Conjunctival discharge may be present
- May have minimal pain

    - More severe with orbital cellulitis and helps to differentiate between the two
- Chemosis (conjunctival swelling)
- Fever

Evaluation

- Detailed ocular exam
    - Anterior and posterior chambers
    - Extraocular motion
    - Pupillary examination
    - CT scan may be needed if unable to differentiate from orbital cellulitis
- CBC and blood culture if age < 5 years
- Culture of eye discharge if present

Treatment options

- Most children need IV antibiotics
- Augmentin (amoxicillin/clavulanate) 45 mg/kg/day divided bid PO for 10–14 days
- Vancomycin
- Rocephin (ceftriaxone)
- Clindamycin
- May use Sanford Guide or other drug databases

Discharge instructions

- Periorbital or preseptal cellulitis aftercare instructions
- Follow up in 24 hours with PCP or ophthalmologist

Orbital Cellulitis

- Most commonly from ethmoid sinusitis spread

Findings and symptoms

- May have toxic appearance
- Proptosis
- Limited extraocular motion
- Diplopia
- Significant pain
- Dark red eyelids
- Decreased vision
- Increased intraocular pressure

Complications

- Meningitis
- Cavernous sinus thrombosis
- Vision loss

Evaluation

- Detailed ocular exam
    - Anterior and posterior chambers
    - Extraocular motion
    - Pupillary examination
    - CT scan may be needed if unable to differentiate from orbital cellulitis
- CBC and blood culture if age < 5 years
- Culture of eye discharge if present

Treatment

- Ceftin (cefuroxime) IV and/or per Sanford Guide or other drug databases
- Admission to hospital

Consult criteria

- All suspected or diagnosed orbital cellulitis patients

Corneal Ulcer or Lesions

- Consult physician

Discharge instructions

- Corneal ulcer aftercare instructions

Iritis

- Photophobia — is consensual (light shined into opened normal eye causes pain in closed affected eye due to pupillary reflex)
- Ciliary flush (red injection at edge of cornea circumferentially)
- Cells and flare in anterior chamber; hypopyon more rare
- Miosis
- 50% associated with systemic disease
- Slit lamp exam helpful

Treatment

- Homatropine eye drops 2–5% 1 drop TID
- Steroid eye drops per ophthalmologist (controversy whether beneficial)
- Biologics have off-label recommendation recently
- Consult physician

Discharge instructions

- Iritis aftercare instructions
- Close ophthalmology follow-up

Corneal Abrasion

- Can detect with direct ophthalmoscopy or fluorescein staining
- No consensual photophobia unless iritis present
- Heals in 24–48 hours
- If corneal pain recurs in 2–3 days, it may indicate sloughing of corneal epithelium

Treatment

- No patching
- Can use local anesthetic eye drops at time of exam only (do not prescribe for home pain control since it is mildly cytotoxic and will prevent healing)
- Narcotics PO prn × 2–3 days
- Antibiotic drops if contact lenses patient — ofloxacin ophthalmic
    - Days 1-2: 1-2 gtt q30min while awake, awaken 4-6 hours after retiring
    - Days 3-7: 1-2 gtt q1hr while awake
    - Days 7-9: 1-2 gtt four times daily until clinical cure

Extensive corneal abrasion

- Homatropine 2% sol 1–2 gtt to achieve cycloplegia (pupil dilation) — may repeat q15 min. × 2 prn
- Can prescribe 1–2 gtt QID up to 3 days

Discharge instructions

- Corneal abrasion aftercare instructions
- Follow up in 2–3 days for recheck with primary care provider or ophthalmologist

Ultraviolet Keratitis (Band Keratitis)

- Usually from welding or tanning beds
- Acular (ketorolac) or Voltaren (diclofenic) eye drops 1 gtt QID for several days until eye corneal pain resolved (not longer than 2 weeks)
- Similar evaluation and treatment as corneal abrasion

Discharge instructions

- Ultraviolet (flash burn) keratitis aftercare instructions

Eye Foreign Body

- Usually a foreign body sensation is the chief complaint
- Anesthetic eye drops with proparacaine or tetracaine immediately relieves symptoms for 15 minutes or so
- Patient may or may not be able to localize the foreign body

Examination

- Evert eyelids as needed to locate the foreign body
- If foreign body is not identified, flush under eyelids with eye irrigation fluids to see if symptoms can be resolved
- If foreign body persists after eye flush, use moistened sterile cotton swab to gently swab under eyelids to see if any foreign bodies are found or the patient's symptoms of foreign body sensation resolve
- Check lacrimal duct opening for retained eyelash

Discharge criteria

- Foreign body removed
- No visual changes or significant residual discomfort

Discharge instructions

- Eye foreign body aftercare instructions

Consult criteria

- Retained intraocular foreign body, discuss with physician
- Significant residual pain post foreign body removal
- Acute visual changes or complaints

Corneal Foreign Bodies

- If an iron containing metallic foreign body is present, a rust ring may develop in a few hours
- Examine anterior and posterior ocular chambers — if abnormal discuss with physician or ophthalmologist
- Fluorescein staining can be used as needed to locate foreign bodies and abrasions
- The Provider may opt to not remove small residual rust rings outside of visual axis, and refer to an ophthalmologist for further treatment in 1–3 days

Removal instructions

- After 3–4 drops of eye anesthetic over 1 minute are instilled into the affected eye and the patient has no further complaints of a foreign body sensation or pain, a sterile moistened cotton swab is used to swab across the foreign body to effect removal
- If the cotton swab does not remove the corneal foreign body, an experienced Provider may use a blunt eye spud or eye burr to remove the foreign body
- Consult a physician if not experienced with using a blunt eye spud or eye burr
- If a metallic foreign body has rusted, a residual rust ring will be left after the majority of the central rust area has been removed with the cotton swab
    - A blunt eye spud or eye burr can be used to remove some of the residual rust left, although it is not unusual to not be able to remove it all
- Fresh rust rings are more difficult to remove and after sterile cotton swabbing the residual rust ring can be left to mature in 1–3 days and the patient can then be referred to an ophthalmologist for follow-up

Discharge instructions

- Corneal foreign body aftercare instructions
- Refer to ophthalmology within 3 days
- Return if pain worsens, or photophobia or visual changes develops

Consult criteria

- Discuss with the physician if the residual rust ring is in the visual axis

Corneal Laceration

- Protective rigid eye shield
- Consult physician and ophthalmologist immediately
- Analgesia and vomiting control IM or IV prn to decrease valsalva

Eyelid Lacerations

Findings to discuss with physician (usually needs referral treatment)

- Tarsal plate involvement
- Eyelid margin
- Tear duct injury
- Orbital septum injury
    - Fat can protrude
- Tissue loss

Globe Injury

- History is important of what patient was doing at time of injury
- Globe injury can be obvious with uveal tissue prolapsing from a wound or pupil, or the eye or papillary shape can be grossly abnormal, or the injury may be subtle
- Small eyelid lacerations can cover or mask perforations of globe
    - Do not close laceration until globe injury is ruled out
- Assess eye motion and visual acuity
    - Visual acuity can be counting fingers at 18 inches or light perception if necessary
    - Critical to avoid pressure on the eye
    - Palpate orbital rims for deformity and crepitus
    - Do not remove any foreign bodies that have penetrated the globe
    - Conjunctival hemorrhage covering 360 degrees of the bulbar conjunctiva can indicate globe rupture

- Assess pupils for size, shape, afferent defect, direct and indirect pupillary light reflex and the red reflex
- Examine anterior chamber
- CT orbital scans are the preferred imaging to evaluate for occult globe injury

Treatment

- Place protective rigid eye shield immediately after assessment with no material touching the eyelids

Disposition

- Consult physician and ophthalmologist immediately
- Analgesia and vomiting control IM or IV prn to decrease valsalva and minimize intraocular pressure increases

Chemical Eye Injuries

Alkali burns most serious

- Causes immediate liquefaction necrosis if the pH is very high
- Penetrates the tissue deeply
- Immediate eye lavage with NS for one hour (Morgan lens)
- Exam after lavage
- Notify physician promptly

Acid burns

- Cause coagulation of proteins which can limit depth of injury
- Can use fluorescein to evaluate cornea (exam after lavage if needed)
- Weak acids burns usually managed as outpatient

Evaluation

- Inspection
- After lavage if strong alkali: fluorescein or slit lamp
- Check visual acuity

Treatment

- Significant burns flush with NS using Morgan lens for 30–60 minutes

- Check pH at 5 and 30 minutes of eye lavage to achieve pH 7.3–7.5
- Mild burns with weak acids can be lavaged less (with or without Morgan lens) depending on symptoms
- Use topical eye anesthetic for pain of examination and treatment as needed
- Gentamicin plus erythromycin or bacitracin ophthalmic ointment tid × 5–10 days or until healed for significant chemical burns
- Mild burns without significant damage can be managed with one topical eye antibiotic ointment
- Narcotics or NSAID's PO prn pain

Discharge criteria

- Mild conjunctivitis and keratitis from weak acid chemical burns
- Discuss with physician all chemical eye injuries

Discharge instructions

- Chemical eye injury aftercare instructions
- Refer to ophthalmologist within 1 day if indicated

Consult criteria

- Alkali burns
- Acid burns of moderate or worse severity
- Visual acuity changes

Glaucoma

- Severe pain, ipsilateral visual defects and may see halos around objects
- Nausea and vomiting common with acute closed angle glaucoma
- Steamy and cloudy cornea
- Increase IOP (normal IOP 10–22 mm Hg)
- Mid-dilated pupil and firm globe
- Consult physician promptly

Orbital Blowout Isolated Fracture

- Orbital wall composed of 7 bones
- Occurs usually with larger object than the orbit (baseball; fist)

- Can result in diplopia

Evaluation

- Neurologic exam
- Extraocular motor exam
- Evaluate for associated ocular injuries (present 20–40% of the time)
- Plain facial (water's view best) or CT head, facial and orbital films
- Ocular anterior and posterior chamber exam
- TM's (tympanic membrane) exam for hemotympanum
- Grasp upper teeth and palate and pull to assess for Lefort fractures (movement noted)
- Dental exam
- C-spine films prn (see Neck Pain Practice Guide)

Treatment

- Most patients can be followed as outpatient with plastic surgeon or ophthalmologist in a timeframe determined by the surgeon
- Discuss with physician
- No nose blowing
- Augmentin (amoxicillin/clavulanate) 500 mg TID PO × 10 days or Levaquin (levofloxacin) 750 mg qday PO × 10 days
- Pediatric Augmentin (amoxicillin/clavulanate) dose — 12.5 mg/kg PO bid × 10 days
- Analgesics PO prn
- Ice prn for swelling
- Tetanus if not up to date (see Tetanus Practice Guide, page 756)

Discharge criteria

- Uncomplicated inferior blowout fracture without extraocular muscle entrapment or other facial fractures or associated conditions

Discharge instructions

- Head injury aftercare instructions
- Orbital blowout fracture aftercare instructions
- Referral to Ophthalmology or plastic surgeon within 7 days

Consult criteria

- Discuss all facial fractures except nasal with physician

Subconjunctival Hemorrhage

- No treatment
- Check PT/INR if on Coumadin (warfarin)
- CBC if constitutional symptoms present

Retinal Detachment

Causes

- Tear in retina

Risk factors

- Near sighted
- Advanced age
- Diabetes
- Sickle cell anemia
- Prior retinal detachment history

Findings and symptoms

- Painless
- Light flashes
- Decreased peripheral vision
- Floaters
- Lowering of curtain over vision in affected eye

Examination includes

- Direct ophthalmoscopy (may need pupils dilated)
- Bedside ultrasound with vascular probe can detect retinal detachment (see Acute Care Ultrasound chapter)

Treatment

- Elevate head of bed for inferior detachment
- Lay flat for superior detachment

Consult criteria

- Consult physician and ophthalmologist promptly

Central Retinal Artery Occlusion

- True emergency

- Usually from emboli
- 90 minutes to restore vision before irreversible damage
- Evaluate for sickle cell anemia and temporal arteritis

Findings

- Sudden loss of vision in one eye
- Pupil reacts consensually
- Afferent defect to light in affected eye (pupil does not constrict)
- Increased intraocular pressure
- Pale fundus
- Dilated pupil
- Retinal artery may have "box cars" appearance
- Macula has enhanced cherry red appearance (different blood supply)

Treatment

- Gentle massage on globe to attempt dislodging emboli
    - Apply direct pressure for 5-15 seconds, then release. Repeat several times
    - Ocular massage can move the embolus further down the arterial circulation and improve perfusion
- Rebreathing bag or mask to increase CO_2
- Hyperbaric oxygen < 2 hours of symptoms, but can be used if vision loss < 12 hours

IOP treatment

- Timoptic (timolol)
- Diamox (acetazolamide)
- Ophthalmology paracentesis of anterior chamber

Consult criteria

- Notify physician immediately
- Ophthalmologist consult immediately

Central Retinal Vein Occlusion

- Rapid and painless vision loss of one eye
    - Slower onset than retinal artery occlusion
    - From thrombosis of central retinal vein

Findings

- Retinal hemorrhages
- Impressive appearance of fundus with bloody engorgement
  - Optic disc edema

Treatment

- Aspirin

Consult criteria

- All central retinal vein occlusion patients
- All patients with acute vision loss

Hyphema and Hypopyon (Blood or Pus in Anterior Chamber)

- Consult physician

Notes

References:

Acute Conjunctivitis: Author: Michael A Silverman; Chief Editor: Barry E Brenner, MD, PhD, FACEP
emedicine.medscape.com/article/797874-overview

Iritis and Uveitis Author: Keith Tsang, MD; Chief Editor: Rick Kulkarni, MD
emedicine.medscape.com/article/798323

[Best Evidence] Islam N, Pavesio C. Uveitis (acute anterior). *Clin Evid (Online)*. November 2009;04:705

Ophthalmology Volume 121, Issue 3, Pages 785-796.e3, March 2014

Levy-Clarke G, Jabs DA, Read RW, Rosenbaum JT, Vitale A, Van Gelder RN. Expert Panel Recommendations for the Use of Anti-Tumor Necrosis Factor Biologic Agents in Patients with Ocular Inflammatory Disorders.*Ophthalmology*. Dec 17 2013

Orbital Fracture in Emergency Medicine Medication
Author: Thomas Widell, MD; Chief Editor: Rick Kulkarni, MD
emedicine.medscape.com/article/825772

Orbital Floor Fractures (Blowout)
Author: Adam J Cohen, MD; Chief Editor: Deepak Narayan, MD, FRCS emedicine.medscape.com/article/1284026

[Best Evidence] Turner A, Rabiu M. Patching for corneal abrasion. *Cochrane Database Syst Rev*. Apr 19 2006;(2):CD004764

Corneal Abrasion Author: Arun Verma, MD; Chief Editor: Hampton Roy Sr, MD
emedicine.medscape.com/article/1195402

Preseptal Cellulitis
Author: Geoffrey M Kwitko, MD, FACS, FICS; Chief Editor: Hampton Roy Sr, MD
emedicine.medscape.com/article/1218009

Fraser SG, Adams W. Interventions for acute non-arteritic central retinal artery occlusion. Cochrane Database of Systematic Reviews 2009, Issue 1. Art. No.: CD001989. DOI: 10.1002/14651858.CD001989.pub2

Hyperbaric oxygenation combined with nifedipine treatment for recent-onset retinal artery occlusion.
Eur J Ophthalmol. 1993; 3(2):89-94 (ISSN: 1120-6721)

Duma SM, Jernigan MV. The effects of airbags on orbital fracture patterns in frontal automobile crashes. Ophth Plast Reconst Surg. 2003;19(2):107-111

Francis DO, Kaufman R, Yueh B, et al. Air bag-induced orbital blow-out fractures. Laryngoscope. 2006;116:1966-1972. (Case series of 150 orbital fractures derived from 2739 crashes in CIREN database)

Hackl W, Fink C, Hausberger K, et al. The incidence of combined facial and cervical spine injuries. J Trauma. 2001;50:41-45

JAMA,310(16):1721-1730

Hordeolum and Stye in Emergency Medicine Treatment & Management Updated: Jul 24, 2018 Author: Michael J Bessette, MD, FACEP; Chief Editor: Gil Z Shlamovitz, MD, FACEP

NOSEBLEED PROTOCOL

When using any protocol, always follow the Guidelines of Proper Use (page 18).

Definition

- Bleeding from nostril, nasal cavity or nasopharynx

Differential Diagnosis

- Nasal foreign body
- Sinusitis
- Barotrauma
- Thrombocytopenia
- Leukemia
- Anticoagulation therapy
- Cocaine abuse
- NSAID use
- ASA use
- Hemophilia
- Von Willebrand's disease
- Trauma

Considerations

- 90% of nosebleeds are anterior
- Most common cause is nose picking
- Hypertension common
- Anticoagulant or antiplatelet agents
- Look for foreign body in young children (suspect if foul smell or unilateral discharge present)
- Posterior Epistaxis
  - Less common than anterior Epistaxis
  - Associated with
    - Elderly
    - Hypertension
    - Atherosclerosis

Evaluation

- Attempt visualization of bleeding
- Use nosebleed tray equipment or otoscope

- Have patient clear blood by forcefully blowing nose
- Use suction prn
- Cocaine intranasally can be used for hemostasis and pain control
    - May use afrin spray with or without pledget
- If bleeding has stopped and site unknown, take moistened cotton swab and gently stroke suspected area to elicit bleeding
- CBC if suspected significant blood loss or patient is tachycardic or orthostatic
- PT/INR if on Coumadin (warfarin). PTT if on heparin or has Von Willebrand's disease or hemophilia

Treatment options

- Control anterior nosebleed by pinching all of nose below nasal bone up to at least 3–10 minutes
    - May apple ice to dorsal nose or pressure under upper lip
- Patients with significant hemorrhage should receive an IV NS 250–500 ml bolus and transfusion as indicated
    - See Bleeding Protocol
    - Continuous cardiac monitoring and pulse oximetry for significant bleeding
- Patients frequently present with an elevated blood pressure
    - Significant reduction can usually be obtained with analgesia and mild sedation alone
    - May treat hypertension if > SBP 180 or DBP > 110 and not decreasing
        - Repeat BP 10–15 minutes initially, before treatment, to see if BP decreases sufficiently without medication
    - Treat initial SBP > 210 or DBP > 120 if actively bleeding
- IV NS if vital signs or CBC reflect significant bleeding (notify physician promptly)

Silver nitrate

- Silver nitrate stick cautery directly on bleeding site for 5–7 seconds, and then in a circle around bleeding site, holding 5–7 seconds each spot, to form a solid eschar

- Then hold 2 dry cotton swabs side by side for 60 seconds over cauterized area with enough pressure to stop any bleeding (usually mild pressure is all that is needed)
- May repeat in places that continue bleeding with more cautery and cotton swabs pressure until bleeding stops

Additional treatments

Use Rapid Rhino anterior or posterior balloons (or similar balloons) if silver nitrate cautery not used or ineffective

- Anterior epistaxis balloons are available in different lengths
- Carboxycellulose outer layer promotes platelet aggregation
- As efficacious as nasal tampons, easier to insert and remove, and more comfortable for the patient
- Soak its knit outer layer with water, insert it along the floor of the nasal cavity aiming down to the level of the ear lobe, and inflate it slowly with air until the bleeding stops.

Merocel packing

- Trim the compressed sponge to fit snugly through the naris
- Moisten the tip with surgical lubricant or topical antibiotic ointment
- Firmly grasp the length of the sponge with a bayonet forceps, spread the naris vertically with a nasal speculum, and advance the sponge along the floor of the nasal cavity
- Once wet with blood or a small amount of saline, the sponge expands to fill the nasal cavity and tamponade the bleeding

Afrin type nasal spray or cocaine pledgets can be used for hemostasis (caution in CAD)

Epistaxis thrombin kit for intranasal application

- Consider Floseal in thrombocytopenic or coagulopathic patients

Tranexamic acid

- Put tranexamic acid used for injection on a pledgelet and allow to be in contact with bleeding site for 20-30 minutes

- Septra DS or sinusitis medication Rx per Sanford Guide or other drug databases for 5–7 days if packing or balloon used

Discharge Criteria

- Successful treatment of anterior bleeding
- Hemodynamically stable
- No respiratory distress

Discharge instructions

- Nosebleed or epistaxis aftercare instructions
- Packing removal in 2–3 days
- Refer to ENT or primary care provider in 2–3 days
- Antibiotic ointment twice a day for 7–10 days for cautery or after packing removed — gently applied

Consult Criteria

- Unable to stop bleeding
- Posterior nasal bleeding or packing
- Significant blood loss per CBC or vital signs abnormalities
- Tachycardia or orthostatic vital signs
- Coagulopathy secondary to Coumadin (warfarin) or other causes
- Bleeding site not identified or not known whether anterior or posterior (if packing not effective then likely is a posterior nosebleed)
- Admit patients with large posterior packing or bilateral long packing for observation and oxygen saturation monitoring
    - Posterior nasal packing is particularly uncomfortable for the patient and promotes hypoxia and hypoventilation
    - Failure to admit and appropriately monitor all patients who require large posterior packing (i.e. nasostat or large gauze packing) may result in mortality

Vital signs and age consult criteria

- Adult HR > 105
- SBP < 90 or relative hypotension (SBP < 105 with history of hypertension)
- Pediatric heart rate
    - 6–8 years ≥ 130
    - 9–12 years ≥ 125
    - 13–15 years ≥ 115
    - 16 years or older ≥ 110

Lab consult criteria

- Acute hemoglobin decrease of > 1 gm
- Hemoglobin < 10 gm
- Thrombocytopenia
- INR > 1.2
- PTT > 1.2 times normal

Notes

References:

Acute Epistaxis Author: Ola Bamimore, MD; Chief Editor: Steven C Dronen, MD, FAAEM
emedicine.medscape.com/article/764719

Brinjikji W, Kallmes DF, Cloft HJ. Trends in Epistaxis Embolization in the United States: A Study of the Nationwide Inpatient Sample 2003–2010. *J Vasc Interv Radiol*. May 3 2013

ENT EMERGENCY PROTOCOL

When using any protocol, always follow the Guidelines of Proper Use (page 18).

Ludwig's Angina

Definition

- Cellulitis (occasionally abscess) involving submandibular and sublingual spaces

Considerations

- Mortality has declined to < 10% since penicillin was introduced
- Can result in elevation of tongue to obstruct airway
- Increased association with diabetes; SLE; neutropenia; alcoholism
- Polymicrobial infection is usual
- Infection of 2nd and 3rd molars most common cause — 80% of cases
- Is a clinical diagnosis
- Assess airway status — may need anesthesia or ENT if difficult intubation likely
- Ability of tongue to be protruded beyond vermillion border excludes sublingual space infection

Signs

- Bilateral submandibular swelling - All (firm floor of mouth)
- Elevated or protruding tongue - 19/20
- Fever - 9/10
- Increased WBC - 17/20
- Recent dental extraction or toothache - 8/10
- Neck swelling - 7/10
- Dysphagia - 5/10
- Trismus - 5/10
- Neck pain - 1/3
- Respiratory (stridor; dyspnea; tachypnea) - 7/20
- Dysphonia and dysarthria - 1/5

Evaluation

- Is a clinical diagnosis
- Airway management takes precedence over testing
- CT scanning best modality if needed
- Soft tissue neck and panorex useful when CT not available
- CBC
- BMP

Treatment options

- Antibiotics effective
  - Penicillin + Flagyl (metronidazole)
  - Unasyn
  - Clindamycin
- Surgery
  - Needed 20–65% of time
  - If abscess identified
- Airway management if needed
  - Endotracheal intubation
  - Cricothyroidotomy by physician
  - Notify physician immediately if suspected airway compromise

Complications

- Aspiration
- Mediastinitis
- Pneumonia
- Empyema
- Bacteremia
- Septic emboli
- Pericarditis
- Cavernous sinus thrombosis
- Cerebral abscess

Consult criteria

- All Ludwig's angina cases
- If imminent airway concern, notify physician immediately

Angioedema of Oropharyngeal Area

Considerations

- Affects deeper tissues
- Localized non-pitting edema
- 25% of population experiences urticaria or angioedema during lifetime
- Localized swelling resolves in several days
- Typically involves face and upper lip
- GI tract involvement causes
  - Nausea
  - Vomiting
  - Diarrhea
  - Abdominal pain
  - Esophageal involvement can cause chest pain
- Neurologic involvement rare
- Upper respiratory involvement responsible for mortality

Types of angioedema

- Histamine mediated
  - Allergic/immunogenic
- Bradykinin mediated
  - ACE inhibitors
  - Hereditary
    - Decreased C1 esterase inhibitor (or poorly functioning C1 esterase inhibitor) allowing overproduction of bradykinin
      - Cyroprecipitate may help (contain C1 esterase inhibitor)
  - Acquired
  - Bradykinin metabolized mainly by angiotensin converting enzyme
- Physically induced
- Idiopathic

Predictors of need for airway intervention

- Increased age
- Tongue swelling
- Oropharynx swelling
- Odynophagia
- Hoarseness/voice change

Signs

- Respiratory distress
- Stridor
- Voice changes
- Dysphagia

Causes

- Hereditary angioedema (HAE)
- Angiotensin converting enzyme inhibitors (ACE) around 70% of patients
  - Increased incidence in African-Americans and women
  - Most occur in first week of therapy
    - But can occur anytime

Treatment options

- Medical management usually suffices
- Stop offending agent if known — ACE inhibitor most common
- Examining the airway may precipitate airway obstruction in advanced oropharyngeal angioedema if aggressive
  - Double set-up with ET tube and cricothyrotomy equipment if patient in distress

Histamine mediated angioedema (allergic)

- Epinephrine
  - Caution if history of coronary artery disease
  - Adult: 0.3–0.5 mg SQ; (if respiratory distress notify physician promptly)
  - Pediatrics: 0.01 mg/kg SQ not to exceed adult dose; give IV or IM (anterior thigh) if respiratory distress present (notify physician promptly)
- Antihistamines (diphenhydramine 50 mg IV/IM) helpful in IgE/histamine mediated (may have pruritus)
  - Benadryl (diphenhydramine) 50 mg PO or IM adult; continue for 5–7 days PO
  - Benadryl (diphenhydramine) 1–2 mg/kg PO or IM pediatrics; continue for 5–7 days PO

    - Pepcid (famotidine) 20–40 mg IV/PO for adult
    - Pepcid (famotidine) 0.25 mg/kg IV/PO for pediatric (NMT 40 mg)
  - Consider steroids
    - Prednisone 40–60 mg PO qday for 5–7 days (> 40 kg)
    - Prednisone/prednisolone 1 mg/kg PO qday (children < 40 kg) for 5–7 days
    - Dexamethasone 10 mg IV
      - Onset of action IV is 1 hour. PO onset of action is 1–2 hours
      - Duration of action is 36–54 hours
      - Dexamethasone 6mg =prednisone 40 mg

Bradykinin mediated (ACE inhibitor induced most common)

  - May respond to fresh frozen plasma or C1 esterase inhibitor concentrate
  - Less responsive to treatment than histamine mediated angioedema with below agents
    - Attempt treatment with
      - Benadryl (diphenhydramine) 50 mg PO or IM adult; continue for 5–7 days PO
      - Benadryl (diphenhydramine) 1–2 mg/kg PO or IM pediatrics; continue for 5–7 days PO
    - Additional treatments if needed
      - Pepcid (famotidine) 20–40 mg IV/PO for adult
      - Pepcid (famotidine) 0.25 mg/kg IV/PO for pediatric (NMT 40 mg)
  - Consider steroids
    - Prednisone 40–60 mg PO qday for 5–7 days (> 40 kg)
    - Prednisone/prednisolone 1 mg/kg PO qday (children < 40 kg) for 5–7 days
- Airway compromise or significant oropharyngeal swelling (notify physician immediately)
  - Epinephrine

- Caution if coronary artery disease history present
- Adult: 0.3 mg SQ; (notify physician promptly)
- Pediatrics: 0.01 mg/kg SQ – do not exceed adult dose (notify physician promptly)
- Oxygen prn

- May respond to fresh frozen plasma (jumbo unit) or C1 esterase inhibitor concentrate

- **Stop ACE inhibitors if currently taking**

Consult physician promptly for posterior oropharyngeal angioedema, respiratory distress or hoarseness

Discharge criteria

- Observation for 4–6 hours
- Discharge mild lip or non-oropharyngeal angioedema with normal vital signs and no distress

Discharge instructions

- Angioedema aftercare instructions
- Refer to primary care provider within 1 day if not improving, otherwise 3–4 days if improving

Consult criteria

- Discuss all patients with physician

Barotitis Media and Barosinusitis

- Caused by relative negative pressures from descent during flying usually with a coexistent URI or positive pressures from ascent during diving
- Findings that may be seen
  - Loss of TM (tympanic membrane) landmarks, congestion around umbo, hemorrhage into middle ear

Valsalva maneuver

- On airplane descent can be used to prevent occurrence (nostrils pinched and patient blows against a closed mouth forcing air into Eustachian tubes with tympanic membranes feeling the pressure and subsequently moving – do not perform if vertigo present

Treatment options

- For tympanic membrane congestion only
  - Nasal and oral decongestants
- For hemorrhage into middle ear
  - Adult: prednisone 60 mg PO qday for 6 days then taper over 7–10 days
  - Children: prednisone 1 mg/kg PO for 6 days then taper over 7–10 days (do not exceed adult dose)
- Otitis media antibiotics are prescribed if tympanic membrane perforation or discharge noted
  - Keep ear dry
- Narcotics and/or NSAID's prn for pain

Discharge instructions

- Barotitis or barosinusitis aftercare instructions
- Refer to ENT surgeon if perforation or vertigo present – refer to PCP otherwise
- No altitude traveling till symptoms and findings resolve or scuba diving

Consult criteria

- Discuss with physician immediately any patient with joint pain or swelling, chest pain or dyspnea (order chest x-ray), dizziness, headache, altered mental status or hypotension after diving

Nosebleeds

Considerations

- 90% of nosebleeds are anterior
- Most common cause is nose picking
- Hypertension common
- Anticoagulant or antiplatelet agents
- Look for foreign body in young children (suspect if foul smell or unilateral discharge present)
- Posterior Epistaxis
  - Less common than anterior Epistaxis
  - Associated with
    - Elderly

- Hypertension
- Atherosclerosis

Evaluation

- Attempt visualization of bleeding
- Use nosebleed tray equipment or otoscope
- Have patient clear blood by forcefully blowing nose
- Use suction prn
- Cocaine intranasally can be used for hemostasis and pain control
    - May use afrin spray with or without pledget
- If bleeding has stopped and site unknown, take moistened cotton swab and gently stroke suspected area to elicit bleeding
- CBC if suspected significant blood loss or patient is tachycardic or orthostatic
- PT/INR if on Coumadin (warfarin). PTT if on heparin or has Von Willebrand's disease or hemophilia

Treatment options

- Control anterior nosebleed by pinching all of nose below nasal bone up to at least 5-10 minutes
    - May apple ice to dorsal nose or pressure under upper lip
- Patients with significant hemorrhage should receive an IV line and NS infusion
    - Continuous cardiac monitoring and pulse oximetry for significant bleeding
- Patients frequently present with an elevated blood pressure
    - Significant reduction can usually be obtained with analgesia and mild sedation alone
    - May treat hypertension if > SBP 180 or DBP > 110 and not decreasing
        - Repeat BP 10–15 minutes initially, before treatment, to see if BP decreases sufficiently without medication
    - Treat initial SBP > 210 or DBP > 120 if actively bleeding

- IV NS if vital signs or CBC reflect significant bleeding (notify physician promptly)

Silver nitrate

- Silver nitrate stick cautery directly on bleeding site for 5–7 seconds, and then in a circle around bleeding site, holding 5–7 seconds each spot, to form a solid eschar
    - Then hold 2 dry cotton swabs side by side for 60 seconds over cauterized area with enough pressure to stop any bleeding (usually mild pressure is all that is needed)
    - May repeat in places that continue bleeding with more cautery and cotton swabs pressure until bleeding stops

Additional treatments

Use Rapid Rhino anterior or posterior balloons (or similar balloons) if silver nitrate cautery not used or ineffective

- Anterior epistaxis balloons are available in different lengths
- Carboxycellulose outer layer promotes platelet aggregation
- As efficacious as nasal tampons, easier to insert and remove, and more comfortable for the patient
- Soak its knit outer layer with water, insert it along the floor of the nasal cavity aiming down to the level of the ear lobe, and inflate it slowly with air until the bleeding stops

Merocel packing

- Trim the compressed sponge to fit snugly through the naris
- Moisten the tip with surgical lubricant or topical antibiotic ointment
- Firmly grasp the length of the sponge with a bayonet forceps, spread the naris vertically with a nasal speculum, and advance the sponge along the floor of the nasal cavity

    - Once wet with blood or a small amount of saline, the sponge expands to fill the nasal cavity and tamponade the bleeding

  Afrin type nasal spray or cocaine (caution in CAD) pledgets can be used for hemostasis

  Epistaxis thrombin kit for intranasal application

    - Consider Floseal in thrombocytopenic or coagulopathic patients

- Septra DS or sinusitis medication Rx per Sanford Guide or other drug databases for 5–7 days if packing or balloon used

Discharge Criteria

- Successful treatment of anterior bleeding
- Hemodynamically stable
- No respiratory distress

  Discharge instructions

    - Nosebleed or epistaxis aftercare instructions
    - Packing removal in 2–3 days
    - Refer to ENT or primary care provider in 2–3 days
    - Antibiotic ointment twice a day for 7–10 days for cautery or after packing removed — gently applied

Consult Criteria

- Unable to stop bleeding
- Posterior nasal bleeding or packing
- Significant blood loss per CBC or vital signs abnormalities
- Tachycardia or orthostatic vital signs
- Coagulopathy secondary to Coumadin (warfarin) or DOAC's or other causes
- Bleeding site not identified or not known whether anterior or posterior (if packing not effective then likely is a posterior nosebleed)
- Admit patients with large posterior packing or bilateral long packing for observation and oxygen saturation monitoring

- Posterior nasal packing is particularly uncomfortable for the patient and promotes hypoxia and hypoventilation
- Failure to admit and appropriately monitor all patients who require large posterior packing (i.e. nasostat or large gauze packing) may result in mortality

Vital signs and age consult criteria

- Adult HR > 105
- SBP < 90 or relative hypotension (SBP < 105 with history of hypertension)
- Pediatric heart rate
    - 6–8 years ≥ 130
    - 9–12 years ≥ 125
    - 13–15 years ≥ 115
    - 16 years or older ≥ 110

Lab consult criteria

- Acute hemoglobin decrease of > 1 gm
- Hemoglobin < 10 gm
- Thrombocytopenia
- INR > 1.2
- PTT > 1.2 times normal

Notes

References:

Seidmann MD. Christopher AL. Sarpa JR. Potesta E. Angioedema related to angiotensin converting enzyme inhibitors. Otolaryngology – Head & Neck Surgery. 102:727–31, 1990.

Brown NJ. Ray WA. Snowden M. Griffin MR. Black Americans have an increased rate of angiotensin converting enzyme inhibitor-associated angioedema. Clinical Pharmacology & Therapeutics. 60(1):8–13, 1996 Jul

World Allergy Organization Guidelines for the Assessment and Management of Anaphylaxis
World Allergy Organ J. Feb 2011; 4(2): 13–37.

Acute Epistaxis Author: Ola Bamimore, MD; Chief Editor: Steven C Dronen, MD, FAAEM
emedicine.medscape.com/article/764719

Brinjikji W, Kallmes DF, Cloft HJ. Trends in Epistaxis Embolization in the United States: A Study of the Nationwide Inpatient Sample 2003–2010. *J Vasc Interv Radiol*. May 3 2013

NASAL AND FACIAL FRACTURES PROTOCOL

When using any protocol, always follow the Guidelines of Proper Use (page 18).

Considerations

- The incidence of concomitant major injuries is reported to be as high as 50% in high-impact facial fracture, compared to 21% for lower impact fractures.
- Fractures are more commonly associated with motor vehicle collisions, rather than other blunt trauma
- Airbag deployment considerably decreases the incidence and severity of orbital fractures for front-seat occupants in frontal automobile crashes
- Bleeding control imperative
- Up to 10% of patients with significant blunt facial injuries will also have cervical spine injury
- Blood or edema resulting from the injury can cause upper airway obstruction
- The tongue may obstruct the airway in a patient with a mandibular fracture
- A fractured free-floating maxilla can fall back, obstructing the airway
- Tooth fragments may migrate to the airway

Nasal Fractures

- Most common fracture
- X-rays may miss around 50%

Complications

- Septal hematoma
- Associated orbital wall blowout fractures
- Facial fractures with CSF (cerebrospinal fluid) leak — cribriform plate fracture
- Hyphema
- Retinal detachment
- Subconjunctival hemorrhage

CSF rhinorrhea

- Cribriform plate fracture
- Increased by leaning forward
- Increased with jugular compression
- Ring sign (2 rings formed when CSF placed on filter paper) — blood inner circle and CSF clearer ring outer
- Dipstick findings — CSF glucose > 30mg%

Evaluation options

- Physical examination
- Clear nares of blood
- Evaluate for septal hematoma
- CT facial bones if suspected facial fractures
- CT head injury protocols
- C-spine films prn (see Neck Pain Protocol)
- Plain nasal films not usually needed but can be ordered
- CBC if significant blood loss suspected or tachycardia/hypotension
- Tympanic membranes for hemotympanum
- Eye exam of anterior and posterior chambers if suspected eye injury or complaints
- Excessive tearing may indicate nasolacrimal duct injury — if suspected instill fluorescein in eye and exam posterior pharynx (with Wood's light if needed) to see if dye flows into pharynx through intact duct

Treatment options

- Epistaxis controlled with pinching nares together for 2–5 minutes
- Septal hematoma needs immediate drainage
  - Can be drained with 18 gauge needle after cocaine topical anesthesia
  - Rolled cotton swab can help decompress hematoma
  - Packing after drainage for 3–5 days
  - Antibiotics to prevent sinusitis (same as otitis media antibiotics)
- Analgesics prn
- Tetanus if not up to date (see Tetanus Protocol, page 756)

Discharge criteria

- Simple nasal fractures

Discharge instructions

- Nasal fracture aftercare instructions
- Refer to ENT within 7–10 days
- Head injury instructions
- No nose blowing with facial fractures for 1 week

Consult criteria

- Septal hematoma
- Associated facial fractures
- Other associated injuries
- Significant blood loss

Orbital Blowout Fractures

- Orbital wall composed of 7 bones
- Occurs usually with larger object than the orbit (baseball; fist)
- Can result in diplopia

Evaluation

- Neurologic exam
- Extraocular motor exam
- Plain facial (water's view best) or CT orbital films
- CT head injury protocols
- Ocular anterior and posterior chamber exam
- TM's (tympanic membrane) for hemotympanum
- Grasp upper teeth and palate and pull to assess for Lefort fractures (movement noted)
- Check orbital rim for step off and for malar flattening
- Dental exam
- C-spine films (see Neck Pain Protocol)
    - In any fall facial fracture (especially elderly)

Treatment

- Antibiotics (same as sinusitis treatment)
- Analgesics prn
- Tetanus if not up to date (see Tetanus Protocol)

Discharge criteria

- Uncomplicated inferior blowout fracture without extraocular muscle entrapment or other facial fractures or associated conditions
- Head injury instructions should be given to competent alert patient or family member or similar person

Discharge instructions

- Head injury aftercare instructions
- Orbital blowout fracture aftercare instructions
- Referral to Ophthalmology or plastic surgeon within 7 days

Consult criteria

- Discuss all facial fractures except uncomplicated nasal fracture with physician
- Vision changes
- EOM entrapment
- Referral to Ophthalmology within 7 days

Mandible dislocation

- May be traumatic or spontaneous
- Unilateral dislocation the mandible is tilted
- Bilateral dislocation patient appears to have an underbite
- Teeth cannot be closed
- Mandible films or panorex

Treatment

- Prep skin and inject 2% lidocaine if desired for masseter spasm and pain

Facing patient technique

- Back of head supported by wall if possible
- Pad thumbs gauze taped on
- Place thumbs on lower posterior molars
- Lock elbows and push down on lower molars with bending knees and using your weight

Behind patient technique

- May need conscious sedation
- Place padded thumbs **behind** last molar
- Grab mandible anteriorly and push caudally

Syringe technique

- 5 or 10cc syringe placed across posterior molars and patient instructed to bite down and roll syringe back and forth
    - 30 of 31 patients had success with this method

Mandible Fracture

- Third most common facial fracture
- 20–40% of mandibular fracture patients have associated injuries
- Children age 4–11 years at risk for facial growth disturbance if fracture missed
- The tongue may obstruct the airway in a patient with a mandibular fracture
- Tooth fragments can become may migrate to the airway

Findings

- Facial asymmetry
- Malocclusion of teeth
- Paresthesia to lower lip or gums indicate inferior alveolar nerve damage
- Blood in mouth suggests open fracture
- Jaw may deviate to side of fracture

Evaluation

- Airway exam — notify physician immediately if any airway concerns
- Dental exam
- Neurologic exam
- Plain mandible films or panorex
- CT mandible if the plain films not helpful in suspected fracture
- CT head if per head injury protocols or abnormal neurologic exam
- Chest x-ray if missing teeth cannot be located
- C-spine films (see Neck Pain Protocol)
    - In any fall facial fracture (especially elderly)

Treatment

- Dental antibiotics choices
    - Pen VK 500 mg PO qid × 7–10 days

- Cleocin (clindamycin) 300 mg PO qid × 7–10 days
- Erythromycin 250 mg PO qid × 7–10 days

- Tetanus if not up to date (see Tetanus Protocol)
- See Dental Injury Protocol

Discharge criteria

- Simple nondisplaced mandible fractures
- Soft diet
- Analgesics prn

Discharge instructions

- Mandible fracture aftercare instructions
- Referral to oral surgeon within 1–4 days
- Head injury instructions

Consult criteria

- Discuss all mandible fractures with physician or oral surgeon

Notes

References:

Orbital Fracture in Emergency Medicine Medication
Author: Thomas Widell, MD; Chief Editor: Rick Kulkarni, MD
emedicine.medscape.com/article/825772

Orbital Floor Fractures (Blowout)
Author: Adam J Cohen, MD; Chief Editor: Deepak Narayan, MD, FRCS emedicine.medscape.com/article/1284026

Bartkiw TP, Pynn BR, Brown DH. Diagnosis and managment of nasal fractures. Int J Trauma Nurs. 1995;1:11–18. (Review article)

Duma SM, Jernigan MV. The effects of airbags on orbital fracture patterns in frontal automobile crashes. Ophth Plast Reconst Surg. 2003;19(2):107–111

Francis DO, Kaufman R, Yueh B, et al. Air bag-induced orbital blow-out fractures. Laryngoscope. 2006;116:1966–1972. (Case series of 150 orbital fractures derived from 2739 crashes in CIREN database)

Hackl W, Fink C, Hausberger K, et al. The incidence of combined facial and cervical spine injuries. J Trauma. 2001;50:41–45

Gorchynski J, Karabidian E, Sanchez M. The "syringe" technique: a hands-free approach for the reduction of acute nontraumatic temporomandibular dislocations in the emergency department. J Emerg Med. 2014;47(6):676-681. (Prospective convenience sample, multicenter study

DENTAL INJURY PROTOCOLS

When using any protocol, always follow the Guidelines of Proper Use (page 18).

Considerations

- Injury to primary teeth common in toddlers
- Older children dental injuries commonly from sports
- Assess for other injuries
- Primary tooth eruption from 7 months to 2–3 years of age
- Malocclusion of teeth is a mandible or maxilla fracture until proven otherwise

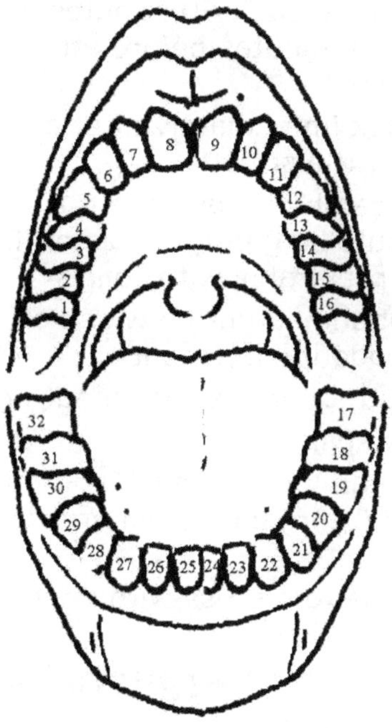

Tooth Fractures

- Ellis class 1: enamel injured only
- Ellis class 2: dentin involved
- Ellis class 3: pulp involved (bloody dental tissue seen)

Dental Avulsions of Permanent Teeth

- 1% loss of successful reimplantation of avulsed tooth per minute that tooth is not replaced in socket
- More than 15 minutes out of socket has poor salvage rate
- After 60 minutes of being out of socket there usually is no salvage rate
- Avulsed teeth should be handled by crown only
- Put in either Hank's solution, milk, or normal saline as a temporizing measure
    - Tooth can be held in buccal mucosa side of mouth if no other means to keep it stored, making sure not to swallow it
- Leave the socket alone as much as possible.
- If extraoral time is 20–60 minutes, soak in Hanks solution for 30 minutes before attempting reimplantation
- Put tooth back immediately after aspirating any clot and irrigating the socket
- If the tooth can be replaced in the prehospital setting, the root should be gently rinsed off first to remove any debris (preferably with saline)
    - The root should not be wiped off as this removes the periodontal ligament
- Apply a mouth guard (sports mouth guard acceptable)
    - Coe Pak splinting
- Antibiotics: Pen VK 500 mg PO qid for 10 days and see dentist or oral surgeon within one day for further treatment
- It is preferable to discuss with dentist at time of injury

Dental Avulsions of Primary Teeth

- Leave out of mouth

Gingival Lacerations

- Heal well
- Reapproximate with chromic or Vicryl sutures
- Antibiotics are not indicated

Lip and Intraoral Lacerations

- Repair from inside out then close skin

- Use absorbable sutures intraorally
- Line up vermillion border if involved
- Antibiotics are not indicated
- Refer to Laceration Protocol

Evaluation

- Dental history important to know to determine if teeth worth saving
- Time of injury important
- Palpate and lightly percuss teeth (should be a ping sound normally)
- Remove blood clots
- Check for intraoral lacerations and any through and through involvement
- Check facial bones for looseness (Lefort fractures) by pulling forward on palate or upper maxillary rim
- Plain x-rays for
  - Bony abnormalities
  - Aspirated teeth
  - Foreign bodies (tooth fragments) in lacerations
- Panorex films if available
- CT of facial bones may be needed for more extensive injury
- Check posterior molar's occlusion are normal
- Refer to Head Injury Protocols

Treatment

- Enamel fractures do not require immediate treatment
- Class 2 fractures
  - Cover with Dycal (calcium hydroxide paste)
- Class 3 fractures
  - Anesthetize tooth
  - Immediate covering with Dycal
  - Antibiotics
    - Adult
      - Pen VK 500 mg PO qid × 10 days
      - Clindamycin 300 mg PO tid × 10 days
      - Amoxicillin 500 mg PO tid × 10 days
    - Weight adjustment of above antibiotics for pediatrics

- Analgesics prn
- Loose teeth are referred to dentist and prescribe a soft diet
    - Chlorhexidine rinses
- Can use mouth guard to splint very loose teeth
    - Coe Pak splinting
- Move displaced teeth into position post local anesthesia
- Tetanus prophylaxis: (High risk = every 5 years; Low risk = every 10 years)
    - Tetanus IG 250–500 units if high risk and less than 3 tetanus or unknown history of immunizations previously in life — usually with the elderly
- Refer to health department or primary care provider to complete tetanus primary vaccination series if < 2 vaccines given in past
    - See Tetanus Protocol (page 756)

Discharge Criteria

- Ellis class 1 and 2 fractures
- Primary tooth avulsions
- Mildly loose teeth
- Refer to dentist or oral surgeon
    - Ellis class 2 fractures within 24 hours for primary dental avulsions and loose teeth
    - Ellis class 3 fractures dental referral ASAP, no more than next day if possible
- Give avulsed teeth that are not reimplanted to patient to take to dentist

Consult Criteria

- Displaced teeth
- Avulsed permanent teeth
- It is preferable to discuss with dentist at time of injury
- Discuss with physician or dentist Ellis class 2 and 3 fractures

Notes

References:

Barrett EJ, Kenny DJ. Avulsed permanent teeth: a review of the literature and treatment guidelines.*Endod Dent Traumatol* 1997Aug;13(4):153–163

Krasner P. Modern treatment of avulsed teeth by emergency physicians. *Am J Emerg Med* 1994 Mar;12(2):241–246

ebmedicine.net/topics.php?paction=showTopic&topic_id=543

DENTAL PAIN PROTOCOL

When using any protocol, always follow the Guidelines of Proper Use (page 18).

Differential diagnosis

- Periapical abscess
- Trigeminal neuralgia
- Masticator space infection
- Ludwig's angina
- Retropharyngeal space infection
- Infection after a root canal
- Dental caries

Considerations

- Dental abscess is rare in children
- Abscess can spread more deeply to
    - Bone (osteomyelitis)
    - Cavernous sinus (thrombosis)
    - Maxillary sinus
    - Floor of mouth (Ludwig's angina)
    - Adjacent facial spaces and planes
- Advanced dental disease in children could indicate diabetes mellitus or HIV infection
- Lower third molar most common abscess site followed by other lower posterior teeth
    - Upper teeth uncommon source of dental abscess

Evaluation options

- Usually history and physical exam only
- Percussion tenderness present
- CBC when patient is toxic appearing or cellulitis present
- BMP for tachycardia or history of diabetes or suspicion of undiagnosed diabetes
- Plain films of neck if deeper infections considered
- Panorex
- CT face or neck for suspected deeper infections

- Needle aspiration (remove 1–2 drops of pus if further drainage is to be attempted to leave area large as possible)

Periapical abscess

- Most common dental infection
- Very painful

Treatment options

- I&D with needle if abscess seen
  - Tap water as effective as normal saline for irrigation
- Antibiotics if no pus found or no aspiration performed (choose one below)
  - Pen VK 250 mg PO qid for 7–10 days
  - Clindamycin 150–450 mg PO qid for 7–10 days
  - Metronidazole 500 mg PO bid for 7–10 days
  - Azithromycin 5 day dose pak
  - Erythromycin 250 mg PO qid for 7–10 days
- NSAID's prn
- Hydrocodone prn up to 5 days

Discharge criteria

- Nontoxic patient
- Most dental pain patients

Discharge instructions

- Warm salt water rinses very frequently for 1–5 days. Hold in mouth for several minutes as tolerated
- Warm compresses to painful area several times a day
- Follow up with dentist within 48 hours

Consult criteria

- Deep space infection diagnosed or suspected
- Fever
- Potential for airway compromise
- Immunocompromised
- Systemic involvement

Notes

References:

Dental Abscess Empiric Therapy

Author: Jane M Gould, MD, FAAP; Chief Editor: Thomas E Herchline, MD emedicine.medscape.com/article/2060395

HealthPartners Dental Group guideline for diagnosing and treating endodontic emergencies. Minneapolis (MN): HealthPartners; 2009 Sep 1. 11

Trauma

Section Contents

When using any protocol, always follow the Guidelines of Proper Use (page 18).

MOTOR VEHICLE ACCIDENT PROTOCOL

When using any protocol, always follow the Guidelines of Proper Use (page 18).

Considerations

- Leading cause of death ages 1–37 years
- Complete exam important even when single isolated injury suspected
- Initial assessment critical in determining life threatening processes
- Comorbidities should be addressed
- Liver and spleen most common intra-abdominal injuries followed by small and large intestine in blunt abdominal trauma
- Cervical and lumbar strains common in minor MVA
- Seatbelt marks may indicate deeper injuries
- Early coagulopathy in trauma from shock and tissue damage
    - Activated protein C and t-PA released

Evaluation

- Patients seen by the practitioner should have minor injuries only
- Patients on spine boards can be moved carefully if no evident spinal cord injury
    - Log roll patient off spine board within 60 minutes of arrival with team of 4 persons with 1 person maintaining inline cervical immobilization to prevent pressure tissue damage from board
- Notify physician immediately for Glasgow scale < 15

Primary survey

- Airway
- Breathing
- Circulation/bleeding
- Disability (neurologic exam)
- Exposure/environment (expose patient and hypothermia evaluation)

- Contact physician immediately if any serious findings found on primary survey
- Significant hemorrhagic vital sign findings, contact physician immediately
  - See Permissive hypotension section below (consult physician immediately)

Secondary survey

- Complete physical exam
- Palpate and inspect all body areas
- Complete neurovascular exam

AMPLE mnemonic for historical key elements

A – Allergies
M – Medications
P – Past history
L – Last meal
E – Events leading to presentation

Estimated Blood and Fluid losses (adults)

	Class I	**Class II**	**Class III**	**Class IV**
Blood loss (cc)	Up to 750	750–1000	1500–2000	> 2000
Blood loss %	Up to 15%	15–30%	30–40%	> 40%
Pulse rate	< 100	> 100	> 120	> 140
Blood pressure	Normal	Normal	SBP < 90	SBP < 70
Capillary refill	Normal	Normal	Delayed	Absent
Pulse pressure	Normal/incr	Decreased	Decreased	Decreased
Respiratory rate	14–20	20–30	30–40	> 35
Urine output (cc/hr.)	> 30	20–30	5–15	Negligible
Mental status	Anxious	Anxious	Confused	Lethargic

(Derived from Advanced Trauma Life Support)

Lethal triad for bleeding (each contributes to the others)

- Hypothermia
- Acidosis
- Coagulopathy (frequently too much crystalloid without blood product replacement)

Imaging and Lab Tests (As indicated by exam, history, and mechanism of injury)

- C-spine

- Extremities
- Chest x-ray
    - Deep sulcus sign may indicate pneumothorax when one is not seen in periphery
        - Costophrenic angle deeper than normal
- CT head and C-spine
- CT abdomen/pelvis; chest if indicated (physician should be involved)
- See Acute Care Ultrasound chapter

Lab if indicated

- CBC
- BMP
- LFT's
- U/A
- Type and screen or cross

Treatment Options

- Analgesics prn
    - Dilaudid (hydromorphone) 0.5 mg IV or 1–2 mg IM
    - Stadol (butorphanol) 0.5–1 mg IV or 1–2 mg IM
    - Toradol (ketorolac) 30 mg IV or 60 mg IM (if no bleeding possibility present)
        - Do not use Toradol (ketorolac) if creatinine is elevated
- NSAID's or PO narcotics prn (outpatient treatment)
- Tetanus prophylaxis: (High risk = every 5 years; Low risk = every 10 years) Tetanus IG 250–500 units at different site if high risk and less than 3 tetanus or unknown history of immunizations previously in life — usually with the elderly
- Refer to health department or primary care provider to complete tetanus primary vaccination series if < 2 vaccines given in past
    - See Tetanus Protocol (page 756)

Blood/fluid replacement for hemorrhage

- PRBC's/FFP/platelets 1:1:1 ratio

Permissive hypotension

- Administering 2 liters of crystalloid in hypotensive trauma patients worsens coagulopathy and should be replaced by permissive hypotension

- Normotensive patients receive no fluid resuscitation
- Hypotensive patients have fluid withheld until SBP approaches 80 mm Hg, at which point 250 – 500 ml boluses of blood or plasma are given to maintain SBP between 80 – 90 mmHg
- Avoid > 500 ml of NS for acute blood loss and shock before blood products transfusion started if possible
    - NS used if blood products not readily available
- Avoid hypertension
- Use blood warmer
- Uncrossed match blood for hemorrhagic shock if needed emergently
- Tranexamic acid 1 gm/10 minutes then 1 gm over 8 hours given within first 3 hours of trauma

  OR

  10 mg/kg IV followed by infusion of 1mg/kg/h
- Use lab to guide ongoing resuscitation after initial resuscitation if available

Head Trauma

Considerations

- Loss of consciousness (LOC), amnesia, headache, vomiting and seizures have low sensitivity and specificity for detecting intracranial injury
- Cervical spine exam and evaluation important
- Skull films mainly replaced by CT evaluation of head trauma
- Evaluate for significant maxillofacial injuries

Concussion definitions

Grade 1 concussion

- Transient confusion
- No LOC

- Duration of mental status abnormalities < 15 minutes

Grade 2 concussion

- Transient confusion
- No LOC
- Duration of mental status abnormalities > 15 minutes

Grade 3 concussion

- Loss of consciousness

Evaluation

- CT per head injury protocols
- Evaluate for other injuries, especially C-spine
- Retinal exam: for hemorrhages
- Detailed neurologic exam

ENT exam

- Check for hemotympanum
- CSF rhinorrhea
- Battle's sign
- Cranial nerve palsy

CT head scanning rules (choose)

Nexus 2 CT Head Rule (age 1 or greater)

- Any positive below then perform head CT
- Age ≥ 65 years
- Coagulopathy
- Evidence of significant skull fracture
- Scalp hematoma
- Neurologic deficit
- Abnormal behavior
- Altered level of alertness
- Persistent vomiting

New Orleans CT criteria (for ordering CT brain)

- Normal neurologic exam and one of the following
    - Decreased GCS
    - Headache
    - Vomiting
    - Age > 60
    - Persistent anterograde amnesia

  - Drug-alcohol intoxication
  - Visible trauma above the clavicle
  - Seizure

Canadian CT Head Rule

- Any positive below then perform head CT
- GCS < 15 at 2 hours after injury
  - Suspected or open skull fracture
  - Signs of basilar skull fracture
  - Vomiting ≥ 2 episodes
  - Age ≥ 65 years
  - Pre–impact amnesia ≥ 30 minutes
  - Dangerous mechanism

Pecarn Algorithm Age < 2 years

- Order CT head if any positive
  - Abnormal GCS
  - Palpable skull fracture
  - Signs of altered mental status
  - Occipital, parietal or temporal scalp hematoma
  - History of loss of consciousness ≥ 5 seconds
  - Severe mechanism
  - Not acting normally

Pecarn Algorithm Age ≥ 2 years for pediatric head trauma

- Order CT head if any positive
  - Abnormal GCS
  - Palpable skull fracture
  - Signs of altered mental status
  - History of loss of consciousness
  - History of vomiting
  - Severe mechanism
  - Severe headache

Discharge criteria

- Stable condition
- Normal neurologic exam
- No other significant trauma
- No radiologic abnormalities

Discharge instructions

- Head injury aftercare instructions
- Tylenol (no ASA or NSAID's for 36 hours)
- Avoid more potent analgesics so progression of symptoms can be detected
- Return for any neurologic changes
- Follow up with primary care provider or neurologist

Consult criteria

- Age ≥ 70 or < 2 years of age
- Bleeding potential
- Concussions
- Dementia
- Persistent vomiting
- Severe persistent headache
- Focal neurologic deficits
- Inadequate home observation

Neck Trauma

Penetrating neck trauma

- Consult physician unless very superficial laceration
- Do not explore Zone 2 penetrating deep injuries
    - Angle of mandible to cricoid cartilage
    - Consult physician

Cervical spine trauma

- Leave cervical collar on until patient examined and cleared
- Plain C-spine x-ray 3 views

Exclusionary criteria for C-spine films

- No neurologic deficit
- No distracting injuries
- No evidence of intoxication
- Normal mentation
- No posterior midline tenderness

CT C-spine indications

- Moderate to high risk of cervical fracture
- Significant mechanism of injury

- Fracture on plain C-spine films
- Neurologic deficit or complaint
- Inadequate plain C-spine films
- Severe neck pain with normal plain C-spine films
- Patient will not move neck actively (on their own) without external support of patient's hands ("head in hand sign")
- Obtunded patients
- Facial fractures

Flexion-extension plain films

- Significant pain with negative plain and CT imaging in subacute patients only
- Evaluation for ligamentous instability

Treatment

- C-spine cleared: analgesics and ice packs

Discharge criteria

- Benign cause of neck pain

Discharge instructions

- Neck injury aftercare instructions
- Refer to primary care provider or neurosurgeon within 3 days if not improving
- Avoid discharging with cervical collar if possible

Consult criteria

- Cervical fracture or dislocation/subluxation
- Neurologic deficit or complaint
- Significant pain
- Significant mechanism of injury

Extremity Trauma

- Refer to specific protocols

Lacerations and Cutaneous Wounds

- Refer to Laceration and Cutaneous Wound Protocol

Discharge Criteria for MVA

- No significant injury that needs admission or acute consultation

Discharge Instructions for MVA

- MVA aftercare instructions
- Refer to appropriate physician specialty within 7–10 days as needed

Consult Criteria for MVA

- As in above sections
- Notify physician immediately for suspected severe trauma or bleeding
- Significant injuries or mechanism of injury should be seen by physician initially and throughout length of stay
- Severe pain
- Moderate abdominal pain
- Refer to General Patient Criteria Protocol (page 22)
- Hemorrhage from more than minor simple laceration
- Fractures
- Dislocations
- Neurovascular injuries
- Tendon injuries

Notes

References: Advanced Trauma Life Support

Hemorrhagic Shock Author: John Udeani, MD, FAAEM; Chief Editor: John Geibel, MD, DSc, MA emedicine.medscape.com/article/432650

ACEP Clinical Policy: Neuroimaging and Decisionmaking in Adult Mild Traumatic Brain Injury in the Acute Setting

Head Trauma Treatment & Management

Author: David W Crippen, MD, FCCM; Chief Editor: John Geibel, MD, DSc,
emedicine.medscape.com/article/433855

Closed Head Trauma
Author: Leonardo Rangel-Castilla, MD; Chief Editor: Allen R Wyler, MD emedicine.medscape.com/article/251834

NEJM. 2019;380:763

LACERATION AND CUTANEOUS WOUND PROTOCOL

When using any protocol, always follow the Guidelines of Proper Use (page 18).

Considerations

- Scalp lacerations with arterial bleeding can cause shock
  - Suture initially instead of pressure dressings if significant arterial bleeding present
- Tap water is a safe and cost effective means of wound flushing
- Tissue adhesives, adhesive strips, staples, and hair apposition are cost-effective techniques for wound closure
- Wounds closed with absorbable sutures do not have worse cosmetic outcomes
- Most traumatic wounds do not require antibiotic prophylaxis.
- Patients with high-risk bite wounds should receive prophylactic antibiotics

Anesthetics

- There are two major types of local anesthetics: amides and esters — little cross reactivity
- Maximum safe doses of local anesthetics
  - Lidocaine plain — 4.5 mg/kg
    - Lidocaine with epinephrine — 7 mg/kg
  - Marcaine plain — 2 mg/kg
    - Marcaine (bupivacaine) with epinephrine — 3 mg/kg

Duration of anesthesia

- Lidocaine without epinephrine lasts 15 minutes locally
  - Regional block lasts longer
- Lidocaine with epinephrine lasts 2–3 hours (avoid in end-circulation areas: fingers, toes, etc.)
- Marcaine (bupivacaine) lasts 90 minutes to 12 hours

Local anesthetic tips

- If lidocaine mixed with NaHCO3 in 9:1 ratio (90% lidocaine and 10% NaHCO3) it will yield a pH closer to body pH that will not burn with injection
- Warming local anesthetic to body temperature decreases pain of injection
- Topical tetracaine in wound for 20–30 minutes decreases pain of injection and may by itself be superior to local anesthetic injection

Increased infection risk with

- Foreign body
- Crush injury
- Human or animal bite

Lacerations

Sutures

Nonabsorbable (nylon; polypropylene)

- Retains strength > 60 days; low tissue reactivity
- Use 6′0 on face
- Use 4′0 on rest of body
- May use 3′0 on very high tension areas except on face

Absorbable

- Synthetic is less reactive
- Synthetic has increased strength vs. cat gut
- Wound retains 50% of strength in < 1 week to 2 months
- Plain 5′0–6′0 gut sutures can be used to close the skin margins on children's facial lacerations
    - Avoid using plain gut in high tension areas
    - Vicryl retains strength to 21 days which is too long for external skin closure on facial lacerations
- Vicryl rapide may be used for oral lacerations
- Plain gut retains strength for 4–5 days

Deep sutures

- Helps relieve skin tension
- Decreases dead space and hematoma formation
- May improve cosmetic outcomes
- Recommend liberal use of deep sutures to approximate skin edges before closure with either skin sutures or tissue adhesives

Staples

- Considered for scalp; trunk; extremity lacerations
- When saving time is essential

Tissue adhesives (Dermabond)

- Reduces the need of suturing in up to 1/3 of lacerations
- Sloughs in 7–10 days
- Not to use if skin margins cannot be manually approximated or held together without a lot of tension
- Use 3–4 coats
- Keep out of laceration
- Caution: too much applied can cause too much heat to be released from the exothermic reaction
- Can be removed with bathing, petroleum or antibiotic gel, or acetone if rapid removal necessary
- May take shower after 24 hours, but avoid bathing or swimming until the adhesive sloughs — usually within 7 days

Evaluation

- Assess for other injuries
- X-ray for foreign bodies or fractures as indicated by history and exam
- Ultrasound may be used to detect foreign bodies depending on level of experience
- Record neurovascular exam prior to anesthesia
- Examine and document any deeper structures involvement
- Tendon involvement or injuries, consult physician

- High pressure injection injuries, consult physician promptly

Treatment Options

Sutures

- On face use 6'0 nylon or equivalent
- Use nylon 4'0 or equivalent on rest of body
- Nylon 3'0 can be used for high tension body lacerations (not on face)
- Vicryl or equivalent absorbable sutures used for deeper layers or intraoral
- Plain 5′0–6′0 gut can be used on children's facial lacerations to avoid later suture removal (or vicryl rapide)

Wound preparation

- All foreign material needs to be removed as much as possible
- Flush lacerations deeply with 0.1% betadine sol. (diluted betadine), NS or municipal tap water
    - PSI 5–8 flush is sufficient and superior to high pressure flush, as long as foreign material is removed
    - Flush with at least 50–100 ml/cm of laceration
- Municipal potable tap water is safe and effective to flush wounds (if doubt of water quality then use sterile flush)
    - May have lower infection rate than other methods of flush
- Hemostasis by direct pressure
    - Elevation of extremity helpful with point pressure to stop persistent extremity bleeding

Closure techniques

- Keep wound margins flat or everted with the closure (corner suture may be used for V or X shaped laceration)
- Avoid wound margin inversion
- Partial muscle injury can be closed by using fascia of muscle
- Lacerations with high risk of infection may need to be left partially or fully open

- Steri–strips or tissue adhesive can be used as indicated

Simple Suture

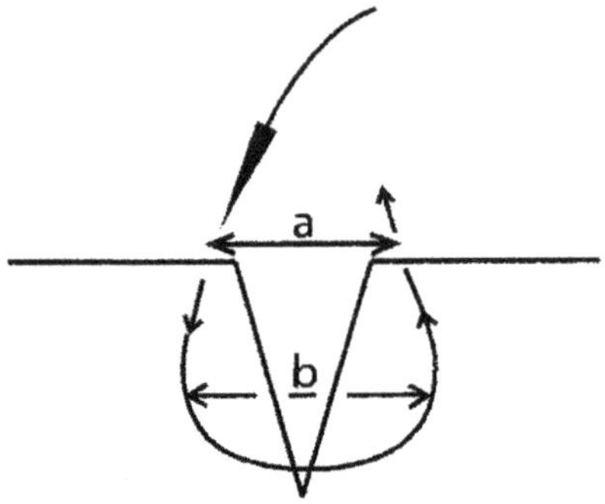

The distance of line (a), the skin entry and exit points, is less than line (b) at the base of the laceration.

- This creates wound eversion which is cosmetically desirable.
- Wound inversion creates a shadow in the laceration site after healing.

Vertical Mattress Suture

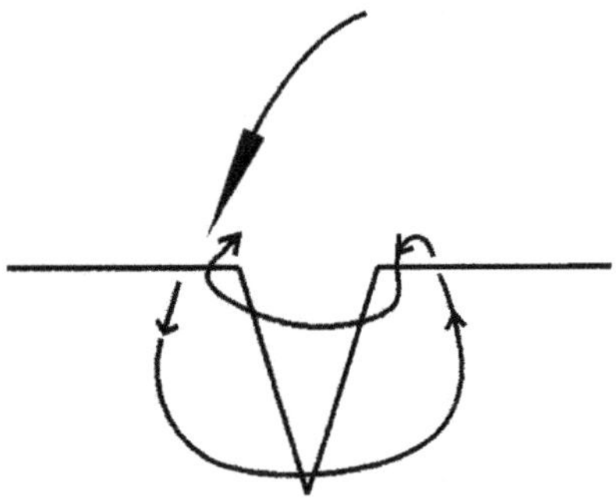

Vertical mattress is used for high tension wounds and when laceration margin eversion is needed.

Antibiotics for

- Tendon or bone involvement
- Septic contamination
- Animal/human bites

Aftercare

- Laceration aftercare instructions

- Sutured or stapled lacerations keep clean and gently cleansed after 24–48 hours
- Sutured or stapled lacerations should be protected with nonadherent dressing for 48 hours
- Air dry lacerations after 48 hours of dressing (cover dressing when in contaminated environment)
- Sutured or stapled laceration infection incidence may be reduced with topical antibiotic ointments
- Splint if there is a fracture or tendon injury and prn otherwise
- No antibiotics for clean, simple lacerations that are not animal or human bites

Suture and Staple Removal

- Face 3–5 days
- Neck 4–6 days
- Scalp and trunk 7–10 days
- Upper extremity 10–14 days
- Lower extremity 14–21 days
- Joints 10–21 days

Consult criteria

- Wounds beyond the practitioner's ability to treat
- See General Consult Criteria below

Skin tears

- Common among elderly and long term steroid therapy
- Skin tears can be closed with tissue adhesive if within 8 hours

Class 1 skin tear

- No tissue loss
- Close with surgical tape
- Cover with nonadherent dressing

Class 2 skin tear

- Partial tissue loss
- Manage with absorbent dressings (petroleum based, hydrogels, foams, or hydrocolloids, etc.) for 5–7 days
  - Change daily if needed
  - Use elastic tubular nets to hold in place

Class 3 skin tear

- Complete tissue loss
- Manage same as Class 2 skin tear

Discharge instructions

- Skin tear aftercare instructions
- Follow up with primary care provider or surgeon within 2–5 days as needed

Consult criteria

- Large amount of tissue loss

Plantar puncture wounds

- Rate of cellulitis 2–10%
  - Usually staph or strep
  - Use dicloxicillin or Sanford Guide or other drug databases
- Cleaning alone may be effective
- If foreign body suspected, use plain x-rays if radiopaque, or CT or ultrasound scan otherwise if needed
- Punctures through sweaty moist tennis shoes carries risk of pseudomonas osteomyelitis
  - May prescribe antipseudomonal antibiotic such as Cipro (ciprofloxacin)
- Frequent cleansing and topical antibiotic as treatment at home
- Do not core out puncture wound

Discharge instructions

- Puncture wound aftercare instructions
- Close follow-up within 2–3 days for suspected deep punctures

Consult criteria

- Neurovascular or bone injury

Subungual hematomas

- Treat with nail trephination (burr hole)
- Nail may be removed for disruption of nail or surrounding nail folds

Discharge instructions

- Subungual hematoma aftercare instructions

General Consult Criteria

- Open fracture

- Neurovascular or tendon injuries or deficits
- Muscle bundle totally severed
- Practitioner is uncomfortable repairing laceration
- Human or animal bites

Vital signs and age consult criteria

- Adult heart rate > 100
- SBP < 90 or relative hypotension (SBP < 105 with history of hypertension)
- Pediatric heart rate
    - 0–4 months ≥ 180
    - 5–7 months ≥ 175
    - 8–12 months ≥ 170
    - 1–3 years ≥ 160
    - 4–5 years ≥ 145
    - 6–8 years ≥ 130
    - 9–12 years ≥ 125
    - 13–15 years ≥ 115
    - 16 years or older ≥ 110

Lab consult criteria

- Acute hemoglobin decrease of > 1 gm
- Hemoglobin < 10 gm unless chronic and stable
- Thrombocytopenia
- INR > 1.5 if checked

Notes

Emergency management of skin and soft tissue wounds : an illustrated guide Ernest N Kaplan; Vincent R Hentz

Weiss EA, Oldham G, Lin M, et al. Water is a safe and effective alternative to sterile normal saline for wound irrigation prior to suturing: a prospective, double-blind, randomised, controlled clinical trial. BMJ Open. 2013;3(1):1-6. (Randomized controlled trial; 663 patients)

Liu JX, Werner JA, Buza JA 3rd, et al. Povidone-iodine solutions inhibit cell migration and survival of osteoblasts, fibroblasts, and myoblasts. Spine (Phila Pa 1976). 2017. (In vitro study

ebmedicine.net/topics.php?paction=showTopic&topic_id=55
8

Bleeding Protocol

When using any protocol, always follow the Guidelines of Proper Use (page 18).

Considerations

- Active hemorrhage may be apparent or unsuspected
- Scalp lacerations with arterial bleeding can cause shock
    - Suture initially instead of pressure dressings with significant arterial bleeding
- Medical therapy can precipitate or worsen bleeding
- Early coagulopathy in trauma from shock and tissue damage
    - Activated protein C and t-PA released

Estimated Blood and Fluid losses (adults)

	Class I	Class II	Class III	Class IV
Blood loss (cc)	Up to 750	750–1000	1500–2000	> 2000
Blood loss %	Up to 15%	15–30%	30–40%	> 40%
Pulse rate	< 100	> 100	> 120	> 140
Blood pressure	Normal	Normal	SBP < 90	SBP < 70
Capillary refill	Normal	Normal	Delayed	Absent
Pulse pressure	Normal/incr	Decreased	Decreased	Decreased
Respiratory rate	14–20	20–30	30–40	> 35
Urine output (cc/hr)	> 30	20–30	5–15	Negligible
Mental status	Anxious	Anxious	Confused	Lethargic

(Derived from Advanced Trauma Life Support)

Lethal triad for bleeding (each contributes to the others)

- Hypothermia
- Acidosis
- Coagulopathy

Evaluation

- CBC
- PT/INR/PTT if on anticoagulant or have comorbid conditions contributing to bleeding
- Type and screen or cross depending on level of hemorrhage

Treatment

- Direct pressure of bleeding site for 2–5 minutes if actively bleeding when possible
- Tourniquet for exsanguination from extremities where direct pressure ineffective (notify physician immediately)

Blood/fluid replacement for hemorrhage

- PRBC's/FFP/platelets 1:1:1 ratio (recommendations range from 4:1:1 to 1:1:1)
  - 1:1:1 ratio yields estimated hematocrit of 29%, platelet count of 90,000 and coagulation factors 62% of whole blood
- Avoid > 1 liter of isotonic fluids for acute blood loss before blood products transfusion started if possible
- Avoid hypertension
- Target systolic blood pressure of 80-90 mm Hg until major bleeding stopped
- Target Hgb of 7-9 g/dl after termination of major bleeding
- Pediatric: 20 cc/kg IV NS bolus, start blood and plasma for continued hypotension and bleeding (notify physician promptly)
- Use blood warmer
- Uncrossed match blood for hemorrhagic shock if needed emergently
- Tranexamic 1 gm/10 minutes then 1 gm every 8 hours
  - Give within first 3 hours of trauma

    OR

  10 mg/kg followed by infusion of 1 mg/kg/hour
- Use lab to guide ongoing resuscitation after initial resuscitation

Reversal of anticoagulation

Elevated INR for patient on warfarin (vitamin K antagonists)

- INR 4.5–10 without bleeding — no vitamin K treatment
  - Hold warfarin until in therapeutic range
- INR > 10 without bleeding give oral vitamin K
  - Hold warfarin until in therapeutic range

- INR 2–3 will be normal after holding warfarin for 4–5 days
  - Warfarin half-life is 1.5–2 days
- For major bleeding — see below

Warfarin

- Major bleeding give 4 factor prothrombin complex concentrate if available over FFP
- Vitamin K 10 mg IV over 10 minutes (not faster than 1 mg/minute) or IM/SQ/PO prn Coumadin (warfarin) therapy — may take 24–48 hours to affect INR
- **FFP** 10–15mL/kg – FFP unit usually is 250 mL
- Prothrombin complex concentrate
  - Kcentra
- FEIBA 500 units (Factor VIII inhibitor bypassing activity) when INR was < 5 or 1,000 units of FEIBA when INR was ≥ 5

Heparin

- Protamine 1 mg IV for each 100 units of heparin given to reverse anticoagulation prn
  - Do not exceed 50 mg in a single dose

Timing for dosage

- Heparin given
  - < 30 minutes ago — protamine 1U/100U heparin
  - 30–60 minutes — protamine 0.75U/100U heparin
  - 60–120 minutes — protamine 0.5U/100U heparin
  - > 120 minutes give protamine 0.25U/100U heparin

Low Molecular Weight Heparin

- Last dose < 4 hours give protamine 1 mg for each 1 mg of enoxaparin
  - If bleeding continues give ½ the dose in 4 hours
- Last dose 4–8 hours ago give 0.5 mg for each 1 mg of enoxaparin

t-PA

- No universal accepted guideline (empirical)
- Cryoprecipitate 0.15 U/kg if fibrinogen < 150 mg/dL

- Tranexamic acid 1000 mg IV/10minutes (inhibits plasminogen activation)
- Platelet transfusion for platelet count < 100,000 or platelet dysfunction suspected

Dabigatran (thrombin inhibitor)

- Half-life 14–16 hours
- Praxbind (idarucizumab) is reversal agent (for life threatening bleeding or uncontrolled bleeding)
- Supportive care
- Activated charcoal if dabigatran taken within past 2 hours
- Hemodialysis

Other direct Xa inhibitors (DOAC'S)

- Rivaroxaban half-life ~ 5 - 13 hours
    - Andexxa — Coagulation factor Xa recombinant, inactivated-zhzo (for life threatening bleeding or uncontrolled bleeding)
- Apixaban half-life ~ 8 - 15 hours
    - Andexxa — Coagulation factor Xa recombinant, inactivated-zhzo (for life threatening bleeding or uncontrolled bleeding)
- Consider PCC (Kcentra prothrombin complex concentrate or recombinant activated factor VII) if Andexxa not available for life threatening bleeding (not a specific antidote)
- Normal PT rules out significant clinical effect

Admission Criteria

- Massive ingestion of anticoagulant
- Long acting anticoagulant
    - Hydroxycoumadin > 0.05 mg
    - Indandione > 5 mg
    - Warfarin > 0.5 mg/kg
- Rapid or severe increase in PT
- Any significant bleeding
- Risk of falls

Discharge Criteria

- Bleeding without effect on vital signs or hemoglobin level
- Further significant bleeding unlikely
- No coagulopathy

Consult Criteria

- Refer to General Patient Criteria Protocol (page 22)
- Significant bleeding (notify physician promptly)
- Adult tachycardia
- SBP < 90 or relative hypotension (SBP < 110 with history of hypertension)
- Pediatric heart rate
  - 0–4 months ≥ 180
  - 5–7 months ≥ 175
  - 8–12 months ≥ 170
  - 1–3 years ≥ 160
  - 4–5 years ≥ 145
  - 6–8 years ≥ 130
  - 9–12 years ≥ 120
  - 13–15 years ≥ 115
  - 16 years or older ≥ 100

Notes

References:

Advanced Trauma Life Support

Saver JL. Stroke 2007;38(8):2279–2283

French KF, et al. Neurocrit Care 2012;17(1):107–111

Fugate JE, et al. Mayo Clin Proc, epub, April 28 2014

Hirsh J, Warkentin TE, Shaughnessy SG, et al. Chest 2001;119:64S-94S

Borgman J Trauma 2007: 63; 805

Chest 2012;141(2_suppl):e152S-e184S
JEM, Vol. 45, pg. 467

https://reference.medscape.com/drug/eliquis-apixaban-999805#5

https://reference.medscape.com/drug/xarelto-rivaroxaban-999670#5

https://reference.medscape.com/drug/pradaxa-dabigatran-342135#5

Hemorrhagic Shock in Emergency Medicine Guidelines
Updated: May 06, 2016 Author: William P Bozeman, MD; Chief Editor: Trevor John Mills, MD, MPH

Rossaint R, Bouillon B, Cerny V, Coats TJ, Duranteau J, Fernández-Mondéjar E, et al. The European guideline on management of major bleeding and coagulopathy following trauma: fourth edition. *Crit Care*. 2016 Apr 12. 20 (1):100

JEM, epub, 3/20319

Burn Protocol

When using any protocol, always follow the Guidelines of Proper Use (page 18).

Considerations

- In children consider child abuse
- Electrical burns may be much worse than suspected
- Evaluate airway and pulmonary system with enclosed building fire or with facial burns
- Consider possible carbon monoxide and cyanide poisoning in enclosed areas
- Difficult to tell difference between deep second degree burn and third degree burn
- Second degree deep partial thickness burn can become a third degree burn
- Body surface area (BSA) of burn use rule of 9's or the palmer surface of patient is approximately 1% BSA
- Rule of nines for BSA burned is for patients ≥10 years of age
- Depth of burn frequently underestimated
- Size of burn frequently overestimated
- Carbon monoxide (CO) has affinity for hemoglobin 230 times that of oxygen
    - Pulse oximetry not accurate in CO poisoning
    - Treat with 100% oxygen

Burn depth

First degree

- Epidermis only; no blisters
- Sensation — painful
- Bleeding on pinprick — brisk
- Appearance — light red and dry
- Blanching to pressure — brisk

Second degree superficial partial thickness

- Dermis involved with blisters
- Sensation — painful
- Bleeding on pinprick — brisk
- Appearance — moist and pink
- Blanching to pressure — slow return

Second degree deep partial thickness

- Dermis involved with blisters
- Sensation — dull

- Bleeding on pinprick — delayed
- Appearance — mottled pink or red; waxy white
- Blanching to pressure — none

Third degree full thickness

- Sensation — none
- No bleeding on pinprick
- Appearance — white, charred and dry
- Blanching to pressure — none

Fourth degree

- Involves muscle, fascia or bone

Thermal Burns

Evaluation

Enclosed space fire with smoke

- Airway evaluation
- O_2 saturation
- CO (carbon monoxide) level
- CBC
- BMP
- Chest x-ray
- Notify physician promptly

BSA burn < 10%

- Physical exam usually all that is needed if no smoke inhalation history or findings

Treatment options

- Clean with soap and water
- Cool burn with cold tap water
    - Decreases pain
    - Decreases depth and extent of injury
    - Do not use ice or ice water

Blister management

- Leave blisters intact ≤ 3 cm in size
    - Heals faster
- Totally debride any ruptured blisters
- May sterilely aspirate blisters > 3 cm

First degree burns

- Aloe vera and NSAIDs can be used for 1st burns

Superficial 2nd degree burns

- Topical antibiotic or absorptive occlusive dressing
  - Absorptive occlusive dressing is less painful and results in faster healing than antibiotic ointment

Deep 2nd and 3rd degree burns

- Topical antibiotic and refer to surgeon
- Silvadene (silver sulfadiazine) ointment qday for 5–7 days (not on face)
- Aquacel dressing superior to plain Silvadene in healing burns and reducing pain and may be used instead (releases silver sulfadiazine slowly)

Parkland formula for IV fluid resuscitation

- 4 ml NS x kg x % BSA burned in 24 hours
  - Give ½ IVF in first 8 hours
  - Give rest of NS in following 16 hours
  - If patient presents, for example, 2 hours after burn, then give first ½ of IVF in 6 hours (8 hours-2 hours)

Tetanus prophylaxis

- Tetanus toxoid (ADT) 0.5 cc IM if last dose > 5 years
- Tetanus immune globulin 250–500 units IM at different site if < 3 or unknown previous tetanus immunizations
- Refer to health department or primary care provider to complete tetanus primary vaccination series if < 2 vaccines given in past
  - See Tetanus Protocol (page 756)

Discharge criteria

- First degree burns
- Second degree superficial burns < 15% in adults and < 10% in children age 10 or less

Discharge instructions for burns

- Burn aftercare instructions
- Wash burn with soap and water qday and change dressing qday for 5–7 days
- Facial burns use triple antibiotic ointment or polysporin ointment 5–7 days
- Antibiotic PO or IM not usually needed

- Pain treatment with NSAID's and/or narcotics prn (hydrocodone, oxycodone)

Consult criteria

- Second degree superficial burns ≥ 10% in adults and 5% or greater in children
- Deep second degree and third degree burns unless extremely small (<2 cm)
- Burns involving hand; joints; perineum; genitalia; face; eyes; ears
- Comorbid conditions such diabetes, immunosuppression
- Circumferential burns
- Age < 12 months
- All inhalation injuries

Electrical Burns

Considerations

- Household electrical injury can be lethal
- Difficult to estimate degree of injury
- Causes tetany of muscles
- Traumatic injuries common (falls)

Compartment syndrome

- From increased pressure in a muscle or other internal compartment
- Not all signs and symptoms are needed to make diagnosis
- High pressures > 8 hours leads to tissue damage
- Normal tissue pressure is < 10 mm Hg
- Capillary blood flow is compromised at > 20 mm Hg
- Intracompartmental pressures > 30 mm Hg or within 10–30 mm Hg of DBP

Signs and symptoms (not diagnostic)

- Pain
  - Out of proportion to injury
  - On passive stretch of muscles
- Pallor
- Paresthesias
- Paralysis
  - Sensory and motor findings are late signs

- Poikilothermia — decreased temperature
- Pulselessness
    - Usually not lost until muscle necrosis has occurred
    - Last sign to develop
- Tense muscle compartment on palpation

Treatment

- Consult physician if suspected
- Keep extremity at level of heart
- Do not use ice if suspected
- Remove cast and padding
- Surgery fasciotomy is usually necessary

Evaluation

- Complete history and physical exam
- Degree of burn and voltage
- Length of time of electrical injury
- Neurologic exam
- EKG and monitor
- CBC
- BMP
- CPK
- U/A for myoglobin if hemoglobin dipstick positive
- Serum myoglobin if U/A positive for hemoglobin

Treatment options

- Treat skin burns same as thermal injuries
- IV NS 200 cc/hr. if significant burn injury or suspicion for significant injury for adults and 2 times maintenance rate for pediatrics
- Tetanus toxoid (ADT) 0.5 cc IM if last dose > 5 years
- Tetanus immune globulin 250–500 units IM different site if < 3 or unknown history of previous tetanus immunizations
- Refer to health department or primary care provider to complete tetanus primary vaccination series if < 2 vaccines given in past
    - See Tetanus Protocol (page 756)
- Pain treatment with NSAID's and/or narcotics prn

Discharge criteria

- Low voltage superficial injury
- Normal lab, EKG and vital signs
- Small burn area

- Follow up with primary care provider or plastic surgeon within 2–3 days

Discharge instructions for burns

- Wash burn with soap and water qday and change dressing qday for 5–7 days
- Burn aftercare instructions
- Facial burns use triple antibiotic ointment or polysporin ointment 5–7 days
- Antibiotic PO or IM not usually needed
- Pain treatment with NSAID's and/or narcotics prn (hydrocodone, oxycodone)

Consult criteria

- Loss of consciousness
- Neurologic abnormalities
- High voltage burns
- Abnormal lab, EKG or vital signs
- Large burns or suspected deep tissue injury
- Uncertainty of the extent of injury
- Suspected compartment syndrome

Chemical Burns

Considerations

- Alkali cause deeper injury
- Acids cause more superficial injury usually, depending on pH

Evaluation

- Usually all that is needed is history and physical exam for minor chemical burns

Treatment

- Remove chemical from skin
- Clean with soap and water
- Flush or soak with NS if alkali burn
- Pain treatment with NSAID's and/or narcotics prn

Hydrofluoric acid (HFl) burns

- Intense pain and tissue damage
- Use copious irrigation followed by calcium gluconate gel
- Subcutaneous calcium gluconate may be needed to relieve pain

- TBSA (total body surface area) burn > 5% needs admission to monitor for the development of hypocalcemia
    - If HFI concentration > 50% then 1% TBSA burn needs admission

Tetanus prophylaxis

- Tetanus toxoid (ADT) 0.5 cc IM if last dose > 5 years
- Tetanus immune globulin 250–500 units IM different site if < 3 or unknown history of previous tetanus immunizations
- Refer to health department or primary care provider to complete tetanus primary vaccination series if < 2 vaccines given in past
    - See Tetanus Protocol

Discharge criteria

- Minor chemical burns

Discharge instructions for burns

- Wash burn with soap and water qday and change dressing qday for 5–7 days
- Burn aftercare instructions
- Facial burns use triple antibiotic ointment or polysporin ointment 5–7 days
- Antibiotic PO or IM not usually needed
- Pain treatment with NSAID's and/or narcotics prn (hydrocodone, oxycodone)

Consult criteria

- Hydrofluoric acid burns
- Abnormal vital signs
- Diabetes or immunosuppression
- Second degree superficial burns ≥ 10% in adults and 5% or greater in children
- Second degree deep and third degree burns
- Burns involving hand, joints, perineum, genitalia
- Comorbid conditions such diabetes, immunosuppression

Vital sign and age consult criteria for all burn types

- Hypotension or relative hypotension (SBP < 105 with history of hypertension)
- Adult heart rate ≥ 110
- Pediatric heart rate

- 0–4 months ≥ 180
- 5–7 months ≥ 175
- 8–12 months ≥ 170
- 1–3 years ≥ 160
- 4–5 years ≥ 145
- 6–8 years ≥ 130
- 9–12 years ≥ 125
- 13–15 years ≥ 115
- 16 years or older ≥ 110

Notes

References:

Guyton AC. Combination of Hemoglobin with Carbonmonoxide. In. Textbook of Medical Physiology. 7th ed. W.B. Saunders Co; 1986:500

Thermal Injury Management

Author: Robert L Sheridan, MD; Chief Editor: Jorge I de la Torre, MD, FACS emedicine.medscape.com/article/1277941

Thermal Burns Author: Richard F Edlich, MD, PhD, FACS, FASPS, FACEP; Chief Editor: Jorge I de la Torre, MD, FACS emedicine.medscape.com/article/1278244

Extremity Disorders

Section Contents

When using any protocol, always follow the Guidelines of Proper Use (page 18).

Extremity Medical Disorder Protocol

When using any protocol, always follow the Guidelines of Proper Use (page 18).

Differential Diagnosis

Painful extremity swelling

- Deep venous thrombosis
- Arterial insufficiency
- Tendonitis, bursitis, and arthritis
- Cellulitis
- Abscess
- Septic arthritis
- Gout
- Radiculopathy
- Peripheral neuropathy

Nonpainful extremity swelling

- Congestive heart failure
- Hepatic cirrhosis
- Post-phlebitic syndrome

General Evaluation

- Complete history and physical exam
- Symptom(s) onset and exacerbating factors
- Associated symptoms
- Neurovascular exam
- Document whether Homan's sign and calf tenderness is positive or negative (Homan's sign not clinically useful, but decreases litigation if documented and is negative regardless of ultimate diagnosis)

Deep Venous Thrombosis (see VTE chapter)

Well's DVT criteria

- One point each:
    - Active cancer

    - Paralysis/recent cast immobilization
    - Recently bedridden > 3 days or surgery < 4 weeks
    - Deep vein tenderness
    - Entire leg edema
    - Calf swelling > 3 cm over other leg
    - Pitting edema > other calf
    - Collateral superficial veins
- Two points — alternative diagnosis less likely

High probability: ≥ 3 points

Moderate probability: 1–2 points

Low probability: 0 points

Evaluation

D-dimer (LIA method) — some methods currently in use not reliable

- Useful if negative at cutoff value to rule out DVT or PE
- Negative D-dimer with low to moderate probability Well's DVT score largely excludes venous thromboembolic disease
- Well's criteria high probability: order ultrasound scan regardless of D-dimer result
- Positive — not as useful as negative result which usually rules out VTE disease
    - Frequently positive with hospitalization in past month
    - Chronic bedridden or low activity state
    - Increasingly positive with age without significant acute disease process
        - D-dimer increases 10 mcg/L for every year over 50 years of age if the upper cutoff is 500 mcg/L (80 year old with d-dimer 700 mcg/L would be in the normal range)
        - If another assay used, then 2% increase/year over age 50 may be used to adjust upper limit for age
- CHF
- Chronic disease processes
- Edematous states

Well's DVT criteria > 1–2 with painful or swollen extremity

- Order D-dimer test (unless patient likely to have positive result regardless of DVT potential)
- Venous Doppler ultrasound of extremity (unless D-dimer negative)
- Coumadin (warfarin) therapy can cause falsely negative D-dimer

Discharge criteria

- Well's DVT criteria low probability
- Negative D-dimer (can be falsely negative with warfarin therapy)
- Negative ultrasound

Discharge instructions

- Leg pain aftercare instructions
- Follow up with primary care provider in 3–5 days if pain persists
- Return if worse

Consult criteria

- DVT diagnosis
- Suspected DVT diagnosis
- Severe pain

Peripheral Arterial Disease

- Pain worse with activity
- Risk factors same as with coronary disease

Ankle brachial index (ABI)

- Systolic blood pressure at ankle divided by systolic blood pressure in arm
- Normal 0.9–1.1
- Worsening PAD yields decreasing ABI
- Diabetes can interfere with test due to calcinosis

Discharge criteria

- Stable claudication
- Pain resolved
- ASA 81–325 mg PO each day
- Smoking cessation

- Refer to surgeon

Discharge instructions

- PAD aftercare instructions
- Follow up with PCP or general surgeon within 3–5 days

Consult criteria

- Continuous pain
- Severe pain as presenting complaint
- Limb discoloration
- Heart rate > 100
- Hypotension
- Absent pulse
- Decreased temperature to touch

Cellulitis and Abscess

- See Cellulitis and Abscess Protocols

Septic Arthritis

Differential diagnosis

- Cellulitis
- Gout
- Bursitis
- Osteomyelitis
- Rheumatoid arthritis
- Soft tissue injury
- Pseudogout

Considerations

- Rapid onset
- Usually one joint infected
- Joint is very painful; hot; red; fluctuant
- Signs of acute systemic illness may be present
- Fever, chills and sweats frequently present
- See Synovial Fluid Analysis if joint fluid obtained

Prosthetic joint infections

- Usually needs surgery and prolonged antibiotic treatment
- Early symptoms

        - Erythema, pain, swelling and delayed wound healing may be present
    - May occur years after surgery
        - May present with chronic pain and prosthesis looseness
    - Suspect if
        - Sinus tract present
        - Drainage from joint
        - Acute onset of pain
        - Chronic pain that develops after prosthetic surgery especially if there was a pain free period after surgery
        - History of wound healing problems or infection after surgery

Evaluation

- History and physical examination
    - Evaluate knee for range of motion as tolerated
- ESR or C-reactive protein (CRP) when diagnosis not clinically evident (significant false positive rate and is nonspecific)
    - Combination of ESR and CRP has better sensitivity and specificity
- CBC
- BMP if diabetic
- Knee films
    - May show other reasons for pain and can be used as a baseline after procedures
- Ultrasound can be considered
- Joint aspiration if provider experienced
- Joint fluid analysis — see specific protocol

Treatment

- Admission to hospital for drainage and antibiotics

Discharge criteria

- Only with physician consent

Consult criteria

- All septic joint or suspected septic joint patients

Gout

Differential diagnosis

- Cellulitis
- Septic arthritis
- Bursitis
- Osteomyelitis
- Rheumatoid arthritis
- Soft tissue injury
- Pseudogout

Considerations

- Crystal uric acid deposits in joints and tissues
- Most common cause of monoarticular arthritis age > 60
- Increased warmth, redness and joint swelling
- First metatarsophalangeal joint of foot 75% of cases — most common
- Joint fluid: 20,000–100,000 WBC; poor string and mucin clot test; no bacteria (pseudogout similar)
- Risk factors
    - Age > 40
    - Hypertension
    - Diuretics
    - Ethanol intake
    - Obesity
- Initially with urate lowering therapy there is an increase in acute gout attacks
    - Patients should be reassured that this is expected and they should not discontinue their new medications

Evaluation

- Clinical evaluation usually all that is needed
- If diagnosis uncertain: CBC, C-reactive protein, x-rays, joint aspiration

Treatment options (monotherapy)

- NSAID's high dose 5–10 days
- Narcotics IM or PO prn
- Prednisone 40–60 mg PO qday × 3–7 days

OR

- Dexamethasone 6 mg PO daily × 3–7 days

  OR

- Depomedrol (methylprednisolone acetate) 80–120 mg IM
- Can consider intra-articular steroids if attack involves 1–2 large joints – if experienced with joint injections
- Colchicine 2 tablets (1.2 mg) with a third tablet (0.6 mg) an hour later, then qday–bid until attack resolves
    - Only for acute attacks < 36 hours
    - Do not use if patient used colchicine within last 14 days
- Allopurinol 50–300 mg PO qday: adjusted for renal function; start after acute episode resolved

Severe attacks use combination of treatments

- Do not stop urate lowering therapy during an acute attack - symptoms would only worsen if it is stopped or adjusted
- Switch to another treatment or add a second treatment is < 20% improvement in pain score within 24 hours, or < 50% improvement in pain score > 24 hours

Discharge criteria

- Uncomplicated acute gout attack

Discharge instructions

- Gout aftercare instructions
- Follow up with primary care provider within 2–3 days if pain persists

Consult criteria

- Uncertain diagnosis
- Fever history or toxicity
- Tachycardia

Radiculopathy

Lumbar radiculopathy (sciatica)

- Complete history and physical examination
- Check reflexes, SLR (straight leg raise), and neurovascular exam

- Spinal cord compression signs
    - Urinary retention with overflow incontinence or voiding
    - Fecal incontinence and decreased rectal tone and perineal sensation (i.e., cauda equina syndrome — see Back Pain Protocol)
- Healthy non-elderly patients without direct blunt trauma usually need no tests
- Elderly frequently need spine films due to higher incidence of vertebral fractures
- Plain back/pelvic films may be needed in falls, MVC's, direct blunt trauma, depending on severity of injury mechanism
- U/A if renal disease suspected or significant injury mechanism
- D-dimer if aortic dissection considered
- CBC, C-RP (or ESR) for fever with isolated vertebral back pain only without associated symptoms or findings

CT scan of spine

- Compression fracture > 30%
- Burst fracture
- Posterior vertebral involvement
- For back pain out of proportion on exam

- MRI for spinal cord findings or symptoms

Treatment options

- NSAID's prn
- Short narcotic course prn for severe pain — avoid Demerol (meperidine)
- Preferable to minimize bed rest (limit bed rest to no more than 1–2 days if possible, unless a fracture is present)
- Avoid heavy lifting
- Muscle relaxants of questionable usefulness

Discharge Criteria

- Uncomplicated presentation and findings with ability to control pain and ambulate

Discharge instructions

- Back pain aftercare instructions

    - Refer to primary care provider
    - If HNP suspected: neurosurgery or orthopedic referral
    - Orthopedic referral for fractures

Consult Criteria

- Severe pain with inability to ambulate
- Progressive neurologic deficits
- Signs of cauda equina syndrome
    - Urinary retention is most common finding in cauda equina syndrome
    - Patients without urinary retention have an approximately 1/10,000 chance of having cauda equina syndrome
    - Normal rectal tone usually excludes cauda equina syndrome
    - Saddle numbness
    - Extreme weakness
- Signs of spinal cord impairment
- Evidence of infectious, vascular, or neoplastic etiologies
- Nontraumatic pediatric back pain
- Fracture
- New onset renal insufficiency or worsening renal insufficiency

Cervical Radiculopathy

Definition

- Compression on cervical spine nerve roots

Considerations

- C7 compression involved 60% of cases
- C6 compression involved 25% of cases
- Younger patients have HNP or injury causing foraminal impingement on nerve root
- Elderly have degenerative changes causing foraminal narrowing and nerve compression

Physical findings

Motor deficits

- C5 — weakness of shoulder abduction

- C6 — weakness of elbow flexion and wrist extension
- C7 — weakness of elbow extension and wrist flexion
- C8 — weakness of thumb extension and wrist ulnar deviation

Sensory dermatomes

- C6 — thumb
- C7 — middle finger
- C8 — little finger
- T1 — inner forearm
- T2 — upper inner arm

Deep tendon reflexes (DTR)

- Biceps DTR tests C5–C6
    - Antecubital fossa
- Brachioradialis reflex test C5–C6
    - Distal radius
- Triceps DTR tests C7–C8
    - Distal triceps tendon posterior and slightly above elbow

Evaluation

- History and physical examination
- Check reflexes, hand grip, shoulder strength and neurovascular exam
- Cervical spine films may be obtained
- Healthy non-elderly patients without direct blunt trauma usually need no tests

Treatment options

- Local ice therapy
- NSAID's
- Hydrocodone or oxycodone prn severe pain
- Semirigid cervical collar for 3–6 weeks
- Physical therapy
- Home exercises

Discharge criteria

- Most patients can be discharged home

Discharge instructions

- Cervical radiculopathy aftercare instructions

    - Referral to neurosurgeon or orthopedic spine surgeon within 7–14 days

Consult criteria

- Incapacitating pain
- Central spinal cord compression symptoms
    - Loss of anal sphincter tone
    - Loss of bladder control
    - Weakness of arms and legs
- Central cord syndrome
    - Arms weaker than legs

Peripheral Neuropathy (PN)

Definition

- Disorder of peripheral nerves

Causes

- Usually as a complication of diabetes or alcoholism
- HIV
- Lyme disease
- Guillain–Barre' syndrome
- Cancer (paraneoplastic syndromes)
- Hypothyroidism
- Herpes zoster
- Acute nerve root compression
- Renal failure
- Heavy metal poisoning (lead, etc.)
- Nutritional deficiency

Evaluation

- Complete history and physical exam
- Motor and sensory exam
    - Gross light touch and pinprick sensation
    - Vibratory sense; deep tendon reflexes
    - Strength testing and muscle atrophy
    - Dorsal pedal and posterior tibial pulses
    - Skin assessment
    - Tinel testing
    - Cranial nerve testing

- Usually no lab testing needed on chronic neuropathy
- Acute neuropathy warrants tests directed at possible causes
  - BMP
  - C-reactive protein
  - CBC
  - Lyme titers if indicated
  - TSH if indicated
  - Lead levels if suspected
  - Chest x-ray if sarcoidosis or lung cancer suspected
  - LP if Guillain–Barre' syndrome suspected

Treatment options

- Symptomatic pain treatment
  - NSAID's
  - Capsaicin cream (depletes and prevents reaccumulation of substance P)
  - Lidocaine tape
  - Gabapentin 900 mg/day initially, then increase as needed every 3 days up to 1800–3600 mg qday
  - Carbamazepine 100–200 mg qday, and may increase slowly up to 1200 mg/day as needed, if above does not work
  - Phenytoin (Dilantin)
  - Amitriptyline
  - Pregabalin
  - Duloxetine (Cymbalta) 60 mg qday
  - Citalopram (Celexa) 20–40 mg qday
- Treatment directed at underlying cause if possible

Discharge criteria

- Stable chronic peripheral neuropathy

Discharge instructions

- Peripheral neuropathy aftercare instructions
- Follow up with PCP or neurologist as needed for chronic PN
- Follow up for acute neuropathy within 1 day

Consult criteria

- Acute neuropathy from a high comorbidity disease process or from an unknown cause

Fibromyalgia

- Widespread chronic musculoskeletal pain and tenderness
- Associated with fatigue, sleep and mood disturbances
- Noninflammatory
- Cause unknown
- Famale most commonly
- Lab testing used to rule out other disorders

Treatment choices

- Mirtazapine 15–30 mg daily
- Amitriptyline 10 mg qHS, increase 5 mg q2weeks
- Desipramine (fewer anticholinergic side effects)
- Duloxetine 20–30 mg qAM, increase to 60 mg if needed (treat exhaustion)
- Pregabalin 30 mg qHS, may increase as tolerated
- Gabapentin 100 mg qHS, may increase slowly over time up to 300 mg to 600 mg tid as needed and tolerated

Nonpainful Extremity Swelling

- Treat underlying condition if feasible
- Elevation
- Compression hose
- Follow up with primary care provider
- Judicious diuretic short term use with caution

General Consult Criteria for Extremity Conditions

- Severe pain
- Acute and progressive arterial insufficiency
- Rapidly spreading rash or cellulitis
- Pain out of proportion to exam
- Crepitus or gas in tissues
- Systemic toxic appearance

- Hypotension or relative hypotension SBP < 105 in patient with hypertension history
- Necrotizing fasciitis or gas gangrene
- Large abscess
- Suspected bony involvement
- Immunocompromised

Vital signs and age consult criteria

- Fever ≥ 101°F (39°C) in cellulitis
- Age < 6 months or > 70 years old
- Adult heart rate ≥ 110
- SBP < 90 or relative hypotension (SBP < 105 with history of hypertension)
- O_2 Sat ≤ 94% on room air
- Moderate dyspnea
- Pediatric heart rate
  - 0–4 months ≥ 180
  - 5–7 months ≥ 175
  - 8–12 months ≥ 170
  - 1–3 years ≥ 160
  - 4–5 years ≥ 145
  - 6–8 years ≥ 130
  - 9–12 years ≥ 125
  - 13–15 years ≥ 115
  - 16 years or older ≥ 110

Lab consult criteria

- Adult: WBC > 15,000 or < 1,000 neutrophils
- Bandemia ≥ 15%
- Acute thrombocytopenia
- Acute anemia

Notes

References:

Osmon DR, et al. Clin Infect Dis 2013 Jan;56(1):1–10

Khanna D, et al. Arthritis Care Res 2012 Oct;64 (10):1447-61

Harrold L. Curr Opin Rheumatol 2013 May;25(3):304-9

Diabetic Neuropathy Author: Helen C Lin, MD;
Chief Editor: Romesh Khardori, MD, PhD, FACP
emedicine.medscape.com/article/1170337

Age-Adjusted D-Dimer Cutoff Levels to Rule Out Pulmonary Embolism: The Adjust-PE Study JAMA 2014;311(11):1117- 1124 doi:10.1001/jama.2014.2135

FRACTURE PROTOCOL

When using any protocol, always follow the Guidelines of Proper Use (page 18).

Considerations

- Complications
    - Neurovascular injury
    - Open fracture
    - Joint involvement
    - Ligament/tendon injury
    - Displaced and angulated
    - Compartment syndrome
    - Fat emboli — long bones
    - Avascular necrosis
    - Osteomyelitis
- Nondisplaced, closed simple long bone fractures usually can be splinted and discharged with orthopedic follow-up
    - Discuss with physician (except for simple nondisplaced torus fractures)

Compartment syndrome

- From increased pressure in a muscle or other internal compartment
- Not all signs and symptoms are needed to make diagnosis
- High pressures > 8 hours leads to tissue damage
- Normal tissue pressure is < 10 mm Hg
- Capillary blood flow is compromised at > 20 mm Hg
- Intracompartmental pressures > 30 mm Hg or within 10–30 mm Hg of DBP

Signs and symptoms (not diagnostic)

- Pain
    - Out of proportion to injury
    - On passive stretch of muscles
- Pallor
- Paresthesias
- Paralysis

    - Sensory and motor findings are late signs
  - Poikilothermia — decreased temperature
  - Pulselessness
    - Usually not lost until muscle necrosis has occurred
    - Last sign to develop
  - Tense muscle compartment on palpation

Treatment

  - Consult physician if suspected
  - Keep extremity at level of heart
  - Do not use ice if suspected
  - Remove cast and padding
  - Surgery fasciotomy is usually necessary

Evaluation

- History of injury
- Past history
- Medication history
- Associated symptoms and complete physical exam
- X-rays of affected areas
- Neurovascular/tendon/ligament exam
- Assess for compartment syndrome
- Assess for open fracture or joint

Vertebral Fractures

Considerations

- Compression fractures commonly seen in the elderly secondary to osteoporosis
- Can be pathologic from cancer
- Point tenderness common at fracture site
- May be caused by high impact

Evaluation

- History and physical examination
- Plain films
- CT scan of affected area may be needed for diagnosis
- CT scan for compression fractures ≥ 30% or any posterior element spinal canal involvement

- CT scan of entire spine for acute neurologic complaints or deficits
- Assess for other injuries
- CBC and U/A for significant mechanism of injury

Treatment options

- Pain control with narcotics usually — PO, IM or IV
    - May try ibuprofen 400–600 mg with acetaminophen 650–1000 mg qid PO prn (more pain relief than hydrocodone 5 mg PO)
- Spine immobilization for neurologic complaints or findings
- Elective vertebroplasty
- Early ambulation as tolerated

Discharge criteria

- Uncomplicated vertebral compression fractures < 30% in osteoporosis patients without significant mechanism of injury
- Patient able to ambulate with or without walker or crutches

Discharge instructions

- Vertebral compression aftercare instructions
- Follow up with neurosurgeon or orthopedic surgeon within 7 days

Consult criteria

- Consult physician for compression fractures > 10%
- Acute neurologic deficits or complaints
- Unable to ambulate
- Uncontrollable severe pain
- Posterior element or spinal canal involvement
- Noncompression–type vertebral fractures
- Significant mechanism of injury

Clavicle Fractures

Considerations

- Most common fracture in children
- 80% middle third
- 15% distal third
- 5% proximal third

- May need CT scan for sternoclavicular injuries
- Patients older than 12 years with more than 2 cm of displacement of fracture fragments should be referred to orthopedics for consideration of operative repair
    - Younger children are excluded due to having more effective remodeling

Treatment

- Sling for middle and distal end fractures for 4–8 weeks; acromioclavicular sprain and separation
- Proximal sternoclavicular fractures and dislocations, consult physician
- Posterior sternoclavicular dislocation — notify physician promptly if available
    - May have stridor or respiratory distress
    - May have venous congestion of head or neck or affected arm

Posterior sternoclavicular dislocation treatment

- 3–4 inch roll between scapula and spine to extend or open up affected sternoclavicular joint
- Abduct affected shoulder to 90° and extend shoulder to 15° and apply traction with assistant holding trunk still
- If above fails, maintain traction and manually grasp clavicle and pull forward
- Consult orthopedic surgeon for sternoclavicular dislocations

- NSAID's (very effective in children); narcotics prn

Discharge criteria

- Uncomplicated clavicle fracture

Discharge instructions

- Clavicle fracture aftercare instructions
- Referral to orthopedics or PCP within 7–10 days

Consult criteria

- Immediate physician consultation for suspected posterior sternoclavicular joint dislocation
- Neurovascular injury

Scapular Fractures

Considerations

- Can occur with significant trauma to trunk and other injuries
- Evaluate for associated injuries
- Type 1: body of scapula
- Type 2: coracoid and acromion
- Type 3: neck and glenoid
- Shoulder x-rays needed
- CT may be needed if going to surgery for repair

Treatment options

Type 1

- Sling
- Analgesics
- Consult physician

Type 2 and 3

- Per physician and orthopedic consultation

Discharge criteria

- Uncomplicated Type 1 scapular fracture

Discharge instructions

- Scapular fracture aftercare instructions
- Follow up with trauma or thoracic surgeon within 5–10 days

Consult criteria

- Type 2 and 3 scapular fractures
- For any significant associated injuries
- Discuss all scapular fractures with physician prior to discharge

Humerus Fractures

Considerations

- Fall on outstretched hand frequent cause
- Usually elderly
- Younger patients with epiphyseal injuries of growth plate
- Shoulder tense and swollen

- Obtain AP and lateral shoulder x-rays
- Evaluate for neurovascular injury
- Proximal humerus – Axillary nerve
- Humeral shaft – Radial nerve

Treatment

- Sling
- Physical therapy
- Narcotics prn
- May try ibuprofen 400–600 mg with acetaminophen 650–1000 mg qid PO prn (more pain relief than hydrocodone 5 mg PO)
- Children can take Tylenol prn

Discharge criteria

- Uncomplicated and minimally displaced proximal closed humerus fracture

Discharge instructions

- Humerus fracture aftercare instructions
- Orthopedic referral within 7 days

Consult criteria

- Orthopedic consultation for severely angulated or comminuted fracture
- Orthopedic consult for pediatric humerus fractures
- Discuss with physician all humerus fractures prior to discharge

Shoulder, Hip, Knee, Wrist, Elbow, and Ankle Dislocations

- Analgesics
- Evaluate for associated injuries
- Consult physician

Rib Fractures – Isolated

Considerations

- First and second rib fractures associated with high impact and significant mechanism of injury

Evaluation

- Complete history and physical examination

- Chest x-ray
- Rib films
- Chest CT scan needed for significant mechanism of injury and/or abnormal vital signs or hypoxia
- Ultrasound can detect subtle rib fractures
- U/A to check for kidney injury in low posterior rib fractures
- Evaluate for associated injuries

Treatment options

- Narcotics prn
- NSAID's prn
    - May try ibuprofen 400–600 mg with acetaminophen 650–1000 mg qid PO prn (more pain relief than hydrocodone 5 mg PO)
- Rib belt not recommended due to causing atelectasis and pneumonia

Discharge criteria

- Simple 1 or 2 rib fractures
- No pulmonary abnormality (pulmonary contusion or pneumothorax)

Discharge instructions

- Rib fracture aftercare instructions
- Follow up with PCP or trauma surgeon within 7–10 days

Consult criteria

- If more than 2 ribs fractured
- Pulmonary abnormality on chest imaging
- Hypoxia or respiratory distress

Forearm Fractures

Torus fractures of distal forearm

- Splint and sling
- Analgesics
- Torus fracture aftercare instructions
- Orthopedic referral within 10 days

Colles, Smith and Barton's fractures

- Consult physician
- Respective fracture aftercare instructions

- OCL sugar tong splint and sling for Colles fracture if discharged
- Analgesics

Radius and ulnar midshaft fractures

- Consult physician

Elbow Fractures

Considerations

- X-ray may or may not show radial head fractures
- Anterior or posterior fat pad sign on x-ray is from blood from fracture or sprain pushing on the fat pad
- Posterior fat pad associated more frequently with fracture

Evaluation

- Elbow x-ray
- Neurovascular examination
- Assess for associated injuries

Treatment options

- Sling
- OCL posterior splint may be needed
- Analgesics prn
- May try ibuprofen 400–600 mg with acetaminophen 650–1000 mg qid PO prn (more pain relief than hydrocodone 5 mg PO)

Discharge criteria

- Nondisplaced simple proximal radius fracture
- X-ray reveals fat pad sign without obvious fracture

Discharge instructions

- Elbow fracture aftercare instructions
- Inform patient and family that the x-ray shows a fat pad sign that may indicate a fracture present, even if no fracture seen at that time
- Follow up with orthopedic surgeon within 10 days

Consult criteria

- Proximal ulnar fracture
- Distal humerus fracture
- Supracondylar fracture
- Neurovascular deficits
- Neurologic complaints

Metacarpal Fractures

Nondisplaced, nonangulated transverse fracture

Evaluation

- X-ray
- Neurovascular exam

Treatment

- Dorsal splint for 3–4 weeks
- Sling
- Analgesics prn

Discharge criteria

- Simple closed fracture

Discharge instructions

- Metacarpal fracture aftercare instructions
- Follow up with orthopedic or hand surgeon within 7–10 days

Consult criteria

- Open fracture
- Neurovascular deficit or complaint

Transverse, angulated and displaced fracture

- Consult physician

Spiral or oblique fracture

- Consult physician

Hip and Femur Fractures

- Consult physician
- Pain control

Patella

Fracture

Nondisplaced with extensor function intact

Evaluation

- Knee x-ray with sunrise view
- Assess neurovascular status

Treatment

- Knee immobilizer
- Analgesics
- Crutches

Discharge criteria

- Closed simple patella fracture with intact extensor function

Discharge instructions

- Patella fracture aftercare instructions
- Orthopedic referral

Consult criteria

- Displaced > 3 mm or extensor function loss

Dislocation

Evaluation

- Same as patella fracture

Treatment

- Reduce dislocation
- Knee immobilizer
- Analgesics

Discharge criteria

- Closed simple reduced patella fracture

Discharge instructions

- Patella dislocation aftercare instructions
- Orthopedic follow-up within 10 days

Consult criteria

- Nonreducible patellar dislocation

Tibial Plateau and Midshaft Fractures

Considerations

- Tibial plateau fractures may be difficult to see on plain x-ray
- CT scan of knee frequently reveals a more extensive fracture than plain film

Evaluation

- Knee or tibial/fibula x-ray
- CT scan of knee may be needed or requested for tibial plateau fractures
- Neurovascular examination
- Assess for associated injuries

Treatment

- Pain control IM or IV
- Splint knee in extension for tibial plateau fracture
- Splint lower leg if needed prior to physician exam

Consult criteria

- Discuss with physician all tibial fractures

Fibula Proximal, Midshaft and Displaced Distal Fractures

Evaluation

- X-ray
- Neurovascular examination
- Assess for associated injuries

Treatment

- Pain control IM or IV
- Splint as needed

Consult criteria

- Discuss these fractures with a physician

Nondisplaced Distal Fibula Fracture

Evaluation

- X-ray
- Neurovascular examination

- Assess for associated injuries
- Ligament examination as tolerated

Treatment

- Walking boot
- Crutches
- Analgesics

Discharge criteria

- Simple closed nondisplaced fibular fracture
- Normal neurovascular examination

Discharge instructions

- Ankle sprain and distal fibular fracture aftercare instructions
- Follow up with orthopedic surgeon within 7–10 days

Consult criteria

- Neurovascular injury
- Open fracture

Knee Strain

- See Knee Soft Tissue Injury Protocol

Foot Fractures and Dislocations

Tarsal or midfoot

- Consult physician
- Analgesics

Metatarsal fractures

Nondisplaced

- Boot
- Crutches
- Analgesics
- Orthopedic referral

Displaced

- Consult physician

Calcaneus fractures

- Posterior splint
- Analgesics prn

- Consult physician

Toe fractures

- Buddy tape to adjacent toe with padding between toes
- Cast shoe
- Significantly displaced fractures consult physician

Consult Criteria

- Acute neurovascular deficits or injury
- Suspected compartment syndrome
- Nonreducible dislocations
- Open fractures, joints or dislocations

Notes

References:

Orthopaedics Primary Care by Chinni Pennathur Ramamurti

Am J Emerg Med 2012;30: 606–614

J Pediatr Orthop 2010;30:307–312

Sternoclavicular Joint Injury Treatment & Management
Author: John P Rudzinski, MD, FACEP; Chief Editor: Rick Kulkarni, MD emedicine.medscape.com/article/828642

Rib Fracture Treatment & Management
Author: Sarah L Melendez, MD; Chief Editor: Rick Kulkarni, MD emedicine.medscape.com/article/825981

Foot Fracture Treatment & Management
Author: Robert Silbergleit, MD; Chief Editor: Rick Kulkarni, MD emedicine.medscape.com/article/825060

Surgical versus conservative interventions for treating fractures of the middle third of the clavicle

Mário Lenza, Rachelle Buchbinder,Renea V Johnston, João Carlos elloti" Flávio Faloppa Cochrane Library 10 MAR 2013

DOI: 10.1002/14651858.CD009363.pub2

Salter Harris Fracture Protocol

When using any protocol, always follow the Guidelines of Proper Use (page 18).

Definition

- Disruption of the cartilaginous plates of the physeal area or growth plate that may or may not involve a fracture of the adjacent bone in children

Salter Pneumonic

- Salter 1 — **S**lip of growth plate
- Salter 2 — **A**bove (fracture extends above growth plate)
- Salter 3 — **L**ow (fracture extends below growth plate)
- Salter 4 — **T**hrough (fracture above and below plate)
- Salter 5 — **E**ntire (crush fracture of growth plate area)
- Salter 6 — **R**ing (injury to the perichondral ring or periosteum)

Considerations

- The cartilage growth plate can be weaker than ligaments in children
- Sprains in children can actually be Salter 1 fractures that are not evident on initial x-ray
- Plain x-rays may depict widening of growth plate as only sign of a fracture
- Comparison x-rays of uninjured opposite extremity can be helpful with Salter 1 fractures
- CT scans may be necessary to delineate degree of injury in severely comminuted Salter fractures
- Growth acceleration (uncommon) or growth arrest can occur with Salter fractures
- Long term follow-up at 6 and 12 months important
- Salter 1 fracture of the great toe with subungual hematoma represents an open fracture

Growth plate (physeal) fractures at increased risk of growth arrest are

- Distal femur
- Distal tibia
- Distal radius and ulna
- Proximal tibia
- Triradiate cartilage — acetabulum in children

Evaluation

- History of injury
- Examination for neurovascular and tendon injuries
- Examination for remote undisclosed injuries
- X-ray of injured area
- Comparison x-rays if needed of opposite uninjured extremity

Treatment

- Most Salter 1 and 2 fractures can be treated, if mildly displaced, with reduction if needed and splinting and follow-up in 7–10 days
- Salter 3 and 4 usually require open reduction and fixation
- Salter 5 fractures are rarely diagnosed acutely and treatment is usually delayed because of the delay in diagnosis
- Antibiotics for great toe Salter fractures with subungual hematoma that are discharged — Augmentin (amoxicillin/clavulanate) or cephalosporin
    - Considered an open fracture (preferable to discuss with physician)
- Pain medications as needed

Discharge Criteria

- Nondisplaced Salter 1 and 2 fractures
- Reduced Salter 1 and 2 fractures

Discharge instructions

- Salter Harris fracture aftercare instructions
- Follow up in 7–10 days preferably with orthopedic surgeon

- Instructions in various pediatric "sprains" that could be a nondisplaced Salter 1 fracture

Consult Criteria

- Displaced Salter fractures
- Open Salter fractures
- Neurovascular deficits
- Tendon deficits
- Salter 3–6 fractures

Notes

References:

Salter R, Harris W. Injuries involving the epiphyseal plate. J Bone Joint Surg. 1963 45A: p. 587–621

Orthopaedics Primary Care by Chinni Pennathur Ramamurti

SYNOVIAL FLUID ANALYSIS

When using any protocol, always follow the Guidelines of Proper Use (page 18).

Normal

- Transparent clarity
- Clear color
- WBC < 200/ml
- PMN's < 25%
- Culture negative
- No crystals
- Mucin clot firm
- Glucose approximates blood levels

Noninflammatory

- Transparent clarity
- Yellow color
- WBC 200–2000/ml
- PMN's < 25%
- Culture negative
- No crystals
- Mucin clot firm
- Glucose approximates blood levels
- Associated conditions: rheumatic fever, trauma, osteoarthritis

Inflammatory

- Cloudy clarity
- Yellow color
- WBC 200–50,000/ml
- PMN's > 50%
- Culture negative
- Crystals can be present if gout or pseudogout are etiology
- Mucin clot friable
- Glucose decreased
- Associated conditions: SLE, Lyme disease, gout, pseudogout, spondyloarthropathies

Septic

- Cloudy clarity
- Yellow color
- WBC 25,000/ml to often > 100,000/ml
- PMS's > 50%
- Culture often positive
- No crystals
- Mucin clot friable
- Glucose very decreased
- Fever
- C-reactive protein elevated

Notes

Reference:

Septic Arthritis Surgery Author: Gabriel Munoz, MD; Chief Editor: Harris Gellman, MD
medicine.medscape.com/article/1268369

SHOULDER PROTOCOL

When using any protocol, always follow the Guidelines of Proper Use (page 18).

Shoulder conditions

Impingement syndrome encompasses

- Supraspinatus tendonitis
- Bicipital tendonitis
- Subacromial bursitis

Supraspinatus tendonitis

- Middle aged
- Subacute or chronic pain in shoulder
- Top of shoulder tender distal to acromion
- Abduction beyond 80–120 degrees limited from pain
- X-rays may be normal or show erosions and calcifications in tendon

Bicipital tendonitis

- Pain in anterior shoulder
- Tenderness along long head of biceps and bicipital groove
- Flexion painful with elbow extended
- Rotation restricted by pain
- Flexion against resistant causes pain

Subacromial bursitis

- Least common of shoulder musculotendinous cuff disorders
- Most painful and acute of the 3 impingement disorders
- Any movement of shoulder causes pain
- Shoulder diffusely tender
- May have fever and elevated ESR

Treatment Options

- Severe pain — rest in sling short-term
- Ice packs with severe pain
- NSAID's prn

- Gravity-assisted range of motion pendulum exercises started in hours to days
- Physical therapy
- 1 cc of Depomedrol (methylprednisolone acetate) 40–80 mg/cc or Kenalog (triamcinolone) 10–20 mg/cc mixed with 1 cc of 1–2% plain lidocaine, injected through normal skin if Provider is experienced performing injections

Discharge Criteria

- Uncomplicated case

Discharge instructions

- Shoulder tendonitis and bursitis aftercare instructions
- Referral to primary care provider or orthopedics if pain persists in 7–10 days

Consult Criteria

- Suspected septic shoulder joint

Thoracic outlet syndrome

- Compression of the neurovascular bundle as it passes out of the thoracic outlet above first rib and behind the clavicle
- May be associated with a cervical rib

3 types of thoracic outlet syndrome

Neurologic (most common)

- C8 and T1 roots most commonly affected
- Pain is in medial arm, forearm, and ring and fifth fingers
- Nocturnal paresthesias
- Weakness
- Cold intolerance
- Neck pain (trapezius)
- Occipital headache
- Anterior chest wall pain
- Raynaud's phenomenon

Venous

- Extremity
    - Swelling
    - Cyanosis

- Paresthesias

Arterial (most serious and least common)

- Pain
- Coldness
- Numbness
- Pallor
- Seen in young patients with vigorous activity history
- Seen with emboli

Examination

- Provocative tests not reliable

Elevated arm stress test (EAST)

- Most reliable for all three types
- Arms at 90° to body and elbow flexed 90°
    - Hands opened and closed for 3 minutes
- Symptom reproduction is a positive test

Adson's test

- Palpate both radial arteries while patient turns head side to side
- Loss of pulse positive for arterial type

Testing options

- Chest x-ray for cervical rib and pulmonary disease
- Cervical spine
- Duplex scan of arm

Treatment outpatient options

- NSAID's with or without acetaminophen
- Narcotics prn
- Tricyclic antidepressants for chronic pain

Vascular (arterial and venous) outlet obstruction

- Immediate heparinization
- Emergent vascular surgery consultation

Discharge criteria

- Benign presentation

Discharge instructions

- Thoracic outlet aftercare instructions
- Refer to thoracic surgeon

Consult criteria

- Arterial and venous insufficiency
- Severe pain
- Severe neurologic deficit
- Suspected spinal cord etiology

Rotator Cuff Tear (RCT)

Considerations

- 90% with minimal or no injury
- Tenderness of middle third of shoulder
- Unable to abduct shoulder in massive tears
- Weak abduction and pain with minor tears
- Palpable crepitus with movements
- Painless or tolerable passive abduction
- Atrophy with long standing RCT

Treatment options

- Severe pain — rest in sling short term
- Ice packs with severe pain
- NSAID's prn with or without acetaminophen
- Narcotics prn
- Gravity-assisted range of motion pendulum exercises started in hours to days
- Physical therapy
- Local lidocaine injection 2 cc prn through normal skin (if Provider has experience with injections)
- No steroid injections

Discharge criteria

- Uncomplicated injury

Discharge instructions

- Rotator cuff tear aftercare instructions
- Referral to orthopedics for major RCT tear within 7 days

Consult criteria

- Discuss major tears with physician

Acromioclavicular (AC) Injuries

Acromioclavicular sprain

- Partial tear of capsule of AC joint

- Usually in young or middle aged with injury to AC joint
- AC joint tender and may be slightly swollen
- Attempted abduction > 60 degrees causes pain
- X-rays show normal AC joint

Treatment

- Sling initially
- Early motion encouraged
- Avoid hyperabduction for 3 weeks
- Avoid heavy lifting for 6 weeks
- Ice packs
- NSAID's prn; narcotics prn

Discharge criteria

- Uncomplicated injury

Discharge instructions

- AC sprain aftercare instructions
- Primary care provider or orthopedic follow up within 10–14 days

Acromioclavicular subluxation

- Complete tear of AC joint capsule
- AC joint markedly swollen
- Outer end of clavicle may protrude slightly upward
- Attempted abduction > 60 degrees causes pain
- X-rays without weights may be normal
- X-rays with 10–lb. weights show widened AC joint

Treatment

- Sling initially
- Early motion encouraged
- Avoid hyperabduction > 90 degrees for 3–4 weeks
- Avoid heavy lifting for 2 months
- Ice packs
- NSAID's prn; narcotics prn

Discharge criteria

- Uncomplicated injury

Discharge instructions

- AC injury aftercare instructions
- Primary care provider or orthopedic follow up within 10–14 days

Consult criteria

- Complicated injury
- Neurovascular injury or complaints

Notes

References:

Orthopaedics Primary Care by Chinni Pennathar Ramamurti

Rotator Cuff Disease Author: André Roy, MD, FRCPC; Chief Editor: Rene Cailliet, MD
emedicine.medscape.com/article/328253

Thoracic Outlet Syndrome in Emergency Medicine Clinical Presentation Author: Andrew K Chang, MD; Chief Editor: David FM Brown, MD
medicine.medscape.com/article/760477

SHOULDER AND ARM TRAUMA PROTOCOL

When using any protocol, always follow the Guidelines of Proper Use (page 18).

General Evaluation

- History of injury; past history; medication history
- Associated symptoms and complete physical exam
- X-rays
- Neurovascular/tendon/ligament exam
- Assess for compartment syndrome
- Assess for open fracture or open joint

Acromioclavicular (AC) Injuries

Acromioclavicular sprain

- Partial tear of capsule of AC joint
- Usually in young or middle aged with injury to AC joint
- AC joint tender and may be slightly swollen
- Attempted abduction > 60 degrees causes pain
- X-rays show normal AC joint

Treatment

- Sling initially
- Early motion encouraged
- Avoid hyperabduction for 3 weeks
- Avoid heavy lifting for 6 weeks
- Ice packs
- NSAID's prn; narcotics prn

Discharge criteria

- Uncomplicated injury

Discharge instructions

- AC sprain aftercare instructions
- Primary care provider or orthopedic follow-up within 10–14 days

Acromioclavicular subluxation

- Complete tear of AC joint capsule
- AC joint markedly swollen
- Outer end of clavicle may protrude slightly upward
- Attempted abduction > 60 degrees causes pain
- X-rays without weights may be normal
- X-rays with 10–lb. weights show widened AC joint

Treatment

- Sling initially
- Early motion encouraged
- Avoid hyperabduction > 90 degrees for 3–4 weeks
- Avoid heavy lifting for 2 months
- Ice packs
- NSAID's prn; narcotics prn

Discharge criteria

- Uncomplicated injury

Discharge instructions

- AC injury aftercare instructions
- Primary care provider or orthopedic follow-up within 10–14 days

Consult criteria

- Complicated injury
- Neurovascular injury or complaints

Clavicle Fractures

Considerations

- Most common fracture in children
- 80% middle third
- 15% distal third
- 5% proximal third
- May need CT scan for sternoclavicular injuries

Treatment

- Sling
  - Middle and distal end fractures for 4–8 weeks
  - Acromioclavicular sprain and separation

- Patients older than 12 years with more than 2 cm of displacement of fracture fragments should be referred to orthopedics for consideration of operative repair
    - Younger children are excluded due to having more effective remodeling
- Proximal sternoclavicular fractures and dislocations — consult physician
- Posterior sternoclavicular dislocation — notify physician promptly if available
    - Needs immediate reduction to prevent life threatening complications
    - May have stridor or respiratory distress
    - May have venous congestion of head or neck or affected arm

Posterior sternoclavicular dislocation treatment

- 3–4 inch roll between scapula and spine to extend or open up affected sternoclavicular joint
- Abduct affected shoulder to 90° and extend shoulder to 15° and apply traction with assistant holding trunk still
- If above fails, maintain traction and manually grasp clavicle and pull forward
- Consult orthopedic surgeon for sternoclavicular dislocations

- NSAID's (very effective in children); narcotics prn

Discharge criteria

- Uncomplicated clavicle fracture

Discharge instructions

- Clavicle fracture aftercare instructions
- Follow up with PCP or orthopedic surgeon within 10 days

Consult criteria

- Immediate physician consultation for suspected posterior sternoclavicular joint dislocation

Scapular Fractures

Considerations

- Can occur with significant trauma to trunk and other injuries
- Evaluate for associated injuries
- Type 1: body of scapula
- Type 2: coracoid and acromion
- Type 3: neck and glenoid

Evaluation

- Shoulder x-rays
- Chest x-ray
- CT may be needed if going to surgery for repair

Treatment

Type 1

- Sling
- Analgesics
- Consult physician

Type 2 and 3

- Physician and orthopedic consultation

Discharge criteria

- Uncomplicated Type 1 scapular fracture

Discharge instructions

- Scapular fracture aftercare instructions
- Follow up with trauma or thoracic surgeon within 5–10 days

Consult criteria

- Type 2 and 3 scapular fractures
- For any significant associated injuries
- Discuss all scapular fractures with physician prior to discharge

Humerus Fractures

Considerations

- Fall on outstretched hand
- Usually elderly

- Younger patients with epiphyseal injuries of growth plate
- Shoulder tense and swollen
- Obtain AP and lateral shoulder x-rays
- Evaluate for neurovascular injury
  - Proximal humerus: axillary nerve (test deltoid sensation)
  - Humeral shaft: radial nerve (test for wrist drop and 1st web space sensation loss)

Treatment

- Sling
- Physical therapy
- Narcotics prn
- Ibuprofen 400–600 mg tid–qid with or without acetaminophen 650–1000 mg PO prn adult dosing
- Children may take prn
- Orthopedic referral within 7 days

Discharge criteria

- Uncomplicated and minimally displaced proximal closed humerus fracture

Discharge instructions

- Humerus fracture aftercare instructions
- Orthopedic referral within 7 days

Consult criteria

- Orthopedic consultation for severely angulated or comminuted fracture
- Orthopedic consult for pediatric humerus fractures
- Discuss with physician all humerus fractures prior to discharge

Shoulder (Glenohumeral) Dislocation

Considerations

Anterior dislocation

- Most common: 95–97%
- Axillary nerve most common neurovascular injury
  - Assess with pinprick over lateral shoulder

- Median and ulnar injuries rare
    - Median nerve
        - Decreased sensation to thumb
        - Index and middle finger sensation impaired
        - Thumb opposition weak
    - Ulnar nerve
        - Decreased sensation and weakness of 4th and 5th fingers
        - Abduction and adduction of 4th and 5th fingers very weak or impossible to perform
        - Flexion of the 4th and 5th metacarpophalangeal joints with interphalangeal joints extended is weak or impossible to perform
- Patient holds arm adjacent to body
- Any motion causes severe pain
- Rounded shoulder contour is lost
- Hill-Sachs humeral head deformity present in 50%: no treatment
- Bankart fracture — glenoid rim fracture

Posterior dislocation

- 2–4% of dislocations
- Occurs with seizures, direct anterior shoulder trauma and falls on outstretched hand
- Arm held across chest
- External rotation blocked
- X-ray can be deceptive — less overlap of humeral head and glenoid on AP view

Luxatio Erecta (inferior dislocation)

- 0.5% of glenohumeral dislocations
- Arm held over head
- High complication rate
- 60% neurological injury — most commonly axillary nerve
- Rotator cuff tear > 50%

Evaluation

- Neurovascular exam
- Shoulder x-ray AP and lateral (or Y-view)

Treatment options

- Conscious sedation frequently needed (consult physician)
- Sling for 3–6 weeks in younger patients
- Sling for 1–2 weeks in age > 40 years
- Faster healing and decreased recurrence if arm in 15 degrees external rotation (may be hard to accomplish)
- Aspiration of hemarthrosis and instillation of lidocaine 1% for return visit in 24–48 hours from painful hemarthrosis

Anterior dislocations

External Rotation method

- Patient supine
- Adduct arm and flex 90° at elbow
- Slowly rotate arm externally
- Reduce shoulder before reaching coronal plane

Scapular rotation

- Patient prone
- 5–15 pounds of hanging weights
- Rotate inferior scapula medially and superior scapula laterally

OR

- Patient sitting
- Assistant provides traction on wrist with other hand pushing against chest
- Rotate inferior scapula medially and superior scapula laterally

Traction-counter traction (Modified Hippocratic Technique)

- Sheet over flexed forearm and tied around Provider's waist with counter traction with sheet around axilla by assistant
- Be careful of injuring brachial plexus
- Gentle internal and external rotation with traction by Provider

Stimson technique

- Patient in prone position and secured from falling off table
- Arm hanging off table with axilla and brachial plexus protected
- 20 lb. weights taped or attached to forearm or wrist/hand
- Wait 20 minutes
- Shoulder will usually reduce or will need minimal traction at the 20 minute timeframe
- Can be done without sedation or pain treatment occasionally

Posterior dislocations

- Traction along long axis of arm with anterior pressure on posterior shoulder

Luxatio Erecta (inferior dislocation)

- Overhead traction in upward and outward direction on arm with counter traction towards feet with sheet on injured shoulder

Discharge criteria

- Uncomplicated dislocation

Discharge instructions

- Shoulder dislocation aftercare instructions
- Refer to orthopedic surgeon within 7–10 days
- Wear sling for 3 weeks
- Patients > 50 years need early follow up for early mobilization and to avoid shoulder stiffness

Consult criteria

- Discuss all shoulder dislocations with physician
- Neurovascular injury
- Compartment syndrome
- Orthopedic consult if irreducible dislocation
- Orthopedic consult if associated fracture excluding Hill-Sachs deformity

Notes

References:

Ufberg J, McNamara R. Management of common dislocations. *Clinical Procedures in Emergency Medicine*, 4th ed. pp 946–963

Sternoclavicular Joint Injury Treatment & Management
Author: John P Rudzinski, MD, FACEP; Chief Editor: Rick Kulkarni, MD emedicine.medscape.com/article/828642

Surgical versus conservative interventions for treating fractures of the middle third of the clavicle
Mário Lenza, Rachelle Buchbinder,Renea V Johnston, João Carlos elloti'' Flávio Faloppa Cochrane Library 10 MAR 2013
DOI: 10.1002/14651858.CD009363.pub2

Orthopaedics Primary Care by Chinni Pennathur Ramamurti

Itoi E, Hatakeyama Y, Kido T, et al: A new method of immobilization after traumatic anterior dislocation of the shoulder: a preliminary study, J Shoulder Elbow Surg 2003;12:413–415

Handoll HH, Gibson JN, Madhok R. Interventions for treating proximal humeral fractures in adults. Cochrane Database Syst Rev 2004;4:CD000434. (Systematic review)

Trimmings NP. Haemarthrosis aspiration in treatment of anterior dislocation of the shoulder. *J R Soc Med*1985;78:1023–7

ELBOW PROTOCOL

When using any protocol, always follow the Guidelines of Proper Use (page 18).

Considerations

- Tendonitis is usually from overuse
- "Tennis elbow" is most common elbow complaint orthopedists see

Lateral Epicondylitis ("Tennis Elbow")

- Chronic overuse syndrome
- Occupations that require a rotary motion at the elbow
- Increased with grasping motions (handshake) or twisting motions
- Point tenderness over lateral epicondyle
- X-rays usually normal
- Ice or heat — whichever provides the greatest relief

Treatment options

- Elimination of offending activity
- Rest
- NSAID's prn
- Tylenol prn
- Splinting or "tennis elbow bands"

Discharge criteria

- All uncomplicated cases

Discharge instructions

- Elbow tendonitis aftercare instructions
- Follow with PCP or orthopedic surgeon as needed

Consult criteria

- Orthopedic referral for refractory cases

Medial Epicondylitis

- Less common than lateral epicondylitis
- Tenderness over medial epicondyle

- May be associated ulnar neuritis with loss of sensation over palmar 5th finger and lateral palmar surface of 4th finger

Treatment options

- Similar to lateral epicondylitis
- Oral steroids for 1 week in nondiabetics can be used for ulnar neuritis
- Tylenol prn
- Cock-up brace

Discharge criteria

- All uncomplicated cases

Discharge instructions

- Elbow tendonitis aftercare instructions
- Follow with PCP or orthopedic surgeon as needed

Consult criteria

- Orthopedic referral for refractory cases

Olecranon Bursitis

- Usually a painless cystic swelling
- Can be painful from trauma, infection or cryptogenic cause
- Transudate fluid if aspirated is from chronic inflammation

Treatment options

Nonpainful bursitis

- Sterile lateral bursal aspiration if experienced (avoid bone and joint) — may be as effective with less complications than steroid injection
- 1 cc of 1–2% plain lidocaine mixed with 1 cc Depomedrol (methylprednisolone acetate) 40–80 mg/cc or Kenalog (triamcinolone) 10–20 mg/cc prn if Provider experienced with injections (do not introduce needle into bursa through cellulitis)
- Elbow ace wrapping

Painful bursitis

- Fluid needs evaluation (culture and gram stain)

- Heat if infectious etiology
- Heat or ice if cryptogenic etiology — whichever provides the greatest relief

Traumatic bursitis

- Ice × 2 days
- Elbow ace wrapping
- NSAID's prn; narcotics prn

Discharge criteria

- Nonpainful or minimal painful bursitis
- Not infected

Discharge instructions

- Olecranon bursitis aftercare instructions

Consult criteria

- Infected olecranon bursitis

Nursemaid Elbow

- Peak age 1–4 years
- Toddler pulled up by arm or similar type traction on arm
- Cries for a few minutes and stops usually
- Arm appears normal
- No other history; occasionally no helpful history
- Usually does not need x-ray if history and exam consistent with nursemaid elbow
- X-ray if performed is negative for acute process
- Perform x-ray if unsure of diagnosis

Treatment

- Elbow flexed 90 degrees
- Fully pronate elbow and then supinate
- If performed correctly will feel or hear click
- Patient cries transiently
- Provider leaves room and returns in 5–10 minutes
- Hold an object for toddler to grasp with affected arm to demonstrate resolution or patient moving arm normally

Discharge criteria

- All patients without other concerns (abuse) or other injuries

Discharge instructions

- Nursemaid elbow aftercare instructions

Consult criteria

- If child abuse suspected

Notes

References:

Lateral Epicondylitis

Author: Bryant James Walrod, MD; Chief Editor: Sherwin SW Ho, MD emedicine.medscape.com/article/96969

Orthopaedics Primary Care byChinni Pennathur Ramamurti

Plancher KD, Halbrecht J, Lourie GM. Medial and lateral epicondylitis in the athlete. *Clin Sports Med*. Apr 1996;15(2):283–305

Nursemaid Elbow Author: Wayne Wolfram, MD, MPH; Chief Editor: Richard G Bachur, MD emedicine.medscape.com/article/803026

Weinstein PS, Canoso JJ, Wohlgethan JR. Long-term follow-up of corticosteroid injection for traumatic olecranon bursitis. *Ann Rheum Dis*. Feb 1984;43(1):44–6

Hip Protocol

When using any protocol, always follow the Guidelines of Proper Use (page 18).

Septic Hip

Considerations

- Most common cause of painful hip in infants
- Rapid onset of pain
- Fever
- Elevated ESR and C-reactive protein
- Hip flexed
- All motion of hip resisted
- X-rays show externally rotated hip soft tissue outline

Evaluation

- Neurovascular exam
- Hip and pelvis x-rays
- Hip joint aspiration by specialist if indicated
- Synovial fluid analysis (see Synovial Fluid Analysis as needed)

Treatment

- Orthopedic admission for hip lavage and antibiotics

Consult criteria

- Suspected septic hip joint

Transient Synovitis

Considerations

- Self-limited disease of children age 3–10 years
- Etiology unknown (viral infection etiology postulated)
- Males twice as likely as females to have
- Crying at night in very young
- Antalgic gait or limp
- Usually afebrile; may have low-grade fever

- Hip held in flexion and slight abduction with external rotation
- 1/3 has no decreased hip motion
- Hip may be tender to palpation and painful to passive motion

Evaluation options

- Neurovascular exam
- CBC
- ESR
- Aspiration of hip by specialist if fever > 99.5; ESR > 20; or there is severe pain with movement
- Hip and pelvis x-rays
- Ultrasound as needed

Treatment

- Local heat and massage
- Bed rest for 7–10 days
- No weight bearing
- Close follow-up

Discharge criteria

- Discuss all pediatric hip pain with physician
- Diagnosis firm
- Provide transient hip synovitis aftercare instructions

Consult criteria

- Uncertain diagnosis
- Septic hip suspected

Legg-Calve´-Perthes Disease (Avascular Necrosis of Femoral Head)

Considerations

- Caused by loss of blood supply to hip
- Insidious onset
- Limp often presenting complaint
- Aching in groin and thigh
- Tender over anterior hip joint
- Age 4–10 years most common; range 2–18 years of age

- Male > female prevalence
- 20% bilateral
- Leg externally rotated

Evaluation

- Neurovascular exam
- CBC
- ESR
- Hip and pelvis x-rays
- Ultrasound helpful
- Bone scan diagnostic

Treatment

- NSAID's prn; Tylenol prn
- Non-weight bearing
- Physical therapy twice a week
- Crutches

Discharge criteria

- Most patients
- If adequate pain control is achievable

Discharge instructions

- Legg-Calve'-Perthes Disease aftercare instructions
- Referral to orthopedic surgeon

Consult criteria

- Discuss with physician
- Severe pain not controlled by medications
- Poor social situation not allowing non-weight bearing

Slipped Capital Femoral Epiphysis (SCFE)

Considerations

- Most patients obese
- Male peak age 13–15 years
- Female peak age 11–13 years
- More common in males
- Bilateral hips in 1/3 of cases
- Present with limp
- Pain referred to knee, thigh, groin or hip

- Commonly with leg externally rotated
- Flexion is restricted
- Do not ambulate if SCFE suspected

Evaluation

- Neurovascular exam
- CBC
- ESR
- C-reactive protein
- AP and frog leg lateral views of both hips
- Klein line is a line drawn parallel to lateral femoral neck that does not transect epiphysis; normally it does transect epiphysis in healthy hips

Treatment

- Immobilization
- Non-weight bearing

Consult criteria

- Immediate orthopedic consult

Hip Fracture

Considerations

- Elderly fall most common reason
- Affected leg externally rotated

Evaluation

- Hip and pelvis x-rays
- CT scan if plain hip x-ray without definite fracture but there is high suspicion of hip fracture
- Neurovascular exam
- Assess for other injuries
- Evaluate for acute medical condition if the cause of injury

Treatment

- Pain control

Consult criteria

- All hip fracture patients
- All suspected hip fracture patients

Hip Dislocation

Considerations

- Posterior dislocation most common
- Frequently seen with total hip replacement

Evaluation

- Hip and pelvis x-rays
- Neurovascular exam
- Assess for other injuries or conditions

Treatment

- Pain control

Consult criteria

- Consult physician

Notes

References:

Orthopaedics Primary Care by Chinni Pennathur Ramamurti

Hip Dislocation in Emergency Medicine
Author: Stephen R McMillan, MD; Chief Editor: Barry E Brenner, MD, PhD, FACEP
emedicine.medscape.com/article/823471

Slipped Capital Femoral Epiphysis
Author: Kevin D Walter, MD, FAAP; Chief Editor: Craig C Young, MD emedicine.medscape.com/article/91596

Evidence-based care guideline for conservative management of Legg-Calve-Perthes disease in children aged 3 to 12 years 2010 Oct. NGC:008174

Transient Synovitis
Author: Christine C Whitelaw, MD; Chief Editor: Lawrence K Jung, MD emedicine.medscape.com/article/1007186

KNEE SOFT TISSUE INJURY PROTOCOL

When using any protocol, always follow the Guidelines of Proper Use (page 18).

Differential Diagnosis

- Knee strain
- Anterior cruciate ligament tear or strain
- Posterior cruciate ligament tear or strain
- Medial meniscus tear
- Lateral meniscus tear
- Medial collateral tear or strain
- Lateral collateral tear of stain
- Patellar dislocation

Considerations

- Effusions occurring within 6 hours suggest ligament or cartilage injury
- Grade 1: microscopic ligament injury
- Grade 2: severe stretch with partial tear
- Grade 3: complete ligament disruption

Ottawa Knee Rule for obtaining x-rays (any of the following) for injuries < 24 hours and age > 18

- Inability to bear weight (walk 4 steps) immediately and presently
- Patellar tenderness
- Fibular head tenderness
- Age > 55 years
- Unable to flex knee > 90 degrees

Examination

- Palpate for areas of tenderness
- Check for knee effusion

Lachman's test

- Knee held in 15–30 degree flexion and move tibia forward

- Positive if motion visible; motion more than in uninjured knee
- Suggests anterior cruciate ligament (ACL) tear

McMurray's test

- Flex knee fully
- Rotate externally or internally and extend the knee
- Painful click on extension suggests meniscus injury
    - Internal rotation: lateral meniscus
    - External rotation: medial meniscus

Apley's test

- Patient in prone position
- Knee flexed
- Compression of foot into knee while rotated — suggests meniscus injury
- Distraction of foot from knee while rotated — suggests ligament injury

- Neurovascular exam
- Knee x-ray if indicated
    - Evaluate for fracture, dislocation and effusion

Treatment Options

- Ice
- Elevation
- Knee immobilizer prn
- Crutches prn
- Analgesics: NSAID's, narcotics prn

Discharge Criteria

- Uncomplicated injury

Discharge instructions

- Knee injury aftercare instructions
- Referral to orthopedic surgeon for grade 2–3 ligament injury or suspected meniscus injury suspected within 7–10 days
- Primary care provider follow-up for grade 1–2 sprains and contusions within 7–10 days

Consult Criteria

- Neurovascular injury
- Open joint injury
- Grossly unstable joint

Notes

References:

Orthopaedics Primary Care by Chinni Pennathur Ramamurti

The Ottawa Knee Rule: Examining Use in an Academic Emergency Department West J Emerg Med. Sep 2012; 13(4): 366–372

Knee Examination
Author: Bert Boonen, MD; Chief Editor: Erik D Schraga, MD
emedicine.medscape.com/article/1909230

KNEE DISORDERS PROTOCOL

When using any protocol, always follow the Guidelines of Proper Use (page 18).

Considerations

- Most nontraumatic knee conditions are degenerative or inflammatory
- Blood cultures may be positive in septic arthritis
- Consult physician for acute neurovascular deficits

Synovial fluid analysis

Normal

- Transparent clarity
- Clear color
- WBC < 200/mL
- PMN's < 25%
- Culture negative
- No crystals
- Mucin clot firm
- Glucose approximates blood levels

Noninflammatory

- Transparent clarity
- Yellow color
- WBC 200–2000/mL
- PMN's < 25%
- Culture negative
- No crystals
- Mucin clot firm
- Glucose approximates blood levels
- Associated conditions: rheumatic fever, trauma, osteoarthritis

Inflammatory

- Cloudy clarity
- Yellow color
- WBC 200–50,000/mL
- PMN's > 50%
- Culture negative

- Crystals can be present if gout or pseudogout present
- Mucin clot friable
- Glucose decreased
- Associated conditions: SLE, Lyme disease, gout, pseudogout, spondyloarthropathies

Septic

- Cloudy clarity
- Yellow color
- WBC 25,000/mL to often > 100,000/mL
- PMS's > 50%
- Culture often positive
- No crystals
- Mucin clot friable
- Glucose very decreased
- Fever
- C-reactive protein elevated

Osgood-Schlatter's Disease

Considerations

- Childhood disorder
- Males 10–15 years of age
- Aseptic necrosis within tibial tuberosity
- Pain, swelling and erythema over anterior tibial tuberosity
- Pain during resisted extension
- Pain on kneeling
- Slow onset
- Lateral knee x-ray may or may not show fragmentation of the tibial tubercle
- Clinical diagnosis

Treatment options

- Avoid climbing, running, kicking until pain has resolved
- Initially ice pack 20 minutes every 2–4 hours
- Quadriceps/hip extension exercises once acute episode has resolved
- May use NSAID's for pain
- No steroid injections

Discharge criteria

- All patients usually

Discharge instructions

- Osgood–Schlatter's disease aftercare instructions

Consult criteria

- Orthopedic referral if condition persistent

Prepatellar and Superficial Infrapatellar Bursitis

Considerations

- "Housemaid knee"
- Swelling of involved area

Treatment options

- Avoid kneeling
- Aspirate fluid if experienced with procedure
- May inject 1 cc of triamcinolone 40/cc with 1 cc lidocaine if experienced (do not inject if cellulitis present)
- Ace wrap

Discharge criteria

- Noninfected bursitis

Discharge instructions

- Patellar bursitis aftercare instructions

Consult criteria

- Infected bursitis suspected

Deep Infrapatellar and Anserine Bursitis

Considerations

- Excessive weight bearing may cause
- Pain at rest
- Increased pain with resisted extension
- Pain is felt in knee and may refer to hip, thigh or lower leg
- Swelling may occur
- Tenderness deep to patellar tendon

Treatment options

- Minimize weight bearing
- Avoid climbing, jumping, running, squatting
- Ice packs
- Quadriceps exercise when pain allows
- Range of motion exercises
- Corticosteroid injection prn (if Provider is experienced)
- NSAID's prn; narcotics prn

Discharge criteria

- Noninfected bursitis

Discharge instructions

- Knee bursitis aftercare instructions

Consult criteria

- Infected bursitis
- Orthopedic referral if not resolving

Baker's Cyst

Considerations

- Effusion of semimembranosus bursa
- Predisposes to chronic knee effusion
- Mass behind knee up to 5 × 5 cm
- X-rays may or may not show DJD

Treatment options

- May aspirate if experienced
- Ace wrap prn
- NSAID's prn

Discharge criteria

- Nonseptic joint
- Orthopedic referral

Discharge instructions

- Baker's cyst aftercare instructions

Consult criteria

- Uncertain diagnosis

Chondromalacia Patella

Considerations

- Degeneration of the patellar cartilage
- Any age
- Usually no injury
- Positive Patellar Grind Test — pushing on patella while moving knee into extension causes pain

Treatment options

- Avoid climbing, jumping, running, squatting

Discharge criteria

- Usually most patients

Discharge instructions

- Chondromalacia patella aftercare instructions

Consult criteria

- Orthopedic or primary care provider referral if not resolving

Osteoarthritis (DJD)

Considerations

- Related to increasing age
- Can result from previous injuries or knee surgery
- Knee effusion may be present
- Knee feels like it "gives way" occasionally
- Range of motion limited

Treatment options

- Minimize wear and tear activities
- NSAID's prn; narcotics prn for severe pain — short course
- Oral steroids for 7 days prn if not diabetic
- Knee immobilizer prn
- Crutches or walker prn

Discharge criteria

- Nonseptic knee joint

Discharge instructions

- Knee osteoarthritis aftercare instructions

Consult criteria

- Orthopedic referral for severe knee pain

Gout

Differential diagnosis

- Cellulitis
- Septic arthritis
- Bursitis
- Osteomyelitis
- Rheumatoid arthritis
- Soft tissue injury
- Pseudogout

Considerations

- Crystal uric acid deposits in joints and tissues
- Most common cause of monoarticular arthritis age > 60
- Increased warmth, redness and joint swelling
- First metatarsophalangeal joint of foot involved 75% of the time — most common involved joint
- Joint fluid: 20,000–100,000 WBC; poor string and mucin clot; no bacteria (pseudogout similar)
- Risk factors
  - Age > 40
  - Hypertension
  - Diuretics
  - Ethanol intake
  - Obesity

Evaluation

- Clinical evaluation usually all that is needed
- If diagnosis uncertain may order
  - CBC
  - C-reactive protein
  - X-rays
  - Joint aspiration if experienced Provider

Treatment options

- NSAID's high dose 5–10 days
- Narcotics IM or PO short course prn
- Steroids prn

- Prednisone 40–60 mg PO qday × 3–7 days
  OR
- Dexamethasone 6 mg daily for 3–7 days
  OR
- Depomedrol (methylprednisolone acetate) 80–120 mg IM

- Allopurinol 50–300 mg PO qday — adjusted for renal function; start after acute episode resolved
- Follow up with primary care provider within 2–3 days if pain persists

Discharge instructions

- Gout aftercare instructions

Consult criteria

- Uncertain diagnosis
- Fever or toxicity
- HR ≥ 110

Septic Arthritis

Differential diagnosis

- Cellulitis
- Gout
- Bursitis
- Osteomyelitis
- Rheumatoid arthritis
- Soft tissue injury
- Pseudogout

Considerations

- Onset is rapid
- Usually one joint infected
- Joint is very painful; hot; red; fluctuant
- Signs of acute systemic illness may be present
- Fever, chills and sweats frequently
- C-reactive protein elevated
- Pain and swollen prosthetic knee joint assume septic arthritis until proven otherwise
- See Synovial Fluid Analysis

Treatment

- Admission to hospital for drainage and antibiotics

Discharge criteria

- Only with physician consent

Consult criteria

- All septic joint patients

Notes

References:

Orthopaedics Primary Care by Chinni Pennathur Ramamurti

Pommering TL, Kluchurosky L. Overuse injuries in adolescents. *Adolesc Med State Art Rev*. May 2007;18(1):95–120, ix

Osgood-Schlatter Disease Author: J Andy Sullivan, MD; Chief Editor: Craig C Young, MD emedicine.medscape.com/article/1993268

ANKLE SPRAIN PROTOCOL

When using any protocol, always follow the Guidelines of Proper Use (page 18).

Definition

- Stretching or tearing of the ankle's ligaments

Differential Diagnosis

- Ankle fracture
- Ankle dislocation

Considerations

- 85–90% involves lateral ligaments
- Age < 10 years with traumatic ankle pain and no fracture on x-ray may have Salter type 1 fracture
- Stress testing acutely often limited by pain
- Nonweight bearing for several days has been shown to improve long-term outcomes for all sprains
- Ankle sprain grades
    - Grade 1: Ligament stretching without tearing or instability on exam
    - Grade 2: Some ligament tearing without instability, but more swelling and ecchymosis than grade 1
    - Grade 3: Complete tearing of ligaments with gross instability, marked swelling and ecchymosis and pain

Ottawa Rule for ordering ankle x-rays. Can defer x-ray if no criteria present below

- Bony tenderness distal 6 cm of posterior edge or tip of tibia or fibula, or either malleolus
- Bony tenderness base of 5th metatarsal or navicular bone
- Inability to take 4 unassisted steps at time of injury and when being evaluated
- Performed within 10 days of injury
- Not validated in children

Evaluation

- Assess ankle for instability
- Drawer test — anterior
- Assess inversion and eversion for instability
- Neurovascular exam
- Examine for associated ipsilateral leg injuries
- Examine for other remote injuries
- Evaluate as needed for the cause of injury

Treatment Options

- Ice and elevation
- Mild to moderate sprains can be treated with elastic wrap, air splint or plastic boot.
  - Can be weight bearing or nonweight bearing per Provider's discretion
- Severe sprains (ligament laxity) or severe pain — plastic boot or OCL posterior splint and crutches
- Consider nonweight bearing for 5–10 days to improve long-term outcome
- Nondisplaced distal fibula fractures can be treated with OCL posterior splint or plastic boots and crutches
- NSAID's, Tylenol, or narcotics prn
- May combine NSAID's and acetaminophen prn
- Strengthening exercises
- Aggressive pain-free ROM is recommended

Return-to-play criteria during the recovery phase (3 days to 2 wks. post injury) include the following:

- Full, pain-free active and passive ROM
- No pain or tenderness
- Strength of ankle muscles 70–80% of that on the uninvolved side
- Ability to balance on 1 leg for 30 seconds with eyes closed

Return-to-play criteria during the functional phase (2–6 weeks post injury) include the following:

- Normal ROM of the ankle joint
- No pain or tenderness
- Satisfactory clinical examination

- Strength of ankle muscles 90% of the uninvolved side
- Ability to complete functional examination

Discharge Criteria

- Sprains with intact ankle mortise, closed, with no acute neurovascular deficits
- Potential Salter 1 fractures

Discharge instructions

- Ankle sprain aftercare instructions
- Refer to grade 1 and 2 sprains to primary care provider
    - Permissible to refer to orthopedics
- Refer grade 3 or severe sprains to orthopedics within 7–10 days
- Nonweight bearing for 3 weeks improves outcomes
- Refer potential Salter 1 fractures to PCP or orthopedic surgeon for recheck in 10 days

Consult Criteria

- Grossly unstable ankle joint or disrupted ankle mortise
- Potential open ankle joint
- Acute neurovascular deficits
- Fractures (excluding nondisplaced distal fibula fractures)

Notes

References:

Dowling S, Spooner CH, Liang Y, Dryden DM, Friesen C, Klassen TP, et al. Accuracy of Ottawa Ankle Rules to exclude fractures of the ankle and midfoot in children: a meta-analysis. *Acad Emerg Med*. Apr 2009;16(4):277–87

Ivins D. Acute ankle sprain: an update. *Am Fam Physician*. Nov 15 2006;74(10):1714–20

Ankle Sprain Author: Craig C Young, MD; Chief Editor: Sherwin SW Ho, MD
emedicine.medscape.com/article/1907229

HAND, WRIST, AND DISTAL FOREARM INJURY PROTOCOL

When using any protocol, always follow the Guidelines of Proper Use (page 18).

General Recommendations

Evaluation

- X-ray all orthopedic hand and wrist injuries with mechanism of injury that could cause fractures or dislocations
- Assess neurovascular status and for tendon/ligament deficits

Treatment

- Reduce dislocations if experienced
- NSAID's with or without acetaminophen, or narcotics prn for pain
- Tetanus prophylaxis prn (see Tetanus Guidelines, page 756)

Discharge criteria

- Simple, nondisplaced, nonrotated closed long bone fractures can be splinted and discharged with orthopedic follow-up usually
    - Discuss with physician (except simple nondisplaced torus fractures)
- Simple dislocations that have been reduced

Consult criteria

- Wrist or proximal metacarpal dislocations
- Open injuries
- Acute neurovascular deficits
- Tendon/ligament injuries

Considerations

Complications

- Neurovascular injury
- Open fracture

  - Joint involvement
  - Ligament/tendon injury
  - Displaced and angulated
  - Compartment syndrome
  - Fat emboli — long bones
  - Avascular necrosis
  - Osteomyelitis
- Nondisplaced, closed simple long bone fractures can be splinted and discharged with orthopedic follow-up usually
  - Discuss with physician (except simple nondisplaced torus fractures)

Compartment syndrome

- From increased pressure in a muscle or other internal compartment
- Not all signs and symptoms are needed to make diagnosis
- High pressures > 8 hours leads to tissue damage
- Normal tissue pressure is < 10 mm Hg
- Capillary blood flow is compromised at > 20 mm Hg
- Intracompartmental pressures > 30 mm Hg or within 10–30 mm Hg of DBP

Signs and symptoms (not diagnostic)

- Pain
  - Out of proportion to injury
  - On passive stretch of muscles
- Pallor
- Paresthesias
- Paralysis
  - Sensory and motor findings are late signs
- Poikilothermia — decreased temperature
- Pulselessness
  - Usually not lost until muscle necrosis has occurred
  - Last sign to develop
- Tense muscle compartment on palpation

Treatment

- Consult physician if suspected

- Keep extremity at level of heart
- Do not use ice if suspected
- Remove cast and padding
- Surgery fasciotomy is usually necessary

Human Bite or Clenched Fist Injury

- Augmentin (amoxicillin/clavulanate) preferred antibiotic x 10–14 days
- Need operative irrigation and surgical exploration emergently unless very superficial
- Usually presents late
- Do not perform primary repair of laceration
- Consult physician
- See Human and Animal Bite Protocol

Boxer's Fracture (4th and/or 5th Metacarpal Shaft) and other Metacarpal Fractures

Considerations

- Boxer fractures usually from punching with a closed fist
- No more than 10-15° of angulation in the second and third metacarpals should be accepted without reduction
- No rotational deformity is acceptable

Evaluation

- X-ray
- Assess for neurovascular and tendon injury
- Assess for human teeth injury

Treatment

- Treat with OCL ulnar gutter or boxer's splint
- Most splints leave on for 3–4 weeks
- Sling
- Analgesics
- Fracture splints should be forearm-based and should allow for motion of the interphalangeal (IP) joints
- Splints should extend over the dorsal and palmar aspect of the entire metacarpal being treated

- Generally, the wrist should be placed in 20-30° of extension
    - The metacarpophalangeal (MCP) joints should be immobilized in 70-90° of flexion, with the dorsal aspect of the splint extending to the IP joints; and the volar aspect should end at the distal palmar crease
- Buddy taping the fingers of the involved metacarpal can aid in maintaining rotational control
- After a short period of immobilization, patients may be encouraged to use the fingers on the affected hand to maintain motion

Discharge criteria

- Simple closed Boxer's fracture with < 40 degrees angulation
- Second and third metacarpal fractures ≤ 10–15° of angulation
- No rotational deformity

Discharge instructions

- Boxer's fracture aftercare instructions
- Metacarpal fracture aftercare instructions
- Refer to orthopedic or hand surgeon within 7 days

Consult criteria

- 40 degrees or more of angulation needs reduction (consult physician)
- Greater than 10-15° of angulation in the second and third metacarpals
- Nonreducible dislocations
- Neurovascular compromise
- Loss of ligament or tendon function
- Metacarpal head displaced fractures usually need surgery
- Salter fractures consult physician
- Open fracture
- Human bite

High Pressure Injection Injuries

- Consult physician immediately

- Do not discharge
- Needs surgery usually

Dislocations of the MP Joint

Evaluation

- X-ray
- Assess for neurovascular and tendon injury
- Assess for human teeth injury if in fist fight

Treatment

- May reduce if seen right after injury without x-ray if there is no doubt to diagnosis
- Metacarpal block may not be needed if seen immediately after injury
- Push your thumb on dorsal surface of hand and distally on proximal phalanx to reduce
- Splinting may not be necessary

Discharge criteria

- Closed simple MP joint dislocations that are reduced

Discharge instructions

- MP joint aftercare instructions
- Refer to orthopedic or hand surgeon within 7–10 days

Consult criteria

- Unable to reduce
- Open joint
- Associated fracture

Scaphoid Fracture (or Suspected Scaphoid Fracture)

Considerations

- Most common carpal fracture
- Snuffbox tenderness (with negative x-ray 25% of these patients will have a fracture)
- Complication of avascular necrosis may occur
- High malpractice rewards when fracture missed

Evaluation

- X-ray — may need special views
- Assess for neurovascular and tendon injury

Treatment

- Thumb spica splint and sling if fracture diagnosed or suspected
  - Cast for 12 weeks placed by outpatient referral provider

Discharge criteria

- Closed simple scaphoid fracture
- See Shoulder and Arm Trauma Protocol

Discharge instructions

- Scaphoid fracture aftercare instructions
- Orthopedic or hand surgeon referral within 7–10 days if diagnosed or suspected

Consult criteria

- Open fracture
- Neurovascular, tendon or ligament deficit

Carpal Bone Fractures or Dislocations

- Consult physician (see Scaphoid Fracture above)

Colles and Smith Fractures

Considerations

- Involves distal forearm
- Colles is a dorsal angulation and Smith fracture volar angulation of fracture
- Angulation ≤ 10 degrees can be treated without reduction anatomically
- Intra-articular step-off > 1–2 mm needs orthopedic consultation
- Ulna is usually within 2 mm of radius at wrist
- Treatment varies depending on age and activity level

Evaluation

- X-ray (lateral, AP and oblique)
- Neurovascular examination
- Ligament and tendon examination

Treatment

- Sugar tong splint
- Sling
- Reduction of significant angulation
- Surgery needed commonly

Discharge criteria

- Consult criteria not met
- Simple closed fracture

Discharge instructions

- Colles or Smith fracture aftercare instructions
- Follow up with orthopedic surgeon within 7 days

Consult physician

- Intra-articular step-off > 1–2 mm
- Dorsal tilt 10%
- Volar tilt > 20%
- Radial shortening > 3 mm
- Loss of radial angle
- Neurovascular injury
- Open fracture
- Ligament disruption
- Lunate and perilunate wrist dislocations

Notes

References:

Orthopaedics Primary Care by Chinni Pennathur Ramamurti

Wrist Fracture in Emergency Medicine
Author: Bryan C Hoynak, MD, FACEP, FAAEM; Chief Editor: Rick Kulkarni, MD emedicine.medscape.com/article/828746

Ann of EM, 2015;65:308

Metacarpal Fractures Treatment & Management

Updated: Aug 27, 2018 Author: Thomas Michael Dye, MD; Chief Editor: Harris Gellman, MD

FINGER INJURY PROTOCOL

When using any protocol, always follow the Guidelines of Proper Use (page 18).

General Evaluation and Considerations

- X-ray all finger injuries with mechanism of injury with potential to cause fractures or dislocations
- Assess neurovascular status and for tendon/ligament deficits
- Consult on all open injuries or with acute neurovascular deficits
- Consult on tendon/ligament injuries except as discussed below
- NSAID's or narcotics prn for pain
- Consult for proximal and middle phalanx fractures
- Nondisplaced distal phalange fractures may be splinted in extension and referred to orthopedic or hand surgery

Mallet Finger

- Avulsion of the DIP extensor tendon
- Distal 1 inch foam aluminum splint with joint in full extension for 6 weeks
  - Aluminum strip can be applied either dorsally or volarly
- Can initiate splinting up to 6 weeks post injury
- Surgery only option if injury 2 months old (Refer to orthopedic or hand surgeon)
- Refer to primary care provider, orthopedic or hand surgeon for recent injury

Avulsion of the Flexor Profundus Tendon DIP Joint

- Jamming injury (usually children)
- Palmar middle phalanx and dorsal DIP joint swollen and tender
- Unable to actively flex distal phalanx
- Splint in position of function (normal resting position of an uninjured finger)

- Orthopedic referral for surgery

PIP Joint Dislocation

- Usually from hyperextension injury
- May reduce if seen right after injury without x-ray if there is no doubt about the diagnosis
- Local digital anesthesia may not be needed if seen immediately after injury
- Push distal phalanx back into alignment and x-ray
- Splint in full extension for 3 weeks
- Buddy tape with padding between fingers to adjacent finger
- Refer to orthopedic or hand surgeon

Avulsion of the Central Extensor Slip

- Difficult to diagnose at time of injury because of swelling
- Boutonniere deformity of the PIP joint is frequently a late finding
- Due to forceful PIP joint flexion
- Splint in full extension for 3 weeks if suspected or diagnosed
- Refer to orthopedic or hand surgeon within 7–10 days

Avulsion of the Volar Carpal Plate PIP Joint

- Hyperextension injury or a recently reduced PIP joint dislocation
- Joint movements very painful and limited
- Palmar surface very tender
- Abnormal extension of joint possible on exam
- Splint in full extension for 3 weeks if suspected or diagnosed
- Refer to orthopedic or hand surgeon within 3–7 days

Tear or Avulsion of the Collateral Ligament

- Instability of lateral PIP joint in either direction
- Splint in 15–20 degrees at PIP joint and 70 degrees at MP joint for 3 weeks
- Refer to orthopedic or hand surgeon

Gamekeeper Thumb

- Tenderness over first metacarpal phalangeal joint of thumb
- Rupture of ulnar collateral ligament
- Joint opens up with radial stress > than other uninjured thumb
- Associated avulsion fracture is common
- Thumb spica
- Refer to orthopedic or hand surgeon within 3–7 days

Notes

References:

Orthopaedics Primary Care by Chinni Pennathur Ramamurti

Mallet Finger Author: Roy A Meals, MD; Chief Editor: Harris Gellman, MD emedicine.medscape.com/article/1242305

Phalangeal Fractures Author: Jay E Bowen, DO; Chief Editor: Craig C Young, MD emedicine.medscape.com/article/98322

Mallet Finger Treatment & Management
Updated: Aug 27, 2018 Author: Roy A Meals, MD; Chief Editor: Harris Gellman, MD

Pediatrics

Section Contents

When using any protocol, always follow the Guidelines of Proper Use (page 18).

PEDIATRIC FEVER PROTOCOL

When using any protocol, always follow the Guidelines of Proper Use (page 18).

Definition

- Rectal temperature > 100.4°F (38°C)

Differential Diagnosis

- Viral infections
- Localized bacterial infections
- Bacteremia
- Sepsis
- Urinary tract infection
- Heat illness

Considerations

- Risk of occult bacteremia has declined markedly with pneumococcal and HIB vaccines
- Males < 6 months without a source of fever have a UTI 7% of the time
- Females < 12 months without a source of fever have UTI 8% of the time
- 0–8 weeks of age are at higher risk of bacterial infection — especially 0–4 weeks of age
- Serious bacterial infection (SBI) can occur without fever
- Hypothermia during infection portends a higher risk
- Fever is not dangerous in of itself unless ≥ 105°F (40.6°C)
- Viruses are the most common cause of fever
- Treating fever has no effect on decreasing febrile seizures
- Pneumonia frequently has a normal pulmonary auscultatory exam

Evaluation

Neonates 0–28 days of age

- CBC count, urinalysis, blood culture, urine culture, chest radiography, and diagnostic LP

Children 5–8 weeks of age

- CBC and U/A
- CXR may be obtained especially if respiratory symptoms present
- Lumbar puncture may be omitted if patient appears well, close follow up within 12–24 hours and no antibiotics have been previously given
  - Maintain low threshold for obtaining lumbar puncture

Children 2–24 months of age

- Complete history of fever, any prior treatments and associated symptoms
- Baseline dehydration assessment, see Pediatric Dehydration Protocol
- Assess interaction, feeding and alertness
- Nontoxic patients with viral source of fever may need no further evaluation
- Fully immunized patients including pneumococcal and hemophilus influenza B will not usually need CBC or blood cultures
- CXR
  - O_2 saturation < 95% on room air
  - Tachypnea or respiratory distress
  - WBC ≥ 15,000 with cough
- Fever ≥ 102°F (38.9°C) without source and patient is immunized to pneumococcal disease
  - Consider CXR
  - Cath U/A in males < 6 months; uncircumcised male < 12 months; females < 24 months
- Dehydration > 5% order BMP (See Pediatric Diarrhea Protocol for baseline dehydration assessment and treatment)
- Urinary complaints — order U/A
  - U/A for fever without a clinical source in girls and uncircumcised boys < 2 years of age
  - Final diagnosis of UTI requires a urine culture

- Decreased alertness, toxic appearance or in distress
    - CBC, chest x-ray, blood culture × 1, cath U/A, urine culture — discuss performance of a lumbar puncture with physician

Children > 24 months of age

- Evaluation based on history and physically exam primarily (if fully immunized)
- Specific workup based on clinical findings and suspicion of disease

Pediatric sickle cell disease (SCD) and fever

Admission criteria

- Age < 2 years with hemoglobin SS (HbSS) disease or hemoglobin S–β° (HbS–β°)
    - HbSC or HbS–β+ less likely to have bacteremia and age alone not an admission criteria
- Temperature > 104°F (40°C)
- WBC > 30,000 or < 5,000
    - Both associated with increased bacteremia risk
    - Bandemia > 1,000 with bacterial infection
- Hemoglobin ≥ 2 gms below baseline in HbSS or HbS–β°
- Hemoglobin ≤ 5 gms
- Previous bacteremia or invasion infection
- Indwelling vascular lines
- Signs of systemic toxicity, vital sign instability or serious infection
- Previously treated with clindamycin or vancomycin instead of ceftriaxone
- Presence of SCD manifestations that require inpatient management
    - Acute chest syndrome
    - Painful crisis
    - Aplastic crisis
    - Splenic sequestration

- Concerns about family not able to recognize changes in patient's condition or inability/difficulty for follow–up (Need clear method to contact family if cultures are positive)

Outpatient management

- Patients that do not meet admission criteria can be considered for outpatient management
- Clinically stable
- Specific plan for follow–up the next day
- Recorded working telephone number recorded in chart
- Ceftriaxone 50–75 mg/kg IM or IV daily unless discontinued by medical provider
  - 100 mg/kg if meningitis present or suspected
- Stress oral hydration
- If vomiting occurs then return for further evaluation
- Adequate PO pain medications

Fever Treatment Options

- Fever may be treated; if patient not uncomfortable, it may not need to be treated unless ≥ 104°F (40°C)
- Alternating Tylenol with ibuprofen not officially recommended and may confuse parents increasing toxicity risk through medication error (may lengthen fever control more than a single antipyretic medication alone though)
- Fever ≥ 102°F (38.9°C) without a source and patient is nontoxic and feeding normally (age 2–24 months) who is fully immunized including pneumococcal and hemophilus influenza B
  - Can be treated with Rocephin (ceftriaxone) 50 mg/kg IM
  - Can have no treatment, but needs close follow up within 12–24 hours
- Fever with a source in patient without toxicity or distress
  - Viral: treat symptoms
  - Suspected bacterial infection: appropriate antibiotic
  - May use Sanford Guide or antibiotic database

- Fever with or without a source and patient toxic or in distress
    - Consult physician promptly

Discharge Criteria

- Healthy prior to fever onset
- No significant risk factors (prematurity or comorbid conditions)
- Nontoxic and healthy appearance
- Less than 5% dehydration (serum $CO_2 \geq 18$ if checked)
- Feeding well
- Reliable caregivers and access to follow-up
- WBC < 18,000 and patient appears well

Discharge instructions

- Pediatric fever aftercare instructions
- Return if patient becomes less active or appears worse
- Follow up with primary care provider in 2–3 days if fever persists

Consult Criteria

- Appears toxic, has poor alertness, decreased interaction or in distress
- Fever ≥ 104.5°F (40.3°C)
- Greater than 5% dehydration
- Poor feeding
- No source of fever
- Immunosuppression
- Splenectomy
- Seizure
- Petechiae

Vital signs and age consult criteria

- Fever ≥ 104.5°F (40.3°C)
- Age ≤ 90 days
- O_2 saturation < 95% on room air
- Pediatric heart rate
    - 0–4 months ≥ 180
    - 5–7 months ≥ 175
    - 8–12 months ≥ 170

- Hypotension

Lab and x-ray consult criteria

- WBC ≥ 18,000 or < 3,000; absolute neutrophils < 1,000
- Bandemia ≥ 15%
- Acute thrombocytopenia
- New onset anemia
- Serum CO_2 < 18 mEq/L
- Metabolic acidosis
- Glucose ≥ 200 mg/dL
- Significant pneumonia
- Pleural effusion

Notes

References:

Rudinsky SL, Carstairs KL, Reardon JM, Simon LV, Riffenburgh RH, Tanen DA. Serious bacterial infections in febrile infants in the post-pneumococcal conjugate vaccine era. *Acad Emerg Med*. Jul 2009;16(7):585–90

Emergent Management of Pediatric Patients with Fever
Author: John W Graneto, DO, FACOEP, FACEP; Chief Editor: Russell W Steele, MD
medicine.medscape.com/article/801598

Management of fever in sickle cell disease Author: Zora R Rogers, MD

BENIGN FEBRILE SEIZURE PROTOCOL

When using any protocol, always follow the Guidelines of Proper Use (page 18).

Definition

- A seizure event in infancy or childhood usually occurring between three months and five years of age, associated with fever, but without evidence of intracranial infection or other defined cause

Differential Diagnosis

- Meningitis
- Encephalitis
- Subdural and epidural infections
- Bacteremia and sepsis
- Epilepsy

Considerations

- Affects 2–4% of all children < 5 years of age
- Occurs in early childhood
- Usually occurs in children with systemic viral infection
- Majority last < several minutes
- Rate of serious infections are equivalent to febrile patients without seizures
- Increased rate of febrile seizures on day of DTP vaccination and 8–14 days after MMR vaccination
- Patients with febrile seizure have slightly higher rate of developing epilepsy
- No evidence that treatment with seizure medications decreases future febrile seizures
- No evidence of future cognitive differences in patients with febrile seizures
- Fever treatment does not alter developing febrile seizures
- Mild postictal phase usual
- Occurs in families to some extent

Types

Simple febrile seizure

- Lasts < 15 minutes
- Generalized
- Occurs only once in 24 hours

Complex febrile seizure

- Lasts > 15 minutes
- Focal features at any time
- Recurs within 24 hours

Evaluation

- Complete history and physical exam
- Serum glucose
- Routine labs usually not indicated
- Lab and x-rays if significant comorbid disease suspected (bacterial infection suspected)
- CT head for focal findings
- Lumbar puncture considered for age < 18 months for any of the following
    - History of irritability, decrease feeding, or lethargy
    - Abnormal appearance or mental status after postictal period
    - Signs of meningitis; severe headache
    - Complex febrile seizure
    - Slow postictal clearing of mentation
    - Pretreatment with antibiotics

Treatment Options

- No specific treatment for simple febrile seizure
- Reassure parents
- Treat any serious underlying cause of fever (see Pediatric Fever Protocol or other appropriate protocols)

Complex febrile seizures

- Intubation if airway not secure
- IV NS KVO
- Oxygen
- Lorazepam 0.05–0.1 mg/kg IV prn; may repeat q10–15 minutes prn (NMT 6 mg)
- Diastat (diazepam rectal gel) if no IV available

  - Age up to 5 years: 0.5 mg/kg
  - Age 6–11 years: 0.3 mg/kg
  - Age > 12 years: 0.2 mg/kg
  - Round up to available dose: 2.5, 5, 7.5, 10, 12.5, 15, 17.5, 20 mg/dose
- Midazolam IV/IM/PR/ET/intranasal 0.1–0.2 mg/kg/dose; not to exceed a cumulative dose of 10 mg)

Status epilepticus (beware of "too slow and too low" treatment)

- Lorazepam 0.1 mg/kg IV (NMT 10 mg total dose)
- Cerebyx (fosphenytoin) 15–20 mg/kg IV at 100 mg/minute if no response in 5 minutes to lorazepam or midazolam (Versed)
- Keppra (Levetiracetam) 30-40 mg/kg IV
  - 2-5 mg/kg/minute
  - NMT 2000 mg

Drugs that can be used if lorazepam, midazolam or Cerebyx (fosphenytoin) fail per physician

  - Pentobarbital 1 mg/kg boluses IV to maximum 5 mg/kg per physician
  - Valproic acid 15 mg/kg over 1–5 minutes (NMT 40 mg/kg)
    - 5 mg/kg/hr. drip
  - Phenobarbital 20 mg/kg IV at 100 mg/hr. per physician
  - Propofol 2 mg/kg IV bolus (patient intubated), may repeat if needed and start 5 mg/kg/hr. infusion if necessary

Management of refractory status epilepticus (consult physician immediately)

- Referral to an intensive care unit
- Anesthetic agents such as midazolam, propofol or barbiturates (thiopental, pentobarbital) for generalized convulsive status epilepticus
- Non-anesthetic anticonvulsants such as phenobarbital or valproic acid for nonconvulsive status epilepticus

Discharge Criteria

- Normal neurologic exam
- Simple febrile seizure
- Source of fever can be treated as an outpatient
- All seizures are to be discussed with physician prior to discharge
- Contact primary care physician or provider to alert of visit and arrange follow-up if seen in acute care facility

Discharge instructions

- Benign febrile seizure aftercare instructions
- Return if seizure recurs
- Return if patient appears worse
- Close follow-up within 1 day preferable

Consult Criteria

- Discuss all seizures with physician
- Complex febrile seizure
- Suspected or diagnosed serious underlying infection
- Neurologic abnormality
- History of irritability
- Poor feeding
- Lethargy
- Abnormal appearance or mental status after postictal period
- Signs of meningitis
- Severe headache
- Slow postictal clearing of mentation
- Very recent or concurrent treatment with antibiotics
- Appears toxic, has poor alertness, decreased interaction or distress
- Greater than 5% dehydration
- No source of fever
- UTI — follow UTI Protocol

Vital signs and age consult criteria

- Age < 6 months
- Pediatric heart rate
    - 0–4 months ≥ 180
    - 5–7 months ≥ 175
    - 8–12 months ≥ 170

- Fever ≥ 104.5°F (40.3°C)
- Hypotension

Lab and x-ray consult criteria

- WBC ≥ 15,000 or < 3,000; absolute neutrophils < 1,000
- Bandemia ≥ 15%
- Thrombocytopenia
- New onset anemia
- Metabolic acidosis
- Glucose ≥ 200 mg/dL
- Hyperglycemia with metabolic acidosis (decreased serum CO_2 or elevated anion gap)
- Significant pneumonia
- Pleural effusion

Notes

References:

Brooks M. Intranasal Midazolam Works for Seizure Emergencies in Kids. Medscape Medical News. Nov 5 2013

Pediatric Febrile Seizures Author: Robert J Baumann, MD; Chief Editor: Amy Kao, MD
emedicine.medscape.com/article/1176205

Clinical practice guideline – febrile seizures: guideline for the neurodiagnostic evaluation of the child with a simple febrile seizure. *Pediatrics*. 2011;127;389–394

Pediatric Status Epilepticus Treatment & Management
Updated: Oct 06, 2014
Author: Rajesh Ramachandrannair, MBBS, MD, FRCPC; Chief Editor: Timothy E Corden, MD

Crying Infant Protocol

When using any protocol, always follow the Guidelines of Proper Use (page 18).

Definition

- Crying child that presents without discernible cause of distress

Differential Diagnosis

- Otitis media
- Infant colic
- Viral illness with anorexia
- Dehydration
- UTI
- Corneal abrasion
- Ocular foreign body
- Oropharynx foreign body
- Hair tourniquet syndrome (hair wrapped around toe or penis)
- Brown recluse spider bite
- Clavicle or tibial fracture
- Gastrointestinal prodrome
- GERD
- Intussusception
- DTP reaction
- PSVT
- Intracranial abnormality or infection
- Congenital cardiac disease (check for decreased femoral pulses)
- Child abuse (nonaccidental trauma)

Considerations

- Crying stimulated by
  - Unmet need: hunger; thirst; desire for attention
  - Distress: anger; discomfort; pain
- Often defined by parental perceptions
- Healthy infants: crying levels increase from birth and peaks at 6–8 weeks of life

- Crying follows circadian rhythm — clusters late afternoon or early evening
- Infants that won't stop crying in the exam area is more predictive of serious illness
- Most serious common cause of explained crying is urinary tract infections
- Clinician intuition about severity of illness is important
- Parental concern is a red flag in identifying serious illness
- Normal physical exam and the patient stops crying usually indicates that a serious illness is not present
- Colic (29.5%), acute otitis media (15.5%) and constipation (5.5%) are the most common causes of unexplained crying
- Observational period important to determine if serious illness is present
- Close follow up is important when cause of crying not determined
- Avoid medicating unknown or unclear diagnosis for crying

Colic — recurrent paroxysmal attacks of crying lasting several hours

- Drawing up legs
- Abdomen may appear distended
- Bowel sounds increased
- Flatus may be passed

Colic rules of 3

- Lasting 3 or more hours
- Occurring 3 or more days per week
- Lasting minimum of 3 weeks
- No specific cause identified

Treatment options

- Short trial of hypoallergenic formula
- Stop cow's milk
- Treatments that are not effective
  - Simethicone
  - Lactase enzymes
  - Soy based formula
  - Fiber enriched foods
  - Carrying infant more

- Car ride stimulators
- Chiropractic manipulation

Evaluation

- History and physical exam reveals the majority of causes (71%)
- Consider rectal and genital exam if cause not evident
- Urinalysis and culture is the most helpful screening lab test, especially in the very young
- Tests are aimed at suspected causes of excessive crying
- Evaluate for child abuse and order testing as indicated by exam and history

Treatment Options

- Observe for up to 2–3 hours to see if crying ceases
- Aimed at cause of crying

Discharge Criteria

- Patient stops crying in exam area
- Normal vital signs
- O_2 saturation > 95%
- No serious illness detected
- Cause of crying determined to be benign and can be treated as outpatient
- Contact primary care physician or provider to alert of visit and arrange follow-up

Consult Criteria

- Patient will not stop crying
- O_2 saturation ≤ 94%
- Toxic appearance; poor interaction and activity
- Dehydration
- Poor response to treatment
- Worrisome abdominal tenderness
- Petechial rash
- Altered mental status
- Significant disease causation of crying
- Clinician gut feeling that patient has a serious illness
- Parental concern that a serious illness is present

Vital signs consult criteria

- Pediatric heart rate
  - 0–4 months ≥ 170
  - 5–7 months ≥ 160
  - 8–12 months ≥ 155
  - 1–3 years ≥ 135
- Hypotension

Lab consult criteria

- WBC ≥ 15,000 or < 3,000
- Bandemia ≥ 15%
- Thrombocytopenia
- Serum CO_2 < 18 mEq/L post rehydration
- Initial serum CO_2 < 17 mEq/L

Notes

References:

Barr RG, Paterson JA, MacMartin LM, et al. Prolonged and unsoothable crying bouts in infants with and without colic. J Dev Behav Pediatr. 2005;26(1):14–23

Fahimi D, Shamsollahi B, Salamati P, et al. Excessive crying of infancy; a report of 200 cases. Iran J of Pediatr. 2007;17(3):222–226.

Poole SR, The infant with acute, unexplained, excessive crying. Pediatrics 1991;88(3):450–455

Van den Bruel A, Thompson M, Buntinx F, et.al. Clinician's gut feeling about serious infections in children: observational study. BMJ 2012;345:e6144 (Observational study 3369 children)

URI AND SINUSITIS PROTOCOL

When using any protocol, always follow the Guidelines of Proper Use (page 18).

Definition

- Infection of the nasopharynx, larynx, or sinuses

Differential Diagnosis

- Rhinitis
- Sinusitis
- Laryngitis
- Bronchitis
- Bronchiolitis
- Pneumonia
- Gastroesophageal reflux
- Candidiasis

Considerations

- Sinusitis (rhinosinusitis) is usually viral
- Viral sinusitis difficult to differentiate from bacterial sinusitis early in the course
- Children are 20–100 times more likely to have viral rhinosinusitis then bacterial sinusitis
- Viral rhinosinusitis
    - Congestion
    - Cough
    - Nasal discharge up to 14 days
- Acute bacterial sinusitis is associated with prolonged symptoms lasting more than 10–14 days
- Diagnosis of acute bacterial sinusitis should be made on clinical grounds
- Prescribe antibiotics for worsening sinusitis symptoms or symptoms > 10 days
- Offer observation for an additional 3 days if symptoms not worsening
- CT scan may help in unclear cases. Plain films are rarely helpful
- Antibiotics should not be used to treat nonspecific URI symptoms in previously healthy patients

- Acute bacterial sinusitis does not require antibiotic treatment, especially if symptoms are mild or moderate
- Up to 75% of sinusitis resolves in 1 month without antibiotic treatment
- Severe or persistent moderate symptoms of bacterial sinusitis should receive antibiotic treatment
- Fever not common
- Acute invasive fungal rhinosinusitis
    - Can be caused by Candida, Aspergillus and Phycomycetes species — found in patients with:
        - Diabetes (especially with very high serum glucose levels)
        - Cancer
        - Hepatic disease
        - Renal failure
        - Other immunosuppressive conditions or diseases
- Sinusitis has same pathogens as otitis media

Signs of sinusitis

- Mucopurulent rhinorrhea
- Nasal congestion
- Facial pain, pressure or fullness
- Decreased sense of smell
- Severe headache, malaise, fever
- Pain exacerbation with head movement
- Retro-orbital pain (ethmoid sinus)
- Dental pain (maxillary sinus)
- Ear fullness

Evaluation

- Nasal exam
- Percussion of sinuses for tenderness
- Transillumination for frontal and maxillary sinus opacification
- CBC: severe sinusitis

CT scan indications

- Facial swelling
- Orbital or periorbital swelling
- Visual or mental status changes

- Consider for severe headache

Treatment Options

- Nasal saline for young children
- Antipyretic treatment prn
- Warm compresses to face prn
- Nasal steroids can be considered
- Mucolytics (guaifenesin) can be used to thin secretions — efficacy unknown
- Nasal saline irrigation

Antihistamines and decongestants

- Without benefit
- Can worsen congestion and sinus pain by thickening of mucus and decreasing drainage
- Can use for allergic rhinosinusitis without bacterial infection

Antibiotics — for persistent moderate symptoms or severe symptoms and are the same as for otitis media

Severe symptoms defined as

- Systemic toxicity with fever of at least 102°F and threat of suppurative complications, daycare attendance, age <2 or >65 years, recent hospitalization, antibiotic use within the past month, or immunocompromised state

- Prescribe antibiotics for worsening sinusitis symptoms or symptoms > 10 days
- Offer observation without antibiotics for an additional 3 days if symptoms not worsening
- Augmentin (amoxicillin/clavulanate) 2 g BID or 90 mg/kg/day BID 10–14 days (preferred)
- Amoxicillin 80–90 mg/kg/day PO divided q8–12hr
- Start antibiotics for fever ≥ 102°F (38.9°C) and diagnosis of bacterial sinusitis
- Penicillin allergy can use doxycycline or levofloxacin or moxifloxacin
- May use Sanford guide or antibiotic database

Discharge Criteria

- Uncomplicated rhinosinusitis
- Nontoxic

Discharge instructions

- URI and/or sinusitis aftercare instructions
- Follow up within 10–14 days if symptoms persist

Consult Criteria

- Toxic patients
- Abnormal vision
- Severe headache
- Altered mental status
- Facial swelling
- Vomiting
- Sphenoid sinusitis

Vital signs and age consult criteria

- Fever ≥ 102°F (38.9°C) if felt to be solely from sinusitis
- Age < 2 months
- Adult heart rate ≥ 120
- Pediatric heart rate
  - 0–4 months ≥ 180
  - 5–7 months ≥ 175
  - 8–12 months ≥ 170
  - 1–3 years ≥ 160
  - 4–5 years ≥ 145
  - 6–8 years ≥ 140
  - 9–12 years ≥ 135
  - 13–15 years ≥ 130
- Hypotension
- O_2 saturation < 95% on room air

Lab consult criteria

- WBC ≥ 18,000 or < 3,000
- Bandemia ≥ 15%
- Acute thrombocytopenia

Notes

References:

American Academy of Pediatrics. Subcommittee on Management of Sinusitis and Committee on Quality Improvement. Clinical Practice Guideline: Management of Sinusitis. Pediatrics 2001;108(3):798–808. (Consensus guideline)

Wald ER, Applegate KE, Bordley C, Darrow DH, Glode MP, Marcy SM, et al. Clinical Practice Guideline for the Diagnosis and Management of Acute Bacterial Sinusitis in Children Aged 1 to 18 Years. *Pediatrics*. Jun 24 2013

Acute Sinusitis Author: Itzhak Brook, MD, MSc; Chief Editor: Burke A Cunha, MD
emedicine.medscape.com/article/232670

Clin Infect Dis 2012 Apr;54(8):e72–e112

N Engl J Med 2012; 367:1128–1134

Clin Infect Dis, Vol. 54:e72

OTITIS MEDIA PROTOCOL

When using any protocol, always follow the Guidelines of Proper Use (page 18).

Definition

- Infection of the middle ear with acute onset, presence of middle ear effusion, and signs of middle ear inflammation

Differential Diagnosis

- Bell's palsy
- Dental pain
- TMJ pain
- URI
- Mastoiditis
- Ear canal foreign body
- Barotitis media
- Herpes zoster
- Pharyngitis
- Sinusitis
- Serous otitis media

Considerations

- Viruses 35%; S. pneumoniae 25%; H. influenzea 23%; M. catarrhalis 15%; mixed bacteria 10%
- Most commonly occurs 6–36 months of age
- One-half of patients have fever
- Usually associated with URI
- History can include: earache, irritability, rhinitis, GI symptoms, poor feeding, fever, pulling at ear
- Mild cases resolve without antibiotics 80% of the time within 1 week
- Fever is defined as rectal temperature > 38 °C or 100.4°F; Axillary temperature is unreliable

Treatment considerations

- Antibiotics increases resolution by another 13%
- 50% of patients will have residual middle ear fluid 1 month after antibiotic treatment so rechecking

ears in 10–14 days may be unwarranted unless symptoms continue

- Antihistamines, decongestants, and steroids have no proven effectiveness
- High dose amoxicillin overcomes drug resistance
- Red TM's (tympanic membrane) can also be from fever and crying
- Pneumatic otoscopy most accurate method in diagnosing otitis media
- Otitis media with bulging TM's warrant immediate antibiotic treatment
- Otitis media without bulging TM's will likely clear spontaneously — can delay antibiotics 48–72 hours to see if spontaneous resolution of symptoms occurs
- Antibiotic treatment warranted for age < 6 months or older children > 36 months
- Mastoiditis is the same antibiotic treatment PO as otitis media

Evaluation

- Rectal temperature for age < 3 years unless patient cooperates with oral measurement to nurse's satisfaction
- Feeding, irritability, urine output and fever history
- CBC, chest x-ray, and U/A for fever ≥ 101°F (38.3°C) without a source (no URI symptoms for example)
- BMP for > 5% dehydration
- WBC ≥ 15,000 without a source for fever — get chest x-ray and one blood culture
- Obtain history of recent antibiotic treatment
- Evaluate for TM (tympanic membrane) perforation
- Complete H&P, including nuchal exam

Treatment Options

American Academy of Pediatrics recommendations (February 2013)

- AOM management should include pain evaluation and treatment.
- Antibiotics should be prescribed for bilateral or unilateral AOM in children aged at least 6 months

with severe signs or symptoms (moderate or severe otalgia or otalgia for 48 hours or longer or temperature 39°C or higher) and for nonsevere, bilateral AOM in children aged 6 to 23 months

- On the basis of joint decision-making with the parents, unilateral, nonsevere AOM in children aged 6 to 23 months or nonsevere AOM in older children may be managed either with antibiotics or with close follow-up and withholding antibiotics unless the child worsens or does not improve within 48 to 72 hours of symptom onset
- Amoxicillin is the antibiotic of choice unless the child received it within 30 days, has concurrent purulent conjunctivitis, or is allergic to penicillin. In these cases, clinicians should prescribe an antibiotic with additional β-lactamase coverage.
- Clinicians should reevaluate a child whose symptoms have worsened or not responded to the initial antibiotic treatment within 48 to 72 hours and change treatment if indicated.
- In children with recurrent AOM, tympanostomy tubes, but not prophylactic antibiotics, may be indicated to reduce the frequency of AOM episodes.
- Clinicians should recommend pneumococcal conjugate vaccine and annual influenza vaccine to all children according to updated schedules
- Clinicians should encourage exclusive breastfeeding for 6 months or longer

Antibiotic options

- Amoxicillin 80 mg/kg divided BID–TID for 10 days — preferred first line drug
- Augmentin (amoxicillin/clavulanate) 80 mg/kg divided TID for 10 days
- Zithromax (azithromycin) 10 mg/kg day 1, then 5 mg/kg qday for following 4 days
- Rocephin (ceftriaxone) 50 mg/kg IM × 1 dose (NMT 1,000 mg)
    - Treat qday for 3 days if resistance is suspected
- Septra (trimethoprim/sulfamethoxazole) 0.4 mg/kg BID PO or 0.5 cc/LB BID PO for 10 days
    - Contraindicated in ages < 2 months

- Cefuroxime 30 mg/kg BID for 10 days

  Otitis media with draining PE tubes more effectively treated with otic HC/bacitracin/colistin 5 drops tid for 7 days than oral antibiotics
- May use Sanford Guide or other drug databases

Discharge Criteria

- Uncomplicated otitis media

Discharge instructions

- Otitis media aftercare instructions
- Follow up in 7–10 days if symptoms persist

Consult Criteria

- Toxic patient
- Dehydration > 5% who have not responded to ORT (oral rehydration therapy — see Pediatric Dehydration Protocol)
- Pneumonia
- Age < 2 months
- Fever of unknown etiology

Vital signs consult criteria

- Hypothermia < 95°F (35°C)
- Fever ≥ 104.5°F (40.3°C)
- Pediatric heart rate
  - 0–4 months ≥ 180
  - 5–7 months ≥ 175
  - 8–12 months ≥ 170
  - 1–3 years ≥ 160
  - 4–5 years ≥ 145
  - 6–8 years ≥ 130
  - 9–12 years ≥ 125
  - 13–15 years ≥ 120
  - 16 years or older ≥ 110
  - O_2 saturation < 95% on room air

Lab consult criteria

- WBC ≥ 18,000 or < 3,000
- Bandemia ≥ 15%
- Acute thrombocytopenia

Notes

References:

Pediatrics Vol. 131 No. 3 March 1, 2013

Otitis Media Treatment & Management:
Muhammad Waseem, MD, MS; Glenn C Isaacson, MD, FACS, FAAP; Muhammad Aslam, MD; Orval Brown, MD, Daniel Rauch, MD, FAAP; Glenn C Isaacson, MD, FACS, FAAP, et.al.
Emedicine.medscape.com

PEDIATRIC ASTHMA PROTOCOL

When using any protocol, always follow the Guidelines of Proper Use (page 18).

Definition

- Reversible acute bronchospasm and airway resistance secondary to infectious, allergic, environmental or internal stimuli

Differential Diagnosis

- Panic disorder
- Pneumonia
- Bronchitis
- Bronchiolitis
- Aspiration
- CHF
- COPD
- Anaphylaxis
- URI
- Vocal cord dysfunction
- Laryngospasm
- Epiglottitis
- Croup
- Retropharyngeal abscess

Considerations

- Cough is commonly the first symptom
- Viral URI or allergens or environmental stimuli most common causes of asthma
- Severe episode may have decreased breath sounds without wheezing
- There is evidence that dexamethasone is preferable to prednisone/prednisolone for pediatric patients presenting to the ED with an acute asthma exacerbation
    - A single PO dose of dexamethasone plus PO dose on day 3 to take at home is as effective as 5 day course of prednisone/prednisolone
        - Onset of action IV is 1 hour
        - PO onset of action is 1–2 hours

    - Duration of action is 36–54 hours
  - Dexamethasone causes less vomiting (has antiemetic properties), has improved compliance, and higher parental preference

Peak flow % of predicted (age > 5 yrs. old)

- Mild asthma ≥ 70
- Moderate 40–69%
- Severe < 40%

Principles of Asthma Management

- Recognizing severity of exacerbation
- Using correct therapy
- Identify and treat any precipitants
- Make correct disposition

Evaluation

- Complete history and physical exam
- Assess respiratory effort
- Assess hydration status
- CBC and/or BMP for significant tachycardia and fever
- O_2 saturation measurement
- Consider peak flows before and after aerosols for age 5 years or higher
- Check radiology interpretations if completed prior to discharge if chest x-ray performed

Chest x-ray if

- Pneumonia suspected
- Significant respiratory distress
- Respiratory distress not responsive to aerosols

Treatment Options

- Supplemental oxygen for O_2 Sat < 94% on room air or significant respiratory distress
- Albuterol (with or without atrovent) aerosols up to 3 treatments total every 15–20 minutes prn
  - Nebulized lidocaine solutions 1cc of a 1% solution in 4mL of saline to give 0.25% solution after albuterol treatment for intractable cough may be tried

Additional treatment options if needed for severe exacerbations (notify physician promptly)

- Continuous Albuterol with or without atrovent and notify physician promptly
- Terbutaline 0.25 mg SQ prn q15–20 minutes up to 3 as needed for age ≥ 12 years
- Terbutaline 0.005–0.01 mg/kg SQ q15–20 minutes up to 3 – age < 12 years (NMT 0.4 mg per dose)
- Epinephrine 0.01 mg/kg SQ in children usually not to exceed 0.3 mg per dose up to 3 doses (if severe may give IV or IM)
- MgSO4 (magnesium sulfate) 25–75 mg/kg IV over 10–20 minutes per physician (NMT 2 gm) for children
- MgSO4 (magnesium sulfate) 125–250 mg in 0.3 ml NS aerosol q 20 minutes up to 4 doses as needed (off label use)
  - May combine with albuterol
- May use bipap if needed

Steroid treatment options useful for moderate to severe exacerbations (caution with diabetes)

Effectiveness starts around 3–6 hours after dosing

- Prednisolone 1 mg/kg PO

  OR

- Decadron (dexamethasone) 0.6 mg/kg IV or IM (NMT 20 mg)

Practitioners should consider 2-dose regimen of dexamethasone on day 1 and day 3 as a viable alternative to a 5-day course of prednisone/prednisolone for pediatric asthma

Discharge treatment options

- Albuterol MDI with spacer prn at home (or nebulizer) – give up to 7 puffs in spacer for each treatment as needed
- Albuterol syrup per weight for patients unable to use MDI
- Antibiotics not needed usually
- If bacterial infection suspected, use Sanford Guide or antibiotic database

Discharge systemic steroid treatment (caution if diabetic)

- Prednisolone or prednisone 1 mg/kg PO x 3 days (NMT 60 mg/dose)
- Decadron (dexamethasone) 0.6 mg/kg PO and again on day 3 (NMT 20 mg per dose) — if PO route not usable then IM – preferred over prednisone/prednisolone (see above comment)

Discharge inhaled steroids

- Consider inhaled steroid Rx only after acute exacerbation has resolved
  - Prescribe double dose if already on single strength dose

    OR
  - Advair diskus bid – age > 3 years (combination of long acting beta-agonist and steroid) to be used only after acute exacerbation has resolved
    - Use 100/50 strength dose bid for age 4–11 years
    - Use adult strength for age ≥ 12 years

Discharge Criteria

- Good response to therapy
- Peak flow ≥ 70% predicted if checked (age 5 years or higher)
- O_2 saturation ≥ 94% on room air
- < 5% dehydrated post ORT (oral rehydration therapy) if needed
- Good follow-up and compliance

Discharge instructions

- Follow up in 1–5 days depending on severity of illness and response to treatments
- Provide pediatric asthma aftercare instructions

Consult Criteria

- Insufficient response to treatment
- Work of breathing moderate to severe post Rx
- Wheezing not resolving adequately

- Patient or family of child feels patient is too dyspneic to go home
- Peak flow < 70% predicted if checked
- Moderate respiratory distress
- Age < 6 months
- > 5% dehydration post rehydration
- Poor feeding
- Unable to self-hydrate
- O_2 saturation < 94% on room air post treatment
- Significant comorbid conditions
    - Pediatric heart rate
        - 0–4 months ≥ 180
        - 5–7 months ≥ 175
        - 8–12 months ≥ 170
        - 1–3 years ≥ 160
        - 4–5 years ≥ 145
        - 6–8 years ≥ 130
        - 9–12 years ≥ 125
        - 13–15 years ≥ 120
        - 16 years or older ≥ 110

Notes

References:

Redman E, et al. Arch Dis Children 2013; 98: 916

Williams KW, Â et al. Clin Pediatr 2013;52:30

Keeney GE, et al. Pediatrics March 1, 2014, 133:493–499

Pediatr Emerg Care. 2018 Jan:34:53

Udezue E Lidocaine inhalation for cough suppression *Am J Emerg Med* 2001;19(3):206-7

PEDIATRIC PNEUMONIA PROTOCOL

When using any protocol, always follow the Guidelines of Proper Use (page 18).

Definition

- Infection of pulmonary parenchymal tissue

Differential Diagnosis

- Asthma
- CHF
- Bronchitis
- Bronchopulmonary dysplasia in children with history of prematurity

Considerations

- Number one leading cause of death from infectious disease
- Community acquired causes
    - Strep pneumoniae
    - Mycoplasma pneumoniae
    - H. influenzae
    - Legionella pneumophilia
    - Klebsiella pneumoniae
    - Influenza
- Comorbid conditions
    - Diabetes
    - CHF
    - HIV
    - Immunosuppression
- Signs and Symptoms
    - Cough
    - Sputum production
    - Fever
    - Chills
    - Rigors
    - Dyspnea

- Chest pain
- ***Newborns with pneumonia***
    - Rarely cough
    - More commonly present with poor feeding and irritability, as well as tachypnea, retractions, grunting, and hypoxemia
    - Grunting in a newborn suggests a lower respiratory tract disease
- WBC ≥ 15,000 suggest bacterial infection
- Very high or very low WBC predicts increased mortality

Criteria for Respiratory Distress in Children With Pneumonia (WHO)

Signs of Respiratory Distress

- Age 0–2 months: respiratory rate 60/minute
- Age 2–12 months: 50/minute
- Age 1–5 Years: 40/minute
- Age 5 Years: 20/minute
- Dyspnea
- Retractions (suprasternal, intercostal, or subcostal)
- Grunting
- Nasal flaring
- Apnea
- Altered mental status
- Pulse oximetry measurement 90% on room air

Evaluation

- CBC
- Chest x-ray — may not be needed for suspected CAP in patients that will have outpatient treatment (may be negative even if pneumonia is present)
    - Obtain chest x-ray if patient in respiratory distress or hypoxic and has failed outpatient antibiotic therapy
- ABG if moderate to severe respiratory distress or fatigue
- Blood cultures if toxic or hypotensive and/or patient is to be admitted

Treatment Options

- Oxygen for O2 saturation < 93%
- Viral pneumonia, which is most common type in preschool patients, usually needs no antibiotic treatment unless immunosuppressed
- IV NS/LR or oral rehydration if dehydrated (see Gastroenteritis Protocols for rehydration therapy)

Nontoxic patient treatment that is to be discharged

No chronic cardiopulmonary disease

Age 1–3 months

- Azithromycin 10 mg/kg/1st day PO, then 5 mg/kg/day for 5 days PO

Age 4 months – 5 years

- Amoxicillin 80-90 mg/kg/qday divided into BID dosing x 10 days (first line drug)
  - Or augmentin dosed with same amoxicillin level

OR

- Second line azithromycin 10 mg/kg PO on day 1, followed by 5 mg/kg PO on days 2 through 5 (do not exceed adolescent dosing) for suspected atypical pneumonia

Age 5-15 years

- Amoxicillin 80-90 mg/kg divided into 2 doses (> 40kg: 875 mg PO q12hr or 500 mg PO q8hr for 10-14 days) if bacterial pneumonia suspected

OR

- Augmentin dosed with same amoxicillin level

OR/PLUS

(may combine if clinically needed)

- Azithromycin 10 mg/kg PO on day 1, followed by 5 mg/kg PO on days 2 through 5 for atypical suspected pathogens like mycoplasma (do not exceed adolescent dosing)
  - May use doxycycline age > 7 years of age

- **Maximum amoxicillin total daily dose is NMT 4 gms**

Age ≥ 16 years

- Levaquin 750 mg PO qday X 10 days or azithromycin (Z-pak)
  - Caution using quinolones in children due to possible arthropathy complications

For patients with significant respiratory distress, hypoxemia, toxicity, or are to be admitted:

- IV NS
- IV Zithromax and Rocephin (ceftriaxone)
- Age ≤ 28 days give ampicillin + gentamicin or cefotaxime IV and admission
- Consult physician

Discharge Criteria

- Nontoxic patient
- No respiratory distress
- O2 saturation >93%

Discharge instructions

- Pneumonia aftercare instructions
- Follow up with primary care provider within 1–3 days
- Return if worse

Consult Criteria

- Significant pneumonia
- Patients that the Provider feels need admission
- Significant respiratory distress
- High fever ≥ 104°F (40°C)
- Temperature < 96°F (35.5°C)
- Appears ill or toxic
- Metabolic or respiratory acidosis
- Immunosuppression
- Age < 2 months
- No significant improvement in 48-72 hours
- Failure of outpatient treatment
- Immunizations not up to date

Vital signs and age consult criteria

- Heart rate
    - 0–4 months ≥ 180
    - 5–7 months ≥ 175
    - 6–12 months ≥ 170
    - 1–3 years ≥ 160
    - 4–5 years ≥ 150
    - 6–8 years ≥ 130
    - 7–12 years ≥ 125
    - 12–15 years ≥ 120
    - 16 years or older ≥ 115
- O2 Sat < 94% on room air
- Lab and x-ray consult criteria
    - New onset renal insufficiency or worsening renal insufficiency
    - WBC ≥ 18,000 or < 4,000; Neutrophil count < 1,000
    - Bandemia ≥ 15%
    - Acute thrombocytopenia
    - Anion gap > 18
    - Significant electrolyte abnormally
    - Glucose ≥ 300 mg/dL in diabetic patient
    - Glucose ≥ 200 mg/dL in new onset diabetic patient
    - Hyperglycemia with metabolic acidosis (decreased serum CO2 or elevated anion gap)
    - Pleural effusion
    - Significant pneumonia

Notes

References:

Bradley JS, Byington CL, Shah SS, et al. The management of community-acquired pneumonia in infants and children older than 3 months of age: clinical practice guidelines by the pediatric infectious diseases society and the infectious diseases society of america. *Clin Infect Dis*. 2011 Oct. 53(7):e25-76

Aujesky D, Auble TE, Yealy DM, et al. Prospective comparison of three validated prediction rules for prognosis in community-acquired pneumonia. *Am J Med* 2005; 118:384-92

Mandell LA, Wunderink RG, Anzueto A, et al. Infectious disease society of America/American Thoracic Society consensus guidelines on the management of community-acquired pneumonia. *Clin Infect Dis* 2007: 44(2):S27-72

Bacterial Pneumonia Author: Nader Kamangar, MD, FACP, FCCP, FCCM, FAASM; Chief Editor: Zab Mosenifar, MD emedicine.medscape.com/article/300157

Pediatric Pneumonia Medication Author: Nicholas John Bennett, MBBCh, PhD; Chief Editor: Russell W Steele, MD emedicine.medscape.com/article/967822

Pediatric Pneumonia Clinical Presentation
Updated: Nov 05, 2018 Author: Nicholas John Bennett, MBBCh, PhD, MA(Cantab), FAAP; Chief Editor: Russell W Steele, MD

BRONCHIOLITIS PROTOCOL

When using any protocol, always follow the Guidelines of Proper Use (page 18).

Definition

- Bronchiolitis is an acute infectious disease process of the lower respiratory tract that occurs primarily in young infants, most often in those aged 2–24 months, that may result in obstruction of small airways

Differential Diagnosis

- Asthma
- Pneumonia
- Bronchitis
- Congenital heart disease
- Aspiration
- Foreign body obstruction
- Congestive heart failure
- Bronchopulmonary dysplasia (prematurity history)

Considerations

- Age < 2 years usually
- Fall and spring peaks
- RSV usual cause
- Wheezing and tachypnea usually present
- Hypoxia best predictor of severity of illness
- Variable response to bronchodilators
- Steroids not effective
- Dehydration and poor feeding not uncommon
- Fever usually low grade
- Rhinorrhea and cough frequent
- Apnea more commonly seen in infants < 2 months of age or premature infants
- Hydration treatment helpful possibly

Higher risk

- Prematurity
- Bronchopulmonary dysplasia history
- Cardiac history

Evaluation

- Complete history and physical
- O_2 saturation measurement
- Work of breathing assessment
- Dehydration assessment
- Chest x-ray not routinely be needed unless ill appearing, respiratory distress or underlying cardiopulmonary conditions
- CBC and BMP if moderate to severe respiratory distress or > 5% dehydration
- RSV testing usually not needed unless antibiotics are being considered — positive RSV may stop antibiotic treatment
- RSV testing if admitted, history of prematurity or cardiopulmonary disease history

Treatment Options

- Supplemental O_2 if O_2 saturation < 93%
- Trial with Albuterol aerosol with or without atrovent — may repeat × 2 as needed
    - Controversy whether it is effective
- Oral or IV hydration for dehydration
    - Refer to Pediatric Diarrhea Protocol
- No steroids unless history of asthma

Discharge Criteria

- Feeding well
- Absence of significant respiratory distress
- O_2 saturation ≥ 94% on room air
- < 5% dehydrated post ORT (oral rehydration therapy) if given
- Good follow-up and compliance
- Contact primary care physician or provider to alert of visit if in acute care facility and arrange follow-up

Discharge instructions

- Bronchiolitis aftercare instructions
- Follow up with primary care provider within 1–2 days if seen initially in acute care facility
- Return if symptoms worsen
- Return if activity or feeding decreases

Consult Criteria

- Age < 6 months — discuss with physician
- Significant respiratory distress post treatment or respiratory rate > 60/minute
- Significant chest x-ray infiltrates
- O_2 saturation < 94% on room air post treatment
- Family feels patient is too dyspneic to go home
- > 5% dehydration after any rehydration treatment
- Poor feeding
- Unable to self-hydrate
- Persistent vomiting
- History of apnea
- Significant comorbid conditions
- Toxic appearance
- Respiratory fatigue
- Hypotension
- Heart rate
  - 0–4 months ≥ 180
  - 5–7 months ≥ 175
  - 8–12 months ≥ 170
  - 1–3 years ≥ 160

Notes

References:

Kristjansson S, Lodrup Carlsen KC, Wennergren G, et al. Nebulised racemic adrenaline in the treatment of acute bronchiolitis in infants and toddlers. *Arch Dis Child* 1993;69(6):650–4

Bronchiolitis Author: Lucian Kenneth DeNicola, MD, MS, FAAP, FCCM; Chief Editor: Russell W Steele, MD emedicine.medscape.com/article/961963

Gadomski AM, Scribani MB. Bronchodilators for bronchiolitis. Cochrane Database of Systematic Reviews 2014, Issue 6.

Art. No.: CD001266. DOI: 10.1002/14651858.CD001266.pub4

Al-Ansari K, Sakran M, Davidson BL, El Sayyed R, Mahjoub H, Ibrahim K. Nebulized 5% or 3% hypertonic or 0.9% saline for treating acute bronchiolitis in infants. *J Pediatr*. Oct 2010;157(4):630–4, 634.e1

Croup Protocol

When using any protocol, always follow the Guidelines of Proper Use (page 18).

Definition

- Infection of the upper respiratory tract (trachea) that is usually of a viral etiology and causes varying degrees of obstruction and is usually self-limited

Differential Diagnosis

- Epiglottitis
- Retropharyngeal abscess
- Foreign body in trachea
- Foreign body in esophagus
- Peritonsillar abscess
- Subglottic stenosis
- Tracheomalacia
- Vocal cord paralysis

Considerations

- Most common in 6 months to 6 years of age
- Peak is 2 years of age
- Parainfluenza virus most common, followed by RSV and Influenza
- Seal-like barking cough
- Stridor at rest indicates increased risk
- Can be life threatening
- Drooling may indicate epiglottitis
- Lab tests usually not needed unless patient appears dehydrated or in significant distress
    - Defer blood tests initially when respiratory distress is present
- Imaging not required in mild cases that respond to treatment
- Neck AP & lateral for stridor at rest or significant respiratory distress
    - Consult physician before obtaining films if in significant distress
    - Steeple sign indicative of croup on neck film

- Thumb or vallecula sign (loss of vallecula) indicative for epiglottitis
- Retropharyngeal swelling for retropharyngeal abscess

Severity assessment

Mild severity

- Occasional barking cough
- No audible stridor at rest
- Either no or mild suprasternal or intercostal retractions

Moderate severity

- Frequent barking cough
- Easily audible stridor at rest
- Suprasternal and sternal retractions at rest, with little or no agitation

Severe severity

- Frequent barking cough
- Prominent inspiratory and occasionally expiratory stridor
- Marked sternal retractions
- Agitation and distress

Impending respiratory failure

- Barking cough (often not prominent)
- Audible rest stridor
- Sternal retractions may not be marked (fatigue)
- Lethargy or decreased mentation
- Often dusky appearance if no supplemental oxygen given

Evaluation

- Complete history and physical exam
- Patients can sit on parent's lap for exam
- O_2 saturation measurement
- Assess respiratory effort and for respiratory distress
- Assess for dehydration
- BMP if > 5% dehydrated clinically
- CBC if toxic — hold blood draw if severe respiratory distress

- If drooling or in sniff position consult physician immediately
- Avoid actions that agitate patient

Imaging studies

- Not required in mild cases or that respond to treatment
- Chest x-ray and soft tissue neck films in cases without adequate response to treatment or moderate or greater severity if clinical situation safely permits

Treatment Options

- Humidified oxygen if O_2 saturation < 95%
- Racemic epinephrine if stridor at rest — observe for 2 hours for recurrence of stridor at rest
- Decadron (dexamethasone) 0.6 mg/kg IM (do not exceed 10 mg)

  OR
- Decadron (dexamethasone) 0.15–0.6 mg/kg PO (NMT 10 mg) or prednisolone 1–2 mg/kg PO (NMT 60 mg); Single dosing effective for mild to moderate croup
  - Dexamethasone 0.15 mg/kg as effective as 0.3–0.6 mg/kg
- Consider prednisolone 1–2 mg/kg PO × 5 days
- Avoid steroids in varicella (chickenpox)
- Cool mist vaporizer (or night air) may help
- Antibiotics rarely needed
- Follow up with within 24 hours
- Check radiology interpretations prior to discharge if completed

Discharge Criteria

- Mild croup
- Moderate or severe croup with good response to therapy (discuss with physician)

Discharge instructions

- Croup aftercare instructions
- Refer to primary care provider or notify of visit and arrange follow-up if in acute care facility
- Return if symptoms worsen

Consult Criteria

- Stridor at rest unresponsive to treatment
- Moderate to severe croup post treatment
- Notify physician promptly if "severe" severity assessment or impending respiratory failure
- Dehydration > 5% unresponsive to oral hydration
- Epiglottitis
- Pharyngeal or retropharyngeal abscess
- Suspected foreign body
- O_2 saturation ≤ 95% on room air after treatments
- Moderate to severe respiratory distress
- Significant chest x–ray infiltrates
- Depressed sensorium
- Poor oral intake
- Poor home situation

Vital signs consult criteria

- Pediatric heart rate
    - 0–4 months ≥ 180
    - 5–7 months ≥ 175
    - 8–12 months ≥ 170
    - 1–3 years ≥ 160
    - 4–5 years ≥ 150
    - 6–8 years ≥ 135
- Hypotension
- Age > 7 years or < 5 months

Lab consult criteria

- WBC ≥ 15,000 or < 3,000
- Acute thrombocytopenia
- Bandemia ≥ 15%
- Metabolic acidosis

Notes

References:
Croup Author: Germaine L Defendi, MD, MS, FAAP; Chief Editor: Russell W Steele, MD emedicine.medscape.com/article/962972

Russell KF, Liang Y, O'Gorman K, Johnson DW, Klassen TP. Glucocorticoids for croup. Cochrane Database of Systematic Reviews 2011, Issue 1. Art. No.: CD001955. DOI: 10.1002/14651858.CD001955

Pediatr Emerg Care. 2018 Jan:34:53

PEDIATRIC DEHYDRATION AND GASTROENTERITIS PROTOCOL

When using any protocol, always follow the Guidelines of Proper Use (page 18).

Definition

- Acute inflammatory or infectious process of the stomach and intestines

Differential Diagnosis

- Colitis
- Appendicitis
- Cholecystitis
- Pancreatitis
- Peptic ulcer disease
- GERD
- Biliary colic
- Renal colic
- Bowel obstruction
- Inflammatory bowel disease
- Pyloric stenosis in infants
- Volvulus in infants
- Diabetic ketoacidosis

Considerations

- Degree (%) of acute weight loss indicates degree of dehydration
- Decreased serum CO_2 and increased anion gap are early indicators of dehydration
  - BUN and creatinine rise later
- Vomiting may occur in early gastroenteritis prior to diarrhea
- Vomiting by itself may indicate mechanical obstruction if without fever or diarrhea
- Vomiting with fever only may be from a UTI
- Viral infections are the usual etiology
- Antibiotics not usually indicated

    - Use Sanford guide or antibiotic database prn
- Oral rehydration therapy (ORT) preferred over IV in mild to moderate dehydration

Dehydration assessment

Mild < 5%

- Alert
- Mucous membranes variable dry
- Skin turgor normal
- Fontanel flat
- Blood pressure normal
- Heart rate normal
- Capillary refill < 2 seconds
- Urine output decreased

Moderate 6–9%

- Irritable
- Mucous membranes dry
- Skin turgor variably reduced
- Fontanel depressed
- Blood pressure variably orthostatic
- Heart rate tachycardic
- Capillary refill 2–3 seconds
- Urine output decreased — oliguria

Severe ≥ 10%

- Lethargic
- Mucous membranes dry
- Skin turgor reduced
- Fontanel depressed
- Blood pressure orthostatic or hypotensive
- Heart rate markedly tachycardic
- Capillary refill ≥ 4 seconds
- Urine output decreased — oliguria/anuria

Evaluation

- Detailed history and PE
- Assess patient activity and interactions
- Perform baseline dehydration assessment
- BMP if appears moderate to severely dehydrated

- Lactic acid level and venous pH if in shock or severely dehydrated
- CBC if patient appears less active

  OR

  Pediatric heart rate
  - 0–4 months ≥ 180
  - 5–7 months ≥ 175
  - 8–12 months ≥ 170
  - 1–3 years ≥ 160
  - 4–5 years ≥ 145
  - 6–8 years ≥ 130
  - 9–11 years ≥ 125
  - 12–15 years ≥ 120
  - 16 years or older ≥ 110
- Check U/A if vomiting and fever are only symptoms
- Consider imaging if obstruction suspected
- Stool studies prn

Treatment Options

- < 5% dehydration by weight (or serum CO_2 > 18 mEq/L) small frequent feedings with pedialyte/rehydrate, etc. up to 24 hours
- Zofran (ondansetron) oral chewable tablet in ED for frequent vomiting
  - 2 mg for 8–15 kg; 4 mg for 14–30 kg; 8 mg for > 30 kg
  - Zofran (ondansetron) 2–4 doses can be prescribed for home if indicated

Oral Rehydration Therapy (ORT) for mild to moderate dehydration

- Oral rehydration formula (WHO formula, Rehydralyte or Pedialyte) for above vital signs; mild to moderate dehydration or serum CO_2 14–18 mEq/L
  - 5 cc every 1–2 minutes for small children by caretaker for < 4 hours — start 20 minutes after Zofran (ondansetron) given
  - 5–10 cc every 1–2 minutes for larger children by caretaker for 1–4 hours

    - Hold ORT 10 minutes if vomiting occurs then resume
    - Reassess for urine production, weight gain, improved heart rate and alertness, and absence of severe vomiting
    - Recheck serum CO_2 if initially < 17 mEq/L
    - Mild dehydration give 50 cc/kg in < 4 hours
    - Moderate dehydration give 50–100 cc/kg within 1–4 hours
- Severe dehydration give IV NS or LR bolus 20 cc/kg; may repeat x 2

Exclusion criteria for Oral Rehydration Therapy

- Age < 6 months of age
- Hematemesis
- Bilious vomiting
- Bloody diarrhea
- VP shunt
- Head trauma
- Focal RLQ tenderness (possible appendicitis)
- Severe dehydration
- Patient vomits 3 or more times after starting ORT

IV therapy criteria and treatment for moderate to severe dehydration

- IV NS or LR hydration for CO_2 < 14 mEq/L
- ORT failure
- IV NS/LR 20 cc/kg bolus, may repeat × 2
- Consult physician
- Up to 2 times maintenance IV with D5NS after any vigorous NS rehydration therapy is completed if patient is to be further observed (dextrose clears ketosis faster and decreases return visits)

Home rehydration formula

- In 1 L of water, add 2 level tablespoons of sugar or honey, a quarter teaspoon of table salt (NaCl), and a quarter teaspoon of baking soda (bicarbonate of soda)—add 0.5 cup of orange juice (taste to make sure not more salty than tears)

Discharge Criteria

- Nontoxic patients with mild dehydration
- Patients responding to rehydration with significantly improved vital signs, normal alertness and interaction
- $CO_2 \geq 18$ mEq/L if rechecked
- Improved urine output in mild to moderate dehydration

Discharge instructions

- Pediatric dehydration, gastroenteritis, vomiting or diarrhea aftercare instructions
- Frequent small feedings of 10 cc of pedialyte or rehydrate every 10 minutes at home as needed for continued symptoms
- Resume regular diet (except milk initially) as soon as symptoms start resolving
    - May need to change to soy formula in infants
- Follow up with primary care provider within 1–2 days if symptoms not improving sufficiently at home
- May use dilute apple juice for outpatient treatment of mild gastroenteritis and minimal dehydration

Consult Criteria

- Toxic appearance
- Greater than 5% dehydration post rehydration
- Poor response to treatment
- Persistent vomiting
- Worrisome abdominal tenderness
- Petechial rash
- Seizure

Vital signs consult criteria

- **Pediatric heart rate** — post rehydration therapy
    - 0–4 months ≥ 180
    - 5–7 months ≥ 175
    - 8–12 months ≥ 170
    - 1–3 years ≥ 160
    - 4–5 years ≥ 145
    - 6–8 years ≥ 130

    - 9–12 years ≥ 125
    - 13–15 years ≥ 120
    - 16 years or older ≥ 110
- Hypotension develops or orthostatic vital signs

Lab consult criteria

- Serum CO_2 < 18 mEq/L post rehydration
- Initial serum CO_2 < 17 mEq/L
- WBC ≥ 15,000 or < 3,000
- Bandemia ≥ 15%
- Acute thrombocytopenia

Notes

References:

King CK, Glass R, Bresee JS, Duggan C. Managing acute gastroenteritis among children: oral rehydration, maintenance, and nutritional therapy. *MMWR Recomm Rep*. Nov 21 2003;52:1–16

[Best Evidence] Spandorfer PR, Alessandrini EA, Joffe MD, Localio R, Shaw KN. Oral versus intravenous rehydration of moderately dehydrated children: a randomized, controlled trial. *Pediatrics*. Feb 2005;115(2):295–301

Freedman, S. B et al. Effect of dilute apple juice and preferred fluids versus electrolyte maintenance solution on treatment failure among children with mild gastroenteritis: a randomized clinical trial. JAMA 315, 1966–1974 (2016)

PEDIATRIC DIARRHEA PROTOCOL

When using any protocol, always follow the Guidelines of Proper Use (page 18).

Definition

- Increased fluid content of stool and frequency of bowel movements usually secondary to viral or bacterial infection

Differential Diagnosis

- Inflammatory bowel disease
- Irritable bowel syndrome
- Malabsorption syndromes

Considerations

- Degree (%) of acute weight loss indicates degree of dehydration
- Serum CO_2 and increased anion gap early indicators of dehydration
- BUN and creatinine rise later
- Viruses 70–80% — Bacteria 10–20% — Parasites 5% — Use Sanford Guide or other drug databases prn
- Can be from allergy, food intolerance, malabsorption or inflammatory causes.
- Oral rehydration therapy (ORT) preferred over IV in mild to moderate dehydration.

Dehydration assessment

Mild < 5%

- Alert
- Mucous membranes variable dry
- Skin turgor normal
- Fontanel flat
- Blood pressure normal
- Heart rate normal
- Capillary refill < 2 seconds
- Urine output decreased

Moderate 6–9%

- Irritable

- Mucous membranes dry
- Skin turgor variably reduced
- Fontanel depressed
- Blood pressure variably orthostatic
- Heart rate tachycardic
- Capillary refill 2–3 seconds
- Urine output — oliguria

Severe ≥ 10%

- Lethargic
- Mucous membranes dry
- Skin turgor reduced
- Fontanel depressed
- Blood pressure orthostatic or hypotensive
- Heart rate markedly tachycardic
- Capillary refill ≥ 4 seconds
- Urine output decreased — oliguria/anuria

Evaluation

- Detailed history and PE
- Assess patient activity/interaction
- Perform baseline dehydration assessment
- BMP for moderate to severe dehydration
- Venous pH and lactic acid level if in shock or severe dehydration
- CBC and patient appears less active

  OR

  Pediatric heart rate is

  - 0–4 months ≥ 180
  - 5–7 months ≥ 175
  - 8–12 months ≥ 170
  - 1–3 years ≥ 160
  - 4–5 years ≥ 145
  - 6–8 years ≥ 130
  - 9–12 years ≥ 125
  - 13–15 years ≥ 120
  - 16 years or older ≥ 110
- Check U/A if vomiting and fever only symptoms
- Consider imaging if obstruction suspected
- Stool studies prn (consider rotavirus antigen)

Oral Rehydration Therapy (ORT) for Mild to Moderate Dehydration

- Oral rehydration formula (WHO formula, Rehydralyte or Pedialyte) for above vital signs; mild to moderate dehydration or serum CO_2 14–18 mEq/L
    - 5 cc every 1–2 minutes for small children by caretaker for < 4 hours
    - 5–10 cc every 1–2 minutes for larger children by caretaker for 1–4 hours
    - Hold ORT 10 minutes if vomiting occurs then resume
    - Reassess for urine production, weight gain, improved heart rate and alertness, and absence of severe vomiting
    - Recheck serum CO_2 if initially < 17 mEq/L
    - Mild dehydration give 50 cc/kg in < 4 hours
    - Moderate dehydration give 50–100 cc/kg within 1–4 hours

Severe dehydration give IV NS bolus 20 cc/kg; may repeat × 2 prn

Home rehydration formula

- In 1 L of water, add 2 level tablespoons of sugar or honey, a quarter teaspoon of table salt (NaCl), and a quarter teaspoon of baking soda (bicarbonate of soda)—add 0.5 cup of orange juice (taste to make sure not more salty than tears)

Exclusion criteria for Oral Rehydration Therapy

- Age < 6 months of age
- Hematemesis
- Bilious vomiting
- Bloody diarrhea
- VP shunt
- Head trauma
- Focal RLQ tenderness (possible appendicitis)
- Severe dehydration
- Patient vomits 3 or more times after starting ORT

IV Therapy Criteria and Treatment for Moderate to Severe Dehydration

- IV NS or LR hydration for CO_2 < 14 mEq/L
- ORT failure
- IV NS or LR 20 cc/kg bolus, may repeat × 2 prn
- Consult physician
- Maintenance IV with D5NS (Dextrose decreases return visits)

Antibiotic therapy for bloody diarrhea

- World Health Organization currently recommends empiric antimicrobial therapy in the setting of febrile acute bloody diarrhea in young children
  - Infections by enteropathogenic *E coli*, when running a prolonged course — septra or ceftriaxone
  - Enteroinvasive *E coli*, based on the serologic, genetic, and pathogenic similarities with *Shigella* — septra or ceftriaxone
  - *Yersinia* infections in subjects with sickle cell disease — septra or cipro or ceftriaxone or doxycycline (avoid doxycycline in age <8 years)
  - *Salmonella* infections in very young infants, if febrile or with positive blood culture findings — ceftriaxone
    - Most salmonella infections do not require antibiotics and they may prolong the illness

Discharge Criteria

- Nontoxic patients with mild dehydration.
- Patients responding to rehydration with significantly improved vital signs, normal alertness and interaction
- $CO_2 \geq 18$ mEq/L, with weight gain and improved urine output in mild to moderate dehydration

Discharge instructions

- Pediatric dehydration or diarrhea aftercare instructions
- Frequent small feedings of 10 cc of pedialyte or rehydrate every 10 minutes at home as needed for continued symptoms

- Resume regular diet (except milk initially) as soon as symptoms start resolving
    - May need to change to soy formula in infants
- Follow up with primary care provider within 1–2 days if symptoms not improving sufficiently at home
- May use dilute apple juice for outpatient treatment of mild gastroenteritis and minimal dehydration

Consult Criteria

- Toxic appearance
- Greater than 5% dehydration post rehydration
- Poor response to treatment
- Worrisome abdominal tenderness
- Petechial rash
- More than 1 visit for same episode of diarrhea

Vital signs consult criteria

- **Pediatric heart rate** — post rehydration therapy
    - 0–4 months ≥ 180
    - 5–7 months ≥ 175
    - 8–12 months ≥ 170
    - 1–3 years ≥ 160
    - 4–5 years ≥ 145
    - 6–8 years ≥ 130
    - 9–11 years ≥ 125
    - 12–15 years ≥ 115
    - 16 years or older ≥ 110
- Hypotension develops or orthostatic vital signs

Lab consult criteria

- Serum CO_2 < 18 mEq/L post rehydration
- Initial serum CO_2 < 17 mEq/L
- WBC ≥ 15,000 or < 3,000
- Bandemia ≥ 15%
- Acute thrombocytopenia

Notes

References:

King CK, Glass R, Bresee JS, Duggan C. Managing acute gastroenteritis among children: oral rehydration, maintenance, and nutritional therapy. *MMWR Recomm Rep*. Nov 21 2003;52:1–16

[Best Evidence] Spandorfer PR, Alessandrini EA, Joffe MD, Localio R, Shaw KN. Oral versus intravenous rehydration of moderately dehydrated children: a randomized, controlled trial. *Pediatrics*. Feb 2005;115(2):295–301

Pediatric Dehydration Author: Alex Koyfman, MD; emedicine.medscape.com/article/801012

Diarrhea Author: Stefano Guandalini, MD; Chief Editor: Carmen Cuffari, MD medicine.medscape.com/article/928598

Freedman, S. B et al. Effect of dilute apple juice and preferred fluids versus electrolyte maintenance solution on treatment failure among children with mild gastroenteritis: a randomized clinical trial. JAMA 315, 1966–1974 (2016)

Brief Resolved Unexplained Event (BRUE) Protocol

When using any Protocol, always follow the Guidelines of Proper Use (page 18).

Definition

- Episode that is characterized by some combination of following in patient <1 year of age
  - Apnea (central or obstructive) or altered respiration
  - Color change (cyanotic, pallid, erythematous or plethoric)
  - Change in muscle tone (usually diminished)
  - Choking or gagging
  - Altered level of consciousness
- No other explanation for event
- No other symptoms such as fever, respiratory etc. that could cause the event
- Was labeled in past as Apparent Life Threatening Event

Considerations

- No proven correlation with SIDS
- Is a description of an event and not a diagnosis
- Morbidity is low
- If patient did not move when picked up after event suggests event was significant
- If < 20 seconds could be respiratory pause
- Fluid or vomit present on bed or clothes suggest GERD

Differential diagnosis

- Gastroesophageal reflux disease – 26%
- Pertussis – 9%
- Lower respiratory tract infection – 9%
- Seizure – 9%
- Urinary tract infection – 8%
- Factitious illness including medical child abuse – 3%
- Miscellaneous – 11%

Risk factors

- Age < 60 days
- Gestational age < 32 weeks
- Prior BRUE or multiple episode requiring CPR
- Post–conceptual age < 45 weeks
- Concerning history or physical findings
- Feeding problems
- Respiratory conditions
- Family history of sudden cardiac death

BRUE inclusion criteria

- Duration < 1 minute
- Patient appearance and vital signs returned to normal after event
- Not explained by an identifiable medical condition
- Cyanosis or pallor
- Apnea or irregular breathing
- Change in muscle tone
- Loss or consciousness, lethargy, postictal phase and somnolence

BRUE exclusion criteria

- Duration > 1 minute
- At time of examination
    - Fever or recent fever
    - Tachycardia
    - Tachypnea
    - Low blood pressure
    - Altered mental status
    - Abnormal weight or growth
    - Abnormal head circumference
    - Abnormal muscle tone (hyper or hypotonia)
    - Bruising
    - Abnormal airway sounds
    - Repeat unexplained events
    - Event consistent with a medical condition
    - Acrocyanosis or perioral cyanosis
    - Rubor
    - Breath holding spells
    - Breath holding spells with altered responsiveness
    - Periodic breathing of newborn
    - Seizure activity
    - Muscle tone changes with crying or gagging
    - Eye deviation or nystagmus

- Infantile spasms

Evaluation

- Patients that appear healthy may only need observation before discharge
- As needed for presenting signs and symptoms
  - CBC, CMP, U/A, urine culture (cath specimen), chest x-ray, LP, and ABG

Disposition

Admitting or consulting criteria

- High risk factors patient
- Patient not returned to baseline
- Cardiorespiratory monitoring needed
- Parents not wanting to take patient home
- Discuss with physician all events

Discharge criteria

- Low risk patient
- After observation period, patient with normal appearance and vital signs
- Outpatient close follow up
- Engage in shared decision making with parents

Notes

References:

Brief Resolved Unexplained Events (Apparent Life-Threatening Events)

Updated: Nov 07, 2018

Author: Patrick L Carolan, MD; Chief Editor: Girish D Sharma, MD, FCCP, FAAP

Geriatrics

Section Contents — one protocol

When using any protocol, always follow the Guidelines of Proper Use (page 18).

GERIATRICS PROTOCOL

When using any protocol, always follow the Guidelines of Proper Use (page 18).

Basic Ethical Principles

- Beneficence – act in the patient's best interest
- Autonomy – treatment guided by patient's wishes
- Family responsibility – plays a central role in care of the geriatric patient
- Advance directives – follow wishes of patient and family in care

General Considerations of Elderly

- Live in high density population environments
- May have poor nutritional status
- May have altered immune function
- Have multiple medical problems
- Take multiple medications
- May delay seeking medical evaluation
- Subtle alterations in appearance or behavior may be only indication of serious infections

Pharmacology in the Elderly

Risk factors for adverse drug reactions

- Advanced age and living alone
- Female gender
- Chronic use of medications
- Polypharmacy
- Institutionalization
- Multiple medical problems (especially hepatic or renal insufficiency)

Adverse drug presentations

Confusion

- Anticholinergics
- Antihistamines
- Antidepressants
- Antihypertensives

- Antipsychotics
- Narcotics
- Sedatives
- Digoxin (digitalis)
- Steroids
- NSAID's
- Diuretics

Dementia

- Antihistamines
- Phenothiazines
- Tricyclic antidepressants

Depression

- Sedatives
- Beta-blockers
- Steroids
- Oral diabetic medications
- Ethanol
- NSAID's
- Narcotics

General weakness

- Digoxin (digitalis)
- Diuretics

Nausea

- Digoxin (digitalis)
- Theophylline
- Macrolide antibiotics (erythromycin)
- Iron
- Narcotics
- Steroids
- L-dopa
- ASA

Postural hypotension

- Angina medications
- Hypertension drugs
- Antidepressants
- Antihistamines
- Sedatives
- Beta-blockers

Renal insufficiency

- Digoxin (digitalis)
- Diuretics

Syncope/Near Syncope

- Cardiac drugs
- Hypertension drugs

Urinary incontinence

- Antipsychotics
- Diuretics
- Beta–blockers
- Medications causing fecal impaction
- Sedatives

Urinary retention

- Anticholinergics
- Antihistamines (especially in elderly men with BPH)

Hallucinations

- Anticholinergics

Drugs causing falls

- Antidepressants
- Antihistamines
- Antipsychotics
- Sedatives
- Nitroglycerin

Principles of safe medication usage

- Consider medications as a potential cause for presenting for medical care
- Educate patient about potential adverse reactions
- Obtain drug levels or monitoring tests of medications where appropriate
- Determine compliance and noncompliance of drug use
- Exercise care in prescribing medications that may have an adverse reaction to drugs the patient is currently taking
- Keep refills and number of pills small if appropriate
- Start low and go slow with dosing

- **Do not prescribe atypical antipsychotic medication to dementia patients — use first generation antipsychotic medication such as haloperidol if indicated**

Common Lab Findings in Elderly

- Frequently normal
- Fasting blood glucose: 135–150 mg/dL
- Normal creatinine with evidence of decreased creatinine clearance
- Hemoglobin – women 11 gm/dl; men 11.5 gm/dl
- BUN – up to 28–35 mg/dL

Delirium in the Elderly

- Acute organic brain syndrome manifested by impaired thinking, confusion, deficits in attention, fluctuating course, impaired speech and other symptoms and signs of impaired cognition

Causes of delirium

Medications and substances

- Ethanol
- Anticholinergics
- Antihistamines
- Sedatives
- Narcotics
- Antidepressants
- Lithium
- Neuroleptics
- Tagamet (cimetidine)

Withdrawal

- Ethanol
- Benzodiazepines
- Narcotics

Metabolic

- Electrolyte abnormalities (Na and Ca)
- Hypoglycemia and hyperglycemia
- Acid-base disturbance
- Dehydration
- Hypoxia

- End organ insufficiency – liver, kidney and lungs
- Vitamin deficiency — thiamine, folate
- Fever or hypothermia

Infectious

- Urinary tract infection (most common cause)
- Encephalitis or meningitis
- Pneumonia (second most common cause)
- Sepsis
- Influenza

Neurologic

- Brain tumor
- Subdural hematoma
- Intracerebral hemorrhage
- Seizure disorder
- CVA

Endocrine

- Hyperthyroidism
- Hypothyroidism
- Parathyroid — hyper and hypoparathyroidism

Cardiovascular

- Congestive heart failure
- Arrhythmia
- Acute myocardial infarction

Conditions that mimic delirium

- Dementia
- Depression
- Schizophrenia
- Mania
- Wernicke's aphasia

Evaluation of delirium

- CBC
- BMP
- LFT's
- U/A
- Chest x-ray
- EKG

Ordered as indicated

- Drug levels
- Thyroid studies
- Urine drug screen
- Blood alcohol
- Blood cultures
- CT brain scan
- Lumbar puncture for CSF analysis
- Urine culture

Treatment of delirium

- Treat underlying illness
- Restore any fluid or electrolyte imbalances
- Discontinue unnecessary medication that is contributing to delirium (discuss with physician)

Consult criteria for delirium

- Discuss all cases with physician
- Physician should examine all delirium or acute altered mental status patients

Temporal Arteritis

- True emergency of the elderly
  - Age of onset 50–70 years of age
  - Six times more common in females than in males
- Headache localized over eye or scalp
- Fever, malaise and weight loss are associated symptoms
- Jaw claudication is important associated symptom
- Frequently associated with polymyalgia rheumatica (joint and muscles aches)
- ESR 50–100
- Normal ESR should not dissuade from making the diagnosis of TA as > 15% of biopsy-proven cases have a normal ESR
- C-reactive protein elevated usually
- Vision loss can occur early in course of disease

Treatment

- Prednisone 40–80 mg PO qday or divided bid for several months to one year

- In suspected temporal with normal ESR, treat with steroids

Disposition

- Minimal symptoms can be treated as outpatient
- Severe symptoms or question of eye involvement should be admitted with IV high dose steroid treatment and ophthalmology consultation obtained

Discharge instructions

- Temporal arteritis aftercare instructions
- Follow up with PCP within 1 day
- Return for visual changes

Consult criteria

- Discuss all temporal arteritis cases with physician

Falls in Elderly

Causes

- Environmental or accidental: 30–50% of patients
- Gait, balance, weakness or deconditioning: 10–25% of patients
- Sensation of dizziness: 5–20% of patients
- Syncope: 2–10% of patients
- Orthostatic hypotension: 2–15% of patients
- Drop attacks: 1–10% of patients
- Other: 1–10% of patients

Physical examination

- Orthostatic blood pressures
    - Definition
        - SBP drop 20 mm Hg or DBP 10 mm Hg with assumption of upright posture
        - Sustained HR increase 30 bpm within 10 min of moving from recumbent to nonexertional standing position (or 40 bpm if 12-19 yrs of age)
        - Postural blood pressure changes can occur after standing for 10 minutes and so blood pressure should be checked again

at 10–15 minutes if low orthostatic blood pressure is suspected as cause of the fall
- Orthostatic measurements do not, in isolation, reliably diagnose or exclude orthostatic syncope, nor do they exclude life-threatening causes of syncope
- Orthostatic vital signs are present in up to 40% of asymptomatic patients older than 70 years, and 23% of those younger than 60 years

- Core body temperature
- Skin for evidence of trauma, pallor
- HEENT for vision loss, hearing deficits, cranial nerve deficits, nystagmus
- Neck for carotid bruit, meningeal signs
- Chest auscultation for rales
- Heart for aortic stenosis murmur, arrhythmias
- Extremities for fractures, motion limitations, DJD findings
- Neurologic for altered mental status, focal neurologic deficits, loss of position sense

Lab and x-ray evaluation options as indicated

- CBC
- BMP
- Chest x-ray
- X-ray of injured areas
- U/A
- UDS and blood alcohol
- EKG
- Medication levels
- CT brain scan

Discharge criteria

- Cause of fall benign and no serious injury
- Good social and home support systems if needed

Consult criteria

- Cause of fall requires admission
- New medical condition causing fall
- Significant abnormal lab or imaging study
- Fracture
- See General Patient Criteria Protocol (page 22)

Notes

References:

Delirium Author: Kannayiram Alagiakrishnan, MD, MBBS, MHA, MPH; Chief Editor: Iqbal Ahmed, MBBS, FRCPsych (UK) emedicine.medscape.com/article/288890

American Psychiatric Association. *Diagnostic and Statistical Manual of Mental Disorders, Fifth Edition*. 5th ed. Washington, DC: American Psychiatric Association; 2013

Birkhead NC, Wagener HP, Shick RM. Treatment of temporal arteritis with adrenal corticosteroids: Results in 55 cases in which the lesion was proved at biopsy. *JAMA*. 1975;163:821.

Giant Cell Arteritis Author: Mythili Seetharaman, MD; Chief Editor: Herbert S Diamond, MD emedicine.medscape.com/article/332483

Ann of EM, Vol.655:622

JEM. 2018;55:780

Annals of EM, Vol. 49, pg. 431

Circulation, epub, 3/9/17

Gynecology

Section Contents

When using any protocol, always follow the Guidelines of Proper Use (page 18).

VAGINAL BLEEDING PROTOCOL

When using any protocol, always follow the Guidelines of Proper Use (page 18).

Definition

- Abnormal vaginal bleeding

Differential Diagnosis

- Abnormal Uterine Bleeding (AUB)
- Spontaneous abortion
- Threatened abortion
- Atrophic endometrium (postmenopausal)
- Systemic disorders
- Hypothyroidism
- Vaginal Laceration
- STD's/Cervicitis
- Rectal Bleeding

Structural Causes (PALM)

- Polyp (AUB-P)
- Adenomyosis (AUB-A)
- Leiomyoma (AUB-L)
  - Submucosal myoma (AUB-LSM)
    - Other myoma (AUB-L_O)
    Malignancy
  - Hyperplasia (AUB-M)

Nonstructural Causes (COEIN)

- Coagulopathy (AUB-C)
- Ovulatory dysfunction (AUB-O)
- Endometrial (AUB-E)
- Iatrogenic (AUB-I)
- Not yet classified (AUB-N)

Considerations

- See Pregnancy Complications Protocol if pregnant
- Usually from a benign etiology

- Rule out pregnancy — prior tubal ligation, negative menstrual and sexual histories do not rule out pregnancy
- Causes of bleeding besides pregnancy need evaluation
- Average tampon holds 5–15cc of blood; average pad holds 15–30 cc of blood
- Postmenopausal vaginal bleeding needs to be evaluated for cancer
- Menorrhagia (days of heavy bleeding) may be treated with tranexamic acid 1300 mg PO TID (Max 5 days)

History

- Gestational history
- Last normal menstrual period noted
- Current medications (anticoagulants, hormones)

Evaluation Options

- Pelvic exam (delay for pregnancy > 20 weeks)
- CBC if tachycardia or hypotension present, or worrisome history for significant hemorrhage
- UCG
- Serum quantitative HCG if known to be pregnant
- Rh type if pregnant
- Type and screen if tachycardic
- PT/PTT/INR if indicated
- Type and cross match if hypotensive and notify physician promptly
- Consider transvaginal ultrasonography

Estimated Blood and Fluid losses (adults)

	Class I	Class II	Class III	Class IV
Blood loss (cc)	Up to 750	750–1000	1500–2000	> 2000
Blood loss %	Up to 15%	15–30%	30–40%	> 40%
Pulse rate	< 100	> 100	> 120	> 140
Blood pressure	Normal	Normal	SBP < 90	SBP < 70
Capillary refill	Normal	Normal	Delayed	Absent
Pulse pressure	Normal/incr	Decreased	Decreased	Decreased
Respiratory rate	14–20	20–30	30–40	> 35
Urine output (cc/hr.)	> 30	20–30	5–15	Negligible
Mental status	Anxious	Anxious	Confused	Lethargic

(Derived from Advanced Trauma Life Support)

Treatment Options

Dysfunctional uterine bleeding (DUB) with stable vital signs

- Estrogen 2.5 mg PO QID: add Provera 10 mg qday for 7-10 days when bleeding subsides
- Combination oral contraceptives
    - Nortrel 1/35 one PO bid × 7 days until bleeding stops, then 1 PO qday × 2 weeks
- Provera 10 mg PO qday × 10-30 days
    - Bleeding will resume when hormone therapy is finished
- NSAID's can be used to decrease bleeding and pain

IV NS 250–500cc bolus

- If heart rate ≥ 120
- If SBP < 90
- Avoid > 1 liter of isotonic fluids for acute blood loss before blood products transfusion started if possible
- PRBC's/FFP/platelets 1:1:1 ratio (recommendations range from 4:1:1 to 1:1:1)
- Uncrossed match blood for hemorrhagic shock if needed emergently
- Avoid hypertension
- Target systolic blood pressure of 80-90 mm Hg until major bleeding stopped

- Target Hgb of 7-9 g/dl after termination of major bleeding
    - Tranexamic acid 1 gm/10 minutes minutes then 1 gm over 8 hours
- If SBP < 105 and heart rate ≥ 110 with history of hypertension
- Notify physician promptly

Bleeding profuse and unresponsive to IV fluid management

- Conjugated estrogen (Premarin) 25 mg IV every 4–6 hours until the bleeding stops

Discharge Criteria

- Pregnancy — see Pregnancy Complications Protocol
- Benign vaginal bleeding such as DUB or irregular menses with heart rate ≤ 100, SBP > 90, and SBP ≥ 105 in patients with hypertension history

Discharge instructions

- Vaginal bleeding aftercare instructions
- Referral to OB/GYN within 1–10 days depending on severity of symptoms

Consult Criteria

- Pregnancy or postpartum bleeding — see Pregnancy Complications Protocol
- Ectopic pregnancy or possible ectopic pregnancy
- Fever
- Severe abdominal or pelvic pain
- Purulent vaginal discharge
- Continued heavy vaginal bleeding
- Return visit for same vaginal bleeding episode
- Postmenopausal vaginal bleeding
- Notify physician promptly for significant bleeding

Vital signs and age consult criteria

- Age ≥ 55
- SBP < 90 or relative hypotension (SBP < 105 with history of hypertension)
- Adult heart rate > 100
- Orthostatic vital signs

Lab consult criteria

- Hemoglobin decrease > 1 gm
- Hemoglobin < 10 gms unless stable
- WBC ≥ 15,000
- Bandemia ≥ 15%
- Increased anion gap or metabolic acidosis
- Thrombocytopenia
- Elevated coagulation studies
- Creatinine increase > 0.5 from baseline
- Elevated LFT's

Notes

Reference:

Dysfunctional Uterine Bleeding in Emergency Medicine
Author: Amir Estephan, MD; Chief Editor: Pamela L Dyne, MD emedicine.medscape.com/article/795587

Tranexamic Acid Treatment for Heavy Menstrual Bleeding: A Randomized Controlled Trial Lukes, Andrea S. MD, MHSc; Moore, Keith A. PharmD; Muse, Ken N. MD;
Obstetrics & Gynecology:
October 2010 Volume 116 - Issue 4 - pp 865-875
doi: 10.1097/AOG.0b013e3181f20177

Management of abnormal uterine bleeding associated with ovulatory dysfunction. Practice Bulletin No. 136. American College of Obstetricians and Gynecologists. Obstet Gynecol 2013;122:176–85

Hemorrhagic Shock in Emergency Medicine Guidelines
Updated: May 06, 2016 Author: William P Bozeman, MD; Chief Editor: Trevor John Mills, MD, MPH

PELVIC PAIN PROTOCOL

When using any protocol, always follow the Guidelines of Proper Use (page 18).

Definition

- Female pelvic pain

Differential Diagnosis

- Pelvic inflammatory disease (PID)
- Ectopic pregnancy
- Normal pregnancy
- Ovarian cyst
- Endometriosis
- Ovarian torsion
- Uterine fibroids
- Chronic pelvic pain syndrome
- UTI
- Renal colic

Considerations

- Must be differentiated from GI or urologic causes of pain
- Bilateral tubal ligation does not always prevent pregnancies — order UCG on all BTL patients that would be fertile otherwise

Evaluation

- Pelvic and abdominal exam
- UCG on fertile females
- U/A
- CBC for
  - Fever
  - Tachycardia
  - Hypotension
  - Moderate to severe pain
- BMP for
  - Dehydration
  - Tachycardia

    - Hypotension
    - Diabetes
- C-reactive protein may be helpful for inflammatory disease or PID

Pelvic ultrasound when

- Pregnant
- Suspected ovarian torsion
- Suspected ruptured ovarian cyst with tachycardia
- Suspected tubo-ovarian abscess (TOA)

Pelvic Inflammatory Disease (PID)

Definition

- Spectrum of the female genital tract infection to include uterus, tubes, ovaries and peritoneum

Differential diagnosis

- Ectopic pregnancy
- Normal pregnancy
- Ovarian cyst
- Endometriosis
- Ovarian torsion
- Uterine fibroids
- Chronic pelvic pain syndrome
- UTI
- Renal colic

Considerations

- Common in females of reproductive age
- Gonorrhea and chlamydia are most common causes
- Important to treat sexual partners
- Can lead to tubo-ovarian abscess
- Can lead to infertility, ectopic pregnancy and tubo-ovarian abscess
- Consider admission if patient has never been pregnant
- Usually caused by gonorrhea or chlamydia, but approximately 15% are due to respiratory or enteric organisms that have colonized the lower genital tract

Symptoms and findings

- Can cause peritonitis
- Usually bilateral pelvic pain and tenderness
- Associated with vaginal discharge frequently
- Dyspareunia
- Cervical motion tenderness usually bilateral
- Fever and chills
- Nausea and vomiting

Evaluation

- Pelvic and abdominal exam
- CBC
- UCG (unless hysterectomy history)
- U/A
- Consider RPR
- Consider C-reactive protein
- LFT's if right upper quadrant tenderness for Fitz-Hugh-Curtis syndrome
- Cultures for gonorrhea and chlamydia; wet prep
- Consider pelvic ultrasound if TOA suspected
- CT abdominal/pelvis scan if appendicitis suspected

Treatment options

Outpatient

- Rocephin (ceftriaxone) 250 mg IM

  +

- Doxycycline 100 mg PO BID × 14 days

  +/-

- Flagyl (metronidazole) 500 mg PO BID × 14 days (avoid ethanol)
  - Add Flagyl if evidence or suspicion of vaginitis

    OR

  - The patient underwent gynecologic instrumentation in the preceding 2–3 weeks
- Treatment for sexual partners or refer for treatment for STD
- NSAID's and/or narcotics prn
- Phenergan (promethazine) prn
- May use Sanford Guide or antibiotic database

- Follow CDC recommendations

Inpatient

- Cefotetan 2 gms IV

  +

- Doxycycline 100 mg IV (NMT 100 mg bid)
- Consult physician

Discharge criteria

- Mild to moderate pain
- Does not meet consult criteria

Discharge instructions

- PID aftercare instructions
- Follow up in 3 days to monitor treatment effectiveness
- Return if pain or fever worsens

Consult criteria

- Uncertain diagnosis or toxic appearance
- Suspected pelvic abscess
- Fitz-Hugh-Curtis syndrome (RUQ tenderness and elevated LFT's)
- Pregnancy
- Severe illness (severe pain and vomiting)
- Unable to tolerate PO intake
- Immunodeficiency
- Failure of outpatient therapy
- Return visit for same acute complaint
- Likely noncompliance with outpatient treatment
- Poor follow-up
- Never has been pregnant

Vaginitis

Definition

- Inflammation of the vagina

Differential diagnosis

- 90% of all cases of vaginitis
  - Bacterial vaginosis 40-50%
  - Vaginal candidiasis (or vulvovaginal candidiasis) 20-25%

- Trichomonas vaginalis infection 15-20%

Other less common causes

- Atrophic vaginitis
- Cervical polyp
- Contact dermatitis
- Entamoeba histolytica infection
- Excessive desquamation of normal vaginal epithelium
- Large cervical ectropion
- Lichen sclerosis
- Lichen simplex chronicus
- Vaginal adenosis
- Vaginal cancer
- Vaginal intraepithelial neoplasia
- Vaginal ulcers
- Cervicitis
- Child sexual abuse
- Cystitis, Nonbacterial
- Cytomegalovirus (CMV)
- Foreign Bodies, Rectum
- Herpes simplex
- Pinworms in Emergency Medicine
- Postpartum infections
- Salmonella infection
- Sexual assault
- Ureaplasma infection
- Varicella-zoster virus
- Urinary Tract Infection, Female

Considerations

- Prognosis very good
- Cultures not very useful
- Bacterial vaginosis is not a STD, but can increase susceptibility to STD's
- Avoiding irritants in the vaginal area
    - Perfumes, soaps, and panty liners
    - After swimming or exercise air the area or change the underwear
- Always clean from front to back

History

- Previous episodes
- Sexually transmitted infection
- Sexual activities
- Birth control method
- Last menstrual period
- Douching practice
- Use of personal hygiene products
- Antibiotic use
- General medical history
- Systemic symptoms (e.g., lower abdominal pain, fever, chills, nausea, and vomiting)

Bacterial vaginosis

- May be asymptomatic in 50% of women
- Treat symptomatic patients
- Associated with preterm birth in pregnancy
  - Always treat pregnant females
- Painless usually (pruritus may be present)
- Thin malodorous discharge, pH 5–6

Amsel's Diagnostic Clinical Criteria (wet prep)

- 3 of following
  - Thin white discharge homogenous that coats vaginal walls
  - Clue cells (>20%)
  - pH > 4.5
  - Whiff test of fishy odor before and after adding KOH

Treatment (select one)

- Metronidazole 500 mg orally twice a day for 7 days (no alcohol during and up to 24 hours after)
- Metronidazole gel 0.75%, 1 full applicator (5 gm) intravaginally, daily for 5 days
- Clindamycin cream 2%, 1 full applicator (5 g) intravaginally at bedtime for 7 days
- Clindamycin 300 mg orally twice a day for 7 days
- Clindamycin ovules 100 mg intravaginally once at bed time for 3 days

- Relapse within 3 months use 10–14 days of treatment

Pregnancy

- Metronidazole 500 mg orally twice a day for 7 days (no alcohol during up to 24 hours after)
- Metronidazole 250 mg orally 3 times a day for 7 day
- Clindamycin 300 mg orally twice a day for 7 day
- Pregnant women should have a follow-up visit 1 month after completion of treatment

Disposition

- Usually discharge
- Consider admission in severely ill patients
- Consult OB/GYN or physician as needed
- Follow up with OB/GYN as needed

Vaginal candidiasis (vulvovaginosis)

Yeast normal part of vaginal flora that if overgrows causes symptoms

- Well-demarcated erythema of the vulva
- Satellite lesions (discrete pustulopapular lesions) surrounding the redness
- Vulva, vagina, and surrounding areas may be edematous and erythematous, possibly accompanied by excoriations and fissures
- Adherent cottage cheese–like vaginal discharge may be seen
- Cervix usually appears normal

Treatment uncomplicated disease

- Clotrimazole 1% cream 5 g intravaginally for 7-14 days
- Clotrimazole 100 mg vaginal tablet for 7 days
- Clotrimazole 100 mg vaginal tablet, 2 tablets for 3 days
- Miconazole 2% cream 5 g intravaginally for 7 days
- Miconazole 100 mg vaginal suppository, 1 suppository for 7 days

- Miconazole 200 mg vaginal suppository, 1 suppository for 3 days
- Miconazole 1200 mg vaginal suppository, 1 suppository for 1 day
- Nystatin 100,000 unit vaginal tablet, 1 tablet for 14 days
- Fluconazole 150 mg oral tablet once

Recurrent vaginal candidiasis

- ≥4 episodes in 1 year
- 7-10 days of topical therapy

OR

- 150 mg oral dose of fluconazole every third day for a total of 3 doses (days 1, 4, and 7)
- Maintenance is oral fluconazole 100 mg or 150 mg weekly for 6 months
- **Other medications** that may be used up to 6 months include
  - Ketoconazole 400 mg/day (monitor for liver injury)
  - Clotrimazole 500-mg vaginal suppositories once per wk.

Severe vulvovaginal candidiasis

- 7-14 days of topical azole therapy or 150 mg of oral fluconazole repeated in 72 hours; adjunctive use of nystatin cream or low-potency steroid cream may be beneficial

Pregnant patients

- 7 days of topical agents
  - Fluconazole is contraindicated

Disposition

- Discharge usually
- Admission of signs or symptoms of systemic infection (consult physician)
- Sexual partners should be advised for treatment

Trichomonas vaginitis

Considerations

- Asymptomatic in 50% of females and 75% of men
- Discharge malodorous

- Vaginal or vulvar irritation or itching
- Cervix friable (bleeds easily to swab)
- pH >5.5
- WBC's and mobile trichomonads 60–80%
- 20% reinfected within 3 months
- Sexual partners need treatment

Treatment

- Metronidazole 2 gm orally in a single dose (or 500 mg orally twice a day for 7 days)
    - No alcohol during up to 24 hours after treatment
    - No breast feeding during and up to 24 hours after
- Tinidazole 2 gm orally in a single dose

Treatment failure

- Metronidazole 2 gm PO daily for 3–5 days
- Tinidazole 500mg qid and intravaginal 500mg bid for 14 days

Disposition

- Discharge
- If signs or symptoms of systemic disease consult physician

Ovarian Cysts

Definition

- Fluid filled sac in ovary

Differential diagnosis

- PID
- UTI
- Ovarian torsion
- Appendicitis
- Diverticulitis
- Endometriosis
- Inflammatory bowel disease
- Ovarian cancer

Considerations

- Most asymptomatic and benign
- Cysts < 5 cm usually resolve

- Cysts > 5 cm need referral and follow-up

Evaluation

- Pelvic and abdominal exam
- UCG
- U/A
- CBC for
    - Fever
    - Tachycardia
    - Hypotension
    - Moderate to severe pain
- BMP for
    - Dehydration
    - Tachycardia
    - Hypotension
    - Diabetes

Treatment options

- Pain control if not hypotensive
- Notify physician promptly for bleeding from hemorrhagic cysts or signs of hemorrhagic volume loss
    - Heart rate ≥ 110; SBP < 90; orthostatic vital signs or hypotension
        - IV NS 250–500 cc bolus prn
    - See Bleeding Protocol
- Severe pain order pelvic ultrasound
- Oral contraceptives not effective

Discharge criteria

- Simple ovarian cysts
- Stable vital signs

Discharge instructions

- Ovarian cyst aftercare instructions
- Return if pain worsens or dizziness develops

Consult criteria

- Severe pain
- Fever
- Heart rate ≥ 110; SBP < 90; orthostatic vital signs or hypotension

Endometriosis

Definition

- Endometriosis is the presence of endometrial-like tissue outside the uterine cavity, which induces a chronic inflammatory reaction

Differential diagnosis

- Appendicitis
- Ectopic pregnancy
- Diverticulitis
- Inflammatory bowel disease
- UTI
- PID
- Ovarian cysts
- Ovarian torsion
- Primary dysmenorrhea

Considerations

- Dysmenorrhea
- Heavy or irregular vaginal bleeding
- Pelvic, lower abdominal and lower back pain locations
- 15% of all pelvic pain
- Similar evaluation as ovarian cyst if diagnosis in doubt
- UCG if fertile
- 30–40% of women with be subfertile

Treatment options

- Pain control with NSAID's and/or narcotics
- Provera 10–20 mg qday
- Ortho-Cyclen for one month

Discharge criteria

- Pain controlled
- Stable vital signs

Discharge instructions

- Endometriosis aftercare instructions
- Follow up with primary care provider or gynecologist within 7 days if possible

Consult physician if diagnosis uncertain

- Heart rate ≥ 110
- Orthostatic vital signs
- Fever
- Severe pain

Ectopic Pregnancy

Definition

- Pregnancy outside of uterus

Considerations

- ß-hCG can be < 100 mIU/mL

Differential diagnosis

- Threatened abortion
- Inevitable abortion
- Incomplete abortion
- Missed abortion
- Appendicitis
- Diverticulitis
- Inflammatory bowel disease
- UTI
- PID
- Ovarian cysts
- Ovarian torsion
- Primary dysmenorrhea

Evaluation

- Pelvic and abdominal exam
- Rh type
- CBC
- BMP
- ß-hCG
- Pelvic ultrasound (perform even if ß-hCG < 100 mIU/mL
- Type and screen if vital signs stable
- Type and cross for 2 units PRBC's if hypotensive

Treatment options

- Notify physician promptly

- Notify physician if ectopic pregnancy is possible consideration

IV NS 250–500 cc bolus (avoid > 1000 cc IVF)

- Heart rate ≥ 115 and rupture suspected
- Orthostatic vital signs
- Give blood early if SBP < 80 mmHg or HR > 130 and patient is clearly not stable (see Vaginal Bleeding Protocol)
- Hypotension

Pelvic Pain Consult Criteria

- Dehydration
- Significant blood loss
- Ectopic pregnancy or possible ectopic pregnancy
- Suspected or diagnosed appendicitis or diverticulitis
- Acute surgical abdomen
- Moderate to severe pain of uncertain cause
- Severe pain with any diagnosis
- Return ED visit within 14 days for same acute pelvic pain complaint
- Elevated LFT's
- Any of the above subtopics consult criteria

Vital signs consult criteria

- Pelvic pain that develops hypotension or relative hypotension (SBP < 110 with history of hypertension)
- Heart rate ≥ 110

Lab consult criteria

- WBC > 15,000 or < 3,000
- Bandemia ≥ 15%
- Significant electrolyte abnormally
- Hyperglycemia with metabolic acidosis (decreased serum CO_2 or elevated anion gap)
- Worsening anemia; decrease > 1 gm hemoglobin
- Metabolic acidosis

Notes

References:

Endometriosis Author: Dharmesh Kapoor, MBBS, MD, MRCOG; Chief Editor: Michel E Rivlin, MD emedicine.medscape.com/article/271899

Davis L-J, Kennedy SS, Moore J, Prentice A. Oral contraceptives for pain associated with endometriosis. Cochrane Database of Systematic Reviews 2007, Issue 3. Art. No.: CD001019. DOI: 10.1002/14651858.CD001019.pub2

Endometriosis: diagnosis and management. 2010 Jul. NGC:007969 Society of Obstetricians and Gynaecologists of Canada - Medical Specialty Society

Workowski KA, Berman S. Sexually transmitted diseases treatment guidelines, 2010. *MMWR Recomm Rep*. Dec 17 2010;59:1–110

Pelvic Inflammatory Disease Author: Suzanne Moore Shepherd, MD, MS, DTM&H, FACEP, FAAEM; Chief Editor: Michel E Rivlin, MD emedicine.medscape.com/article/256448

Grimes DA, Jones LB., Lopez LM, Schulz KF. Oral contraceptives for functional ovarian cysts. Cochrane Database of Systematic Reviews 2014, Issue 4. Art. No.: CD006134. DOI: 10.1002/14651858.CD006134.pub5

Counselman FL, et al. Quantitative B-hCG levels less than 1000 mIU/mL in patients with ectopic pregnancy: pelvic ultrasound still useful *J Emerg Med* 1998;16: 699–703

NEJM, 372:2039

emedicine.medscape.com/article/257141
Vaginitis Treatment & Management
Updated: Dec 04, 2018 Author: Hetal B Gor, MD, FACOG; Chief Editor: Michel E Rivlin, MD

Emedicine medscape
Vulvovaginitis Updated: Jan 19, 2018 Author: Jill M Krapf, MD, FACOG; Chief Editor: Christine Isaacs, MD

PREGNANCY COMPLICATIONS PROTOCOL

When using any protocol, always follow the Guidelines of Proper Use (page 18).

Definition

- Processes that interfere with a normal intrauterine pregnancy (IUP) progression

Differential Diagnosis

- Threatened abortion — may present with pain and/or bleeding, closed cervical os, benign exam and no tissue passed
- Inevitable abortion — open cervical os and/or non-viable IUP (such as blighted ovum)
- Incomplete abortion — partial passage of products of conception (POC)
- Missed abortion — fetal death < 20 weeks without passage of POC
- Septic abortion — abortion and infection with pain, fever or foul smelling/purulent discharge
- Preeclampsia — IUP > 20 weeks gestation with hypertension, proteinuria, and/or CNS symptoms or epigastric symptoms and frequently edema with > 1+ pitting edema after 12 hours bedrest; pedal, hands and facial edema and rapid weight gain > 2.7 kg/month (weight gain early sign)
- Eclampsia — preeclampsia with seizures
- Hypertension is 140/90 or rise of SBP 20 and DBP 10 over prepregnancy levels
- HELLP — hemolysis; elevated liver enzymes (twice normal); low platelets (<100K)
- Ectopic pregnancy — occurs 2% of all pregnancies
- Treat all suspected or confirmed influenza pregnant patients up to 2 weeks after delivery with influenza medications

Considerations

- Bleeding occurs in 20–30% of pregnancies in first 20 weeks (50% will have eventual spontaneous abortion)
- Late pregnancy (last 20 weeks) bleeding occurs 3–5%
- 11.5% of patients are pregnant who say it is "not possible" to be pregnant
- 7.5% pregnant with recent "normal period"
- Discrimatory zone where ultrasound usually can visualize the gestation
    - hCG 6000 mIU/mL for transabdominal ultrasound
    - hCG 700–1000 mIU/mL for transvaginal ultrasound
    - Normal pregnancy may be lower than discrimatory zone
    - Ectopic pregnancy may have extremely low hCG of down to 10 mIU/mL

General Evaluation

- Pelvic and abdominal exam
- Complete physical examination
- History of LNMP, amount of bleeding, any POC passed
- CBC
- Serum quantitative HCG
- U/A
- Fetal heart tones – usually 110–160/minute (dependent on gestational age)
- Rh type (if there is vaginal bleeding history or findings)
- Transvaginal ultrasound (usually)
- LFT's if preeclampsia/eclampsia present
- BMP if vomiting and tachycardia present
- Type and screen for significant bleeding or tachycardia
- Type and cross for 2 units PRBC's if hypotensive

  Defer pelvic exam last 20 weeks of gestation if bleeding

Hyperemesis gravidarum and nausea/vomiting of pregnancy

- Hyperemesis gravidarum most severe form of nausea and vomiting in pregnancy, with ketosis and weight loss > 5% of prepregnancy weight

Evaluation options

- Vital signs including orthostatics as needed
- U/A, BMP, magnesium, calcium and serum ketones
- LFT's, amylase/lipase if abdominal pain present
- TSH and T4
- Urine culture
- CBC if abdominal pain/tenderness present
- Hepatitis panel if LFT's elevated
- RUQ ultrasound if gallbladder, liver or pancreas disease suspected

Treatment

- First line: Vitamin B-6 10–25 mg 3–4 times daily with doxylamine 12.5–25 mg 3–4 times daily
    - Diclegis (doxylamine/pyridoxine)
- Ginger capsules 250 mg 4 times daily can be added at this point if the patient is still vomiting
- IV D5LR 1–2 liters over 1–2 hours as needed
- Phenergan 6.25–25 mg IV, metoclopramide 10 mg IV
- Small frequent feedings
- Discontinue prenatal vitamins with iron

Consult criteria

- Persistent vomiting and volume depletion despite treatment
- Abdominal pain or tenderness out of proportion to vomiting
- Weight loss > 5–7.5%

Ectopic pregnancy

- Occurs 2% of pregnancies
- Missed > 40% of time on first visit
- 90% with pain and 50–80% with bleeding
- 30% have atypical presentations
- Normal pelvic exam does not rule out ectopic
- Falling β-HCG does not exclude ectopic pregnancy
- β-HCG normally double every 2 days when < 10,000 mIU/ml with normal pregnancy
- No IUP on ultrasound is suspicious for ectopic pregnancy

- Perform ultrasound on indeterminate β-HCG
    - β-HCG can be < 100 mIU/mL in ectopic pregnancy

Preeclampsia and eclampsia

- IUP > 20 weeks gestation with hypertension and proteinuria
- Can occur up to 4–6 weeks postpartum
- Frequently with pedal and hand edema
- Gestational hypertension is not associated with proteinuria
- Low dose aspirin 81 mg is effective and safe in 2–3rd trimesters in preventing preeclampsia in women with risk factors for preeclampsia
- Notify physician

Risk factors for preeclampsia or eclampsia

- Advanced maternal age > 40 years or young maternal age < 20 years
- First pregnancy
- Prior preeclampsia history
- Chronic Hypertension
- Multiple gestation
- Molar pregnancy
- Diabetes
- Obesity
- Chronic renal disease
- Anti-phospholipid antibody syndrome

Preeclampsia with Severe Features

- SBP > 160 or DBP > 110
- RUQ/epigastric pain
- Hyperreflexia
- Thrombocytopenia (<100K/mL)
- New onset headache or visual disturbances
- Eclampsia
- Dyspnea or pulmonary edema
- Elevated PT and PTT
- LFT's twice normal
- Papilledema
- Creatinine >1.1mg/dL or double from baseline

Eclampsia

- Preeclampsia with seizures

Evaluation

- Cardiac monitoring
- CBC (preeclampsia and eclampsia)
- U/A

CMET (preeclampsia and eclampsia)

- PT and PTT
- DIC panel
- LDH
- Uric acid (is elevated early) — preeclampsia and eclampsia
- OB ultrasound

Treatment options

- Delivery is definitive treatment
- Blood pressure goal of SBP 140–155 mm Hg and DBP 90–100 mm Hg
    - Labetalol 20 mg IV, then 40mg, then 80mg, given q10 min prn (NMT 300 mg)
    - Hydralazine 5–10 mg IV may repeat Q20min prn (NMT 60 mg)
    - Immediate release nifedpine 10-20mg PO, may repeat in 20min if needed

Seizure prophylaxis

- Magnesium sulfate 4–6 gms IV over 20 minutes followed by drip of 1–2 gms IV/hr.
    - Stop MgSO4 (magnesium sulfate)
        - If DTR's are lost
        - For respiratory depression (calcium gluconate 1 gm IV over 10 minutes if needed to reverse magnesium toxicity)
    - Monitor magnesium levels (therapeutic serum level 4-8mg/dl)
    - Caution if renal failure is present

Active seizures

- Give magnesium sulfate 6 gms IV over 5–10 minutes — followed by magnesium drip of 1–2 gms IV per hour

- Dilantin or Ativan can be used for magnesium sulfate failure, avoid polypharmacy (see Adult Seizure Protocol)

Postpartum hemorrhage

Treatment options depending on degree of bleeding (notify physician promptly for significant hemorrhage)

- Oxytocin 20 unit IV at 20-40 mUnit/min (may also be given IM)
- Hemabate 250mcg IM, repeat q15-90 min prn, max 2mg total dose (caution if patient asthmatic)
- Methergine 0.2 mg IM/IV q2-4hr PRN; not to exceed 5 doses, then 0.2-0.4 mg PO q6-8hr PRN for 2-7 days
    - Administer IV only in emergency because of potential for hypertension and CVA (notify physician before giving IV)
        - Administer over >1 minute and monitor BP
- Tranexamic acid 1 gm/10 minutes then 1 gm over 8 hours

    OR

    10 mg/kg IV followed by infusion of 1 mg/kg/hour

Placenta abruption

- Separation of a normally positioned placenta after 20 weeks of gestation and before birth

Signs and symptoms

- Painful vaginal bleeding 80% (dark red commonly)
    - No vaginal bleeding 20%
- Abdominal tenderness 70%
- Uterine tenderness 70%
- Uterus has tetonic contractions 35%
- Shock out of proportion to estimated blood loss
- Fetal distress
- Premature labor

- Fetal death 15 %

Risk factors for placenta abruption

- Previous abruption
- Hypertension or preeclampsia — most common cause
- Diabetes
- Chronic renal disease
- Oligohydramnios, PROM
- Chorioamnionitis
- Trauma - abdominal or rapid deceleration (sheering forces)
- Advance maternal age
- Cocaine use
- Cigarette smoking
- Alcohol use

Evaluation

- CBC
- BMP
- LFT's
- DIC panel
- Type and screen if not in shock
- Type and cross 4 units PRBC's if class 2 or greater hemorrhage (see Bleeding Protocol)
- Transabdominal ultrasound for fetal lie, fluid index, and evaluation of placenta
- Continuous fetal monitoring

Treatment

- 2 large bore IV's of NS
- If class 2 hemorrhage or greater give 250–500 cc NS bolus and consider blood/FFP/platelet transfusion
- See Bleeding Protocol

Consult criteria

- Notify physician and obstetrician promptly

Placenta previa

- Implantation of the placenta near or over the cervical os
- Occurs in the second and third trimesters of pregnancy

- Common cause of pregnancy bleeding

Signs and symptoms

- Painless bright red vaginal bleeding
- Fetal heart tones may be normal
- Bleeding may be intermittent
- Shock can occur

Evaluation

- **Do not** perform digital vaginal or rectal exam (may provoke increased bleeding), speculum exam acceptable
- CBC
- Type and screen
- DIC panel
- Bedside transabdominal ultrasound for fetal presentation, placentation, and fluid index
- Transabdominal or transvaginal ultrasound in radiology if vital signs stable and bleeding amounts judged not to be dangerous
- Continuous fetal monitoring

Consult criteria

- Consult physician and obstetrics

UTI

- **Treat all asymptomatic** and simple cystitis urinary tract infections for 7–10 days
  - Increased incidence of premature rupture of membranes and fetal death if not treated
- Send urine for culture
- No trimethoprim first trimester or sulfa antibiotic last trimester
- Consult for admission on all pyelonephritis patients that are pregnant

Bacterial vaginosis

- Most common cause of vaginal discharge
- Gardnerella vaginalis replaces normal flora
- Risk of preterm labor, premature rupture of membranes and postpartum endometritis if not treated

Criteria – has 3 of 4

- Profuse thin white discharge

- Fishy odor
- pH > 4.5
- Clue cells

Treatment

- All pregnant patients
- All symptomatic nonpregnant patients

Antibiotics

- Metronidazole options 250 mg PO tid × 7 days (avoid 1st trimester)
    - Gel 0.75% 5 gm intravaginally qday × 5 days
- Clindamycin 300 mg PO bid × 7 days

Treatment Options

- Rhogam 300 microunits IM if Rh negative and vaginal bleeding has or is occurring
- IV D5NS rehydration as needed for vomiting of pregnancy (D5 decreases ketosis); No infusion with D5NS > 300 cc/hr.
- IV NS bolus and drip for hemorrhagic compromise (notify physician promptly)
    - No more than 1 liter NS before starting blood transfusion and FFP if possible
    - Give blood:FFP at 1:1 or 2:1 ratio
    - Improved mortality when FFP added
    - See Bleeding Protocol
- Phenergan (promethazine) 6.25 mg IV (25–50 mg IM or PO) or Zofran (ondansetron) 4 mg IV or Reglan 10 mg IV prn
- Narcotics prn (Category B, or C if commonly used in pregnancy)
- Methergine (methylergonovine) 0.2 mg IM prn postpartum or abortion (spontaneous or incomplete) related heavy bleeding
- See Preeclampsia and Eclampsia sections above

Discharge Criteria

- Benign causes of pain of pregnancy (round ligament, etc.)

- Benign pelvic pain and threatened abortion with stable vital signs
- Rehydration with heart rate < 100 in vomiting of pregnancy

Discharge instructions

- Pregnancy aftercare instructions
- Threatened abortions aftercare instructions
- Follow up with OB/GYN provider within 1–3 days
- Return if pain persists or increases
- Return if bleeding recurs or increases

Consult Criteria

- Heart rate ≥ 110
- BP ≥ 140/90
- Intractable vomiting
- Anemia
- Preeclampsia or eclampsia
- Placental abruption
- Placenta previa
- Ectopic or possible ectopic pregnancy
- Any spontaneous abortion (threatened, missed, septic, incomplete)
- Fetal demise
- Significant vaginal bleeding or hypotension or orthostasis (notify physician promptly)
- Late pregnancy bleeding (last 20 weeks)
- Significant pelvic/abdominal pain or headache
- Pyelonephritis

Notes

References:

Hahn SA, Lavonas EJ, Mace SE, Napoli AM, Fesmire FM, American College of Emergency Physicians. Clinical policy: critical issues in the initial evaluation and management of patients presenting to the emergency department in early pregnancy. Ann Emerg Med. 2012 Sep;60(3):381-90.e28

Counselman FL, et al. Quantitative B-hCG levels less than 1000 mIU/mL in patients with ectopic pregnancy: pelvic ultrasound still useful *J Emerg Med* 1998;16: 699-703

Hyperemesis Gravidarum Author: Dotun A Ogunyemi, MD; Chief Editor: Christine Isaacs, MD
emedicine.medscape.com/article/254751

American College of Obstetricians and Gynecologists (ACOG). Nausea and vomiting of pregnancy. Washington (DC): American College of Obstetricians and Gynecologists (ACOG); 2004 Apr. 13 p. (ACOG practice bulletin; no. 52)

Coomarasamy A, Honest H, Papaioannou S, et al. Aspirin for prevention of preeclampsia in women with historical risk factors: a systematic review. *Obstet Gynecol*. Jun 2003;101(6):1319-32

Preeclampsia Author: Kee-Hak Lim, MD; Chief Editor: Ronald M Ramus, MD
emedicine.medscape.com/article/1476919

Postpartum Hemorrhage in Emergency Medicine Medication Author: Maame Yaa A B Yiadom, MD, MPH; Chief Editor: Pamela L Dyne, MD emedicine.medscape.com/article/796785

Lancet 2010;376:23-32

BMJ 2012; 344:e3054

Nausea and vomiting of pregnancy. Practice Bulletin No. 153. American College of Obstetricians and Gynecologists. Obstet Gynecol 2015;126:e12–24.

Vicken P Sepilian, MD, MSc; Chief Editor: Michel E Rivlin, MD emedicine.medscape.com/article/2041923-workup#c8

Clin Infect Dis: epub 12/19/18

Infectious Disease

Section Contents

When using any protocol, always follow the Guidelines of Proper Use (page 18).

SEXUALLY TRANSMITTED DISEASE PROTOCOL

When using any protocol, always follow the Guidelines of Proper Use (page 18).

Definition

- Diseases transmitted by sexual contact

Differential Diagnosis

- Gonorrhea
- PID
- Chlamydia
- Epididymitis
- Orchitis
- Syphilis
- Hepatitis B
- Prostatitis
- Herpes
- Trichomoniasis

Considerations

- Gonococcal and chlamydial disease frequently seen together
- Syphilis — 100,000 new cases per year

Presentations

- Pelvic inflammatory disease (PID)
- Prostatitis (usually age < 35 years)
- Epididymoorchitis
- Bartholin cyst
- Anogenital Warts
- Urethritis
- Vaginitis

Gonococcal Disease

Definition

- Disease spectrum caused by Neisseria gonorrhoeae

Differential diagnosis

- Nonspecific urethritis
- Chlamydial infections
- Strep pharyngitis
- Leucocytoclastic vasculitis (rash)
- Septic arthritis
- Meningitis
- Orchitis
- Epididymitis
- UTI
- Cervicitis
- PID
- Proctitis
- Conjunctivitis

Considerations

- May be disseminated
    - Joints — frequently single and migratory (knee most common)
    - Skin
    - Tenosynovitis
    - Meningitis
    - Endocarditis
- Coexist 25–50% of the time with chlamydial infection
- May coexist with trichomonas and syphilis

Females

- Asymptomatic carriers
- PID — 20% has gonorrhea
    - Cervical motion tenderness
    - Usually bilateral adnexal tenderness
    - RUQ tenderness with elevated LFT's may represent Fitz-Hugh-Curtis syndrome
- Cervicitis
- Associated often with chlamydia and trichomonas

Males

- Severe dysuria
- Purulent urethral discharge
- Proctitis (homosexual relations)
- Pharyngitis

Evaluation

- Sexual and reproductive/menstrual history
- Genital exam usually indicated
- Smear with intracellular gram negative diplococci can be performed
- Culture
- RPR prn

Treatment options

- Follow CDC guidelines
- Analgesics prn
- Rocephin (ceftriaxone) 250 mg IM
- Azithromycin 1gm PO x 1 dose for chlamydia
- Doxycycline 100 mg PO bid × 7 days to cover chlamydia

Discharge criteria

- Nondisseminated gonococcal disease
- Nontoxic patient

Discharge instructions

- STD aftercare instructions
- Return if symptoms persist > 3 days
- Return if worse
- Follow up with health department within 3 days

Consult criteria

- Toxic patient
- Disseminated gonococcal disease (example gonococcal arthritis)
- See General Patient Criteria Protocol (page 22)

Pelvic Inflammatory Disease (PID)

Definition

- Spectrum of the female genital tract infections to include uterus, tubes, ovaries and peritoneum

Differential diagnosis

- Ectopic pregnancy
- Normal pregnancy
- Ovarian cyst
- Endometriosis
- Ovarian torsion
- Uterine fibroids
- Chronic pelvic pain syndrome
- UTI
- Renal colic

Considerations

- Common in females of reproductive age
- Gonorrhea and chlamydia are most common causes
- Important to treat sexual partners
- Can lead to tubo-ovarian abscess
- Can lead to infertility, ectopic pregnancy and tubo-ovarian abscess
- Consider admission if patient has never been pregnant

Symptoms and findings

- Can cause peritonitis
- Usually bilateral pelvic pain and tenderness
- Associated with vaginal discharge frequently
- Dyspareunia
- Cervical motion tenderness
- Fever and chills
- Nausea and vomiting

Evaluation

- Pelvic and abdominal exam
- CBC
- UCG
- U/A
- Wet prep

- Consider RPR
- Consider C-reactive protein
- LFT's if right upper quadrant tenderness for Fitz-Hugh-Curtis syndrome
- Gonorrhea/chlamydia DNA probe
- Consider pelvic ultrasound if TOA suspected
- CT scan if appendicitis also suspected

Treatment options

Outpatient

- Rocephin (ceftriaxone) 250 mg IM

  +

- Doxycycline 100 mg PO BID × 14 days

  +/-

- Flagyl (metronidazole) 500 mg PO BID × 14 days if vaginitis suspected/diagnosed or gynecologic instrumentation in the preceding 2–3 weeks (avoid ethanol)
- Treatment for sexual partners or refer for treatment for STD
- NSAID's; narcotics prn; Phenergan (promethazine) prn
- Follow CDC recommendations

Inpatient

- Cefotetan 2 gms IV

  +

- Doxycycline 100 mg IV NMT 100 mg bid
- Consult physician

Discharge criteria

- Mild to moderate pain
- Does not meet consult criteria

Discharge instructions

- PID aftercare instructions
- Follow up in 3 days to monitor treatment effectiveness
- Return if pain or fever worsens

Consult criteria

- Uncertain diagnosis or toxic appearance
- Suspected pelvic abscess

- Fitz-Hugh-Curtis syndrome (RUQ tenderness and elevated LFT's)
- Pregnancy
- Severe illness (severe pain and vomiting)
- Unable to tolerate PO intake
- Immunodeficiency
- Failure of outpatient therapy
- Return visit for same acute complaint
- Likely noncompliance with outpatient treatment
- Poor follow up
- Never been pregnant

Urethritis and Epididymoorchitis

Definition

- Infection or inflammation of the urethra, epididymis or testicle

Differential diagnosis for epididymoorchitis

- Testicular torsion
- Mumps
- Trauma
- Hernia
- Tumor – usually painless

Considerations

- Gonorrhea and chlamydia are the main causes and coexist 25–50% of the time
- Urethral discharge
- Tender and swollen epididymis and/or testicle

Gonorrhea

- Dysuria
- Thick purulent discharge from urethra
- Gram negative intracellular diplococci

Chlamydia

- Thinner discharge from urethra
- Little to no discomfort

Evaluation

- Sexual history
- Genital exam

- Smear for intracellular gram negative diplococci can be performed
- Urine Culture
- Wet smear
- Gonorrhea/chlamydia DNA probe
- RPR prn

Treatment options

- Follow CDC guidelines
- May use Sanford Guide or other drug databases
- Analgesics prn
- **Gonorrhea**
    - Rocephin (ceftriaxone) 250 mg IM

      +
    - Doxycycline 100 mg PO bid × 7–10 days to cover chlamydia
- **Non-gonococcal Urethritis**
    - Azithromycin 1gm PO x 1 dose

      +
    - Doxycycline 100mg PO bid x 7-10 days

Discharge criteria

- Nontoxic patient

Discharge instructions

- Epididymoorchitis aftercare instructions
- Return if worse
- Follow up with PCP or urologist in 3–7 days

Consult criteria

- Systemic toxicity
- Refer to General Patient Criteria Protocol prn (page 22)

Genital herpes

- See Genital Herpes Protocol
- Obtain HSV culture of lesions
- Treatment can be extended if healing is incomplete after 10 days of therapy
- Acyclovir 400 mg orally three times a day for 7--10 days

OR

- Acyclovir 200 mg orally five times a day for 7--10 days

OR

- Famciclovir 250 mg orally three times a day for 7--10 days

OR

- Valacyclovir 1 g orally twice a day for 7--10 days

Prostatitis

Definition

- Infection or inflammation of the prostate gland

Differential diagnosis

- Prostate cancer
- Urethritis
- Mechanical back pain
- UTI

Considerations

- Gonorrhea and chlamydia are the main causes in men age < 35 years and coexist 25–50% of the time
- Prostate tender (caution with vigorous palpation if fever or toxicity present)
- Age > 35 years usual cause is bacterial
- Nonbacterial prostatitis is inflammatory condition without infection
- Chronic prostatitis
    - Increases risk of UTI and BPH

Acute bacterial prostatitis age > 35 years

- Fever
- Chills
- Perineal prostatic pain
- Dysuria
- Obstructive bladder symptoms
- Low back pain
- Low abdominal pain
- Spontaneous urethral discharge

Evaluation options

- U/A

- CBC
- RPR if STD suspected

Treatment options

Age < 35 years

- Follow CDC guidelines
- Analgesics prn
- Rocephin (ceftriaxone) 250 mg IM

  +

- Doxycycline 100 mg PO bid × 10–14 days
- Treatment for sexual partners or refer for treatment for STD

Age ≥ 35 years

- Septra DS 1 PO bid × 14–28 days
- Quinolone 14–28 days (not recommended for gonorrhea)
- NSAID's and/or narcotics prn

Discharge criteria

- Nontoxic patient
- Refer to General Patient Criteria Protocol prn (page 22)

Discharge instructions

- Prostatitis aftercare instructions
- Return if worse
- Follow up with PCP or urologist in 3–7 days

Consult criteria

- Systemic toxicity
- Urinary retention

Anogenital Warts

- Usually condyloma acuminata
  - Painless pedunculated or sessile wart

Can be secondary syphilis (condyloma lata)

- Highly contagious (wear gloves)
- Smooth, moist flat wart
- Secondary syphilis rash is maculopapular and mimics other diseases
- Painless chancre sore history or finding

- Order RPR

Antibiotic choices for syphilis

- Bicillin LA 2.4 IM
- Doxycycline 100 mg PO × 14 days

Treatment for condyloma acuminata

- Podofilox 0.5% gel or solution bid on wart only for 3 days, rest 4 days, and another cycle of 3 days, repeat up to 4–6 cycles
- Imiquimod 3.75% or 5% cream 3x weekly at bedtime until cleared or max 16 weeks
- TCA (trichloroacetic acid) application
- Cryotherapy
- No treatment as warts frequently resolve may be tried

Discharge criteria

- All nontoxic patients

Discharge instructions

- Venereal wart aftercare instructions
- Refer to health department or PCP within 3–7 days

Consult criteria

- Complicating comorbidities

Syphilis

Definition

- Infection caused by Treponema palladium

Differential diagnosis

- Pityriasis rosea
- Chanchroid
- Condyloma acuminata
- Psoriasis
- Lymphogranuloma venereum
- Herpes simplex

Considerations

Primary syphilis

- Painless chancre (sore) at site of infection

Secondary syphilis

- Occurs 2–10 weeks after primary infection
- Widespread mucocutaneous lesions
- Spreads to liver, joints, muscle, lymph nodes and brain

Latent syphilis

- Asymptomatic
- Can last up to 30 years
    - Early phase within one year of primary infection
    - Late phase after one year of primary infection

Tertiary syphilis

- Noninfectious at this stage
- Irreversible
- Can affect
    - Heart (coronary aneurysms)
    - Aorta
    - Eyes
    - Brain
    - Nerves
    - Bones
    - Joints
- Neurosyphilis develops in 5% of tertiary syphilis
    - Meningovascular type most common
    - Tabes dorsalis (post column of spinal cord with loss of position sense)

Treatment options

Antibiotics choices for primary, secondary or early latent syphilis

- Bicillin LA 2.4 IM
- Doxycycline 100 mg BID PO × 14 days

Antibiotic choices for late latent syphilis

- Bicillin LA 2.4 million units IM qweek × 3 weeks

Discharge criteria

- Primary, secondary or early latent syphilis

Discharge instructions

- Syphilis aftercare instructions
- Refer to health department within 3 days

Consult criteria

- Late latent syphilis
- Neurosyphilis
- Tertiary syphilis
- Pregnancy

Notes

References:

Workowski KA, Berman S. Sexually transmitted diseases treatment guidelines, 2010. *MMWR Recomm Rep*. Dec 17 2010;59:1–110

Update to CDC's Sexually Transmitted Diseases Treatment Guidelines, 2010: Oral Cephalosporins No Longer a Recommended Treatment for Gonococcal Infections. *MMWR Morb Mortal Wkly Rep*. Aug 10 2012;61:590–4

Gonorrhea Author: Brian Wong, MD; Chief Editor: Burke A Cunha, MD emedicine.medscape.com/article/218059

Prostatitis Author: Paul J Turek, MD; Chief Editor: Robert E O'Connor, MD, MPH emedicine.medscape.com/article/785418

Pelvic Inflammatory Disease
Author: Suzanne Moore Shepherd, MD, MS, DTM&H, FACEP, FAAEM; Chief Editor: Michel E Rivlin, MD
emedicine.medscape.com/article/256448

Centers for Disease Control and Prevention, 2015 Sexually Transmitted Diseases Treatment Guidelines

HUMAN IMMUNODEFICIENCY VIRUS (HIV) PROTOCOL

When using any protocol, always follow the Guidelines of Proper Use (page 18).

Definition

- Infection by HIV

Differential Diagnosis

- Cytomegalovirus
- Mononucleosis
- Syphilis
- Influenza
- Meningitis
- Encephalitis
- Viral hepatitis
- Idiopathic thrombocytopenic purpura
- Candidiasis

Considerations

- Three month window between acquiring primary HIV infection and seroconversion
- Life expectancy is extended with HIV infection on current treatment regimens
- CD4 count below 200/µL is considered AIDS-defining in the United States
- CD4 T-cell count reference range, 500-2000 cells/µL
- Because CD4 counts vary, serial counts are generally a better measure of significant changes
- After seroconversion, CD4 counts tend to decrease (~700/µL) and continue to decline over time
- In children younger than 5 years, the CD4 T-cell percentage is considered more important than the absolute count (< 25% is considered to warrant therapy)
- Rate of progression to AIDS and death is related to the viral load

  - Patients with viral loads greater than 30,000/µL are 18.5 times more likely to die of AIDS than those with undetectable viral loads
- With therapy, viral loads can often be suppressed to an undetectable level (< 20-75 copies/mL; optimal viral suppression); complete inhibition of viral replication appears impossible and may be unnecessary

HIV testing

- Fourth-generation test that detects HIV in the blood earlier than antibody tests can; it identifies the viral protein HIV-1 p24 antigen, which appears in the blood before antibodies do
- If this test is positive, an immunoassay that differentiates HIV-1 from HIV-2 antibodies should be performed
  - Faster than they can from the Western blot test
- In patients with positive results on the initial antigen test but with negative or indeterminate results on the antibody differentiation assay, HIV-1 nucleic acid testing should be performed to determine whether infection is present

Department of Health and Human Services (DHHS) guidelines

- Antiretroviral therapy should be initiated in all patients with a history of an AIDS-defining illness or with a CD4 count below 350/µL
- Antiretroviral therapy should be initiated regardless of CD4 count in pregnant patients, patients with HIV-associated nephropathy, and those with hepatitis B virus (HBV) coinfection when treatment of HBV infection is indicated
- Panel divided on initiation of therapy with CD4 counts of 350-500/µL; 55% considered this a strong recommendation, 45% considered it a moderate recommendation
- Panel also divided on initiation of therapy with CD4 counts above 500/µL: half favored initiation in this setting, and half considered treatment initiation optional

HAART (highly active antiretroviral therapy) or cART

- Combination of 2 NRTIs with a NNRTI or Protease Inhibitor or Integrase Inhibitor
- Has significantly increased life expectancy
- Potential for hepatotoxicity
- May cause lactic acidosis
- May cause GI symptoms, rashes, headache and psychiatric disorders
- Pneumonia is usually caused by S. pneumoniae in patients on HAART
- Osteoporosis and osteonecrosis may occur
- Treatment prevents immunosuppressive illnesses and helps prevent CV events, non-HIV related cancers, chronic renal, and chronic hepatic disease

Drug interactions with cART

- Increases concentrations of antiarrhythmia drugs
- Increases levels of anticonvulsants
- Increase concentrations of benzodiazepines
    - Okay to give 1 dose in ED
- Increases rhabdomyolysis risk with statin drugs
- Increases warfarin concentrations

Causes

- Unprotected sexual intercourse
- Anal receptive sexual intercourse is high risk
- Parenteral drug use and needle sharing
- Occupational needle stick
- Contaminated blood product transfusion

Signs, Symptoms, Findings or Processes

- May have no symptoms or physical findings
- Fever
- Fatigue
- Night sweats
- Oral ulcers
- Pharyngitis

- Diarrhea
- Genital ulcers
- Rashes
- Alopecia
- Weight loss
- Headache
- Myalgias
- Lymphadenopathy
- Altered mental status
- Pneumonia
- COPD
- Kidney damage
- Progressive multifocal leukoencephalopathy
- CNS lymphoma
- Anemia
- Sensory neuropathies
- Staph pyomyositis with CD4 < 50 cells/mm^3 (usually in thigh)
- Staph folliculitis
- Psychiatric disorders

Immune reconstitution inflammatory syndrome

- Immune system improves with HAART (cART) and attacks dormant opportunistic infections
- Can worsen autoimmune disorders
- Can manifest as pneumonitis, lymphadenitis, hepatosplenomegaly and hypercalcemia
- Treatment is dependent on opportunistic infection involved
- Discontinuation of HAART is rarely needed

Evaluation

- History of CD4 counts if known
- CD4 count 3 months after cART and then q3–6 months for 2 years, then q12 months if CD4 stable at 300–500 cells/mm^3
  - CD4 > 500 optional testing
- Medication history
- Previous hospitalizations
- Previous infections or cancers

Testing options

- CBC
- LFT's
- U/A if fever or urinary symptoms
- BMP if abnormal vital signs or diabetic
- Stool for ova/parasites and cultures
- STD testing if indicated
- HIV testing offered to patient
- Chest x-ray if respiratory complaints or findings
- CT brain or MRI brain with and without contrast for neurologic complaints or findings

Treatment Options

- Treatment of associated infections
- Discuss AIDS related opportunistic infections or findings with physician
- Antiretroviral treatment per physician or experienced practitioner

Discharge Criteria

- Stable afebrile patient
- Social support systems present
- Pneumonia in HAART patients who are nontoxic, not hypoxic with normal blood pressure and heart rate may be candidates for outpatient treatment
  - Treatment is the same as for typical community acquired pneumonia
  - Discuss with physician

Discharge instructions

- HIV aftercare instructions
- Refer to primary care provider, health department or AIDS clinic for follow-up

Consult Criteria

- Toxic patient
- Altered mental status
- Neurologic deficit
- Respiratory distress
- Fever

- Unable to ambulate
- Vomiting
- Unable to self-hydrate
- Pericardial or pleural effusion
- Significant weight loss
- Acute psychiatric symptoms
- Pneumonitis

Lab consult criteria

- Adult WBC ≥ 13,000 or < 1,000 neutrophils;
- Bandemia
- Acute thrombocytopenia
- Hemoglobin < 10 (unless chronic and stable)
- O_2 Sat ≤ 94% on room air if acute
- Moderate or severe dyspnea

Vital sign and age consult criteria

- Adult heart rate > 100

Notes

References:

CDC Laboratory Testing for the Diagnosis of HIV Infection: Updated Recommendations. Centers for Disease Control and Prevention

Canavan N. New HIV Treatment Guidelines to Cut Millions of Deaths. *Medscape Medical News* [serial online]. Jul 1 2013

Panel on Antiretroviral Guidelines for Adults and Adolescents. Guidelines for the use of antiretroviral agents in HIV-1–infected adults and adolescents. Department of Health and Human Services. January 10, 2011; 1–174. aidsinfo.nih.gov/contentfiles/AdultandAdolescentGL Updated May 1, 2014

[Guideline] Panel on Antiretroviral Guidelines for Adults and Adolescents. Guidelines for the use of antiretroviral agents in HIV-1-infected adults and adolescents. Department of Health and Human Services. October 17, 2017

HIV Infection and AIDS Medication Updated: Sep 12, 2018 Author: Nicholas John Bennett, MBBCh, PhD, MA(Cantab), FAAP; Chief Editor: Michael Stuart Bronze, MD

HIV AND HEPATITIS B POSTEXPOSURE PROPHYLAXIS RECOMMENDATIONS

When using any protocol, always follow the Guidelines of Proper Use (page 18).

Follow your institution's policies and procedures for postexposure prophylaxis if present. Refer to CDC links at the end of this Protocol.

General Wound Guidelines

- Irrigate and clean wound copiously with flushing 1% betadine solution and wash with soap and water for percutaneous injuries and nonintact skin
- Irrigate mucous membranes with water or saline
- Update tetanus as indicated
- The need for tetanus and/or hepatitis B prophylaxis is based on medical history (see Tetanus Protocol, page 756)
- Health care providers should be immunized against hepatitis B
- Hepatitis A prophylaxis may (rarely) need to be considered depending on the source-patient situation
- The need for HIV or chemoprophylaxis (antiretrovirals) is based on an assessment of the risk developed by the Centers for Disease Control and Prevention (CDC)
- HIV PEP indicated in pregnancy—no testing needed

Testing of Source and Exposed Person

Exposed person

- Hepatitis profile
- HIV testing
- Liver function tests
- Serum anti-HBs titers on exposed person if there is a hepatitis B vaccination history

Source patient (if available)

- HIV
- Hepatitis B antigen
- Hepatitis C antibody

- Aspartate aminotransferase/alanine aminotransferase (AST/ALT) and alkaline phosphatase level

Prior to initiating antiretrovirals

- PEP indicated in pregnancy—no testing needed
- CBC count with differential and platelets
- CMP
- Urinalysis with microscopic analysis

Risk of acquiring HIV infection

- 0.3% for percutaneous injuries
- 0.1% for non-intact skin exposure
- 0.09% for mucous membrane exposure
- PEP drops rate of infection 80% if started within 24–36 hours occupational HIV transmission since 1999 in U.S.
- No documented cases of HIV transmission in period between initial HIV infection and formation of detectable HIV antibodies

Higher risk of HIV transmission

- Device has visible blood on it
- Deep injury
- Involving a needle placed in blood vessel
- Hollow bore needle
- Source terminal with HIV infection

Recommended HIV Postexposure Prophylaxis (PEP) for Needlestick Injuries

HIV regimens (Indicated in pregnancy—no pregnancy test needed)

Preferred HIV PEP Regimen for 28 days

- Raltegravir (Isentress) 400 mg PO twice daily plus Truvada, 1 PO once daily (Tenofovir 300 mg and emtricitabine 200 mg)
- Well tolerated usually

Alternative Regimens for 28 days

- May combine 1 drug or drug pair with 1 pair of nucleoside/nucleotide reverse-transcriptase inhibitors

One of these

- Raltegravir (Isentress)
- Darunavir (Prezista) and ritonavir (Norvir)
- Etravirine (Intelence) and Rilpivirine (Edurant)
- Atazanavir (Reyataz) and ritonavir (Norvir)
- Lopinavir/ritonavir (Kaletra)

Combined with one of these nucleoside/nucleotide reverse-transcriptase inhibitors

- Tenofovir and emtricitabine; available as Truvada
- Tenofovir and lamivudine (Epivir)
- Zidovudine (Retrovir; AZT) and lamivudine (Epivir); available as
- Combivir
- Zidovudine (Retrovir; AZT) and emtricitabine (Emtriva)

- Prescribers unfamiliar with these agents/regimens should consult physicians familiar with the agents and their toxicities

Regimen toxicity

- Nephrotoxicity
    - Truvada 1 tablet daily (tenofovir 300 mg+ emtricitabine 200 mg) — dose q48hr if creatinine clearance 30–49 ml/min: avoid with creatinine clearance < 30 ml/min
    - Combivir 1 tablet PO bid (zidovudine 300 mg + lamivudine 150 mg) — avoid use with creatinine clearance < 50 ml/minute
- Hepatotoxicity
- Lactic acidosis
- Read literature for all adverse reactions/contraindications of any HIV antireviral drugs used

Treatment recommendations

Source of unknown HIV status

- Generally no PEP
- Can consider PEP regimen for HIV risk factors

Unknown source (needle from sharps container, for example)

- Generally no PEP
- Can consider in areas in which exposure to HIV infected persons is likely

HIV negative source

- No PEP

Recommended HIV Postexposure Prophylaxis (PEP) for Mucosal Membrane and Nonintact Skin Exposures

Definitions of exposure type

Source of unknown HIV status

- Generally no PEP
- Can consider treatment regimen for HIV risk factors

Unknown source (needle from sharps container, for example)

- Generally no PEP
- Can consider treatment regimen in areas in which exposure to HIV infected persons is likely

HIV negative source

- No PEP

Other body fluids

- Feces, nasal secretions, saliva, sputum, sweat, tears, urine, and vomitus are not considered potentially infectious unless they are visibly bloody

Consultation criteria

Delayed (> 24–36 hours after exposure)

- Interval in which lack of benefit from PEP is undefined

Unknown source

- Use of PEP on case by case basis

Known or suspected pregnancy in exposed person

- Use of optimal PEP not precluded

Breastfeeding in exposed person

- Use of optimal PEP not precluded

Resistance of source virus to antiretrovirals

Toxicity of initial PEP regimen

- Adverse symptoms common with PEP (nausea and diarrhea)
- Symptoms often manageable without changing regimen with GI medications

Hepatitis B Postexposure Prophylaxis

Unvaccinated exposed worker

Source HBsAg positive

- HBIG 0.06 cc/kg IM × 1
- Initiate hepatitis B vaccine series

Source HBsAg negative

- Initiate hepatitis B vaccine series

Source unknown or not available for testing

- Initiate hepatitis B vaccine series

Previously vaccinated

Known responder

- No treatment

Known nonresponder with source HBsAg positive or high risk

- HBIG 0.06 cc/kg IM × 1
- Reinitiate hepatitis B vaccine series

  OR
- HBIG × 2

Antibody response unknown and source HBsAg positive

- Test exposed person
  - If adequate (serum anti-HBs ≥ 10 mIU/cc)
    - No treatment
  - If inadequate (serum anti-HBs < 10 mIU/cc)
    - HBIG × 1
    - Vaccine booster

Antibody response unknown and source unknown or not available for testing

- Test exposed person
  - If adequate titer (serum anti-HBs ≥ 10 mIU/cc)
    - No treatment
  - If inadequate titer (serum anti-HBs < 10 mIU/cc)
    - Vaccine booster
    - Recheck titer in 1–2 months

Notes

References:

http://www.cdc.gov/mmwr/preview/mmwrhtml/rr5011a1.htm#box2

http://www.cdc.gov/mmwr/PDF/rr/rr5409.pdf

http://aidsetc.org/aidsetc?page=cg-301_occupational_pep

http://nccc.ucsf.edu/wp-content/uploads/2014/03/Updated_USPHS_Guidelines_Mgmt_Occupational_Exposures_HIV_Recommendations_PEP.pdf

The clinician managing the exposed person can call the National Clinicians' Post-Exposure Prophylaxis Hotline (PEPline) at 888–HIV-4911 (888–448–4911) at no charge. Service is available 7 days a week, (More information is available at the PEPline website)

emedicine.medscape.com/article/784812

[Guideline] Panel on Antiretroviral Guidelines for Adults and Adolescents. Guidelines for the use of antiretroviral agents in HIV-1-infected adults and adolescents. Department of Health and Human Services. October 17, 2017

Emedicine Medscape HIV Infection and AIDS Medication
Updated: Sep 12, 2018
Author: Nicholas John Bennett, MBBCh, PhD, MA(Cantab), FAAP; Chief Editor: Michael Stuart Bronze, MD

ENDOCARDITIS PROTOCOL

When using any protocol, always follow the Guidelines of Proper Use (page 18).

Definition

- Infection of the endocardial surface of the heart including the heart valves

Considerations

Acute endocarditis

- Usually from Staph aureus or group B strep
- Occurs on normal valves
- More aggressive course
- Related to IV drug abuse
- Valve replacement > 60 days prior

Subacute endocarditis

- Usually from Strep viridans or enterococci
- Less aggressive course
- Valve replacement > 60 days prior

Signs and symptoms

- Fever
- Petechiae
- Heart murmur
- CHF
- Neurologic complaints or findings
- Delirium
- Pericarditis
- Neck pain
- Anemia
- Leukocytosis
- Proteinuria
- Hematuria
- Splenomegaly
- Embolic findings
    - Splinter hemorrhages on nail beds
    - Osler nodes on fingertip pads
    - Roth spots are retinal hemorrhages

  - Janeway lesions are nontender macular rash on palms and soles

Evaluation

- History and physical examination
- Consider in IV drug abuser and fever
- CBC
- Chest x-ray
  - Evaluate for septic emboli, cavitary lesions and infiltrates
- C-reactive protein and ESR (elevated > 90% of patients)
- BMP
- U/A
  - Evaluate for proteinuria and hematuria
- Blood culture q5–10 minutes × 2 sets
- EKG
  - For conduction defects (poor prognostic sign)
- Transesophageal echocardiography

Treatment

- Oxygen prn
- Treat CHF if present
- IV NS as needed

Subacute endocarditis

- Penicillin G 2–3 million units IV q4hr
- Vancomycin for suspected resistant organisms

Acute endocarditis

- Nafcillin 2 gms IV q4hr
- Vancomycin for suspected resistant organisms

Prophylaxis

History of

- Congenital heart disease
- Prosthetic valve
- History of prior endocarditis
- Prophylaxis treatment

Procedural conditions

- Dental procedures
- Abscess I&D

- Incision of respiratory mucosa (tonsillectomy)
- Not recommended for GI or GU procedures

Antibiotic regimens

Adult options

- Amoxicillin 2 gms PO
  OR
- Ampicillin 2 gms IV
  OR
- Cleocin (clindamycin) 600 mg PO or IV
  OR
- Cephalexin 2 gm PO
  OR
- Zithromax (azithromycin) 500 mg PO
  OR
- Rocephin (ceftriaxone) 1 gm IV or IM

Pediatric options

- Amoxicillin 50 mg/kg PO — NMT 2 gms
  OR
- Ampicillin 50 mg/kg IV or IM — NMT 2 gms
  OR
- Cleocin (clindamycin) 20 mg/kg PO — NMT 600 mg

OR

- Zithromax (azithromycin) 15 mg/kg PO — NMT 500 mg
  OR
- Cephalexin 50 mg/kg PO — NMT 2 gm
  OR
- Rocephin (ceftriaxone) 50 mg/kg IV or IM — NMT 1 gm

Consult criteria

- Discuss with physician all endocarditis or suspected endocarditis patients

Notes

References:

Antibiotic Prophylactic Regimens for Endocarditis

Author: Mary L Windle, PharmD; Chief Editor: Rick Kulkarni, MD emedicine.medscape.com/article/1672902

Wilson W, Taubert KA, Gewitz M, Lockhart PB, Baddour LM, Levison M, et al. Prevention of infective endocarditis: guidelines from the American Heart Association: *Circulation*. Oct 9 2007;116(15):1736–54

Adult Severe Sepsis and Septic Shock Protocol

When using any management guideline, always follow the Guidelines of Proper Use (page 18).

For clinical settings that permit the practitioner to perform adult septic shock management and they are trained and experienced to perform those duties

Definitions

Systemic Inflammatory Response Syndrome (SIRS)

- Core temperature > 38° C or < 36° C
- Heart rate > 90/minute unless on beta-blockers
- Respiratory rate > 20/minute or pCO_2 < 32 mm Hg
- WBC > 12,000 or < 4,000 or > 10–15% bands

Sepsis

- Clinical evidence for infection
- 2 or more SIRS criteria met
- New 2016 definition — life-threatening organ dysfunction from dysregulated host response to infection

Severe Sepsis (may be discarded in 2016)

- Evidence for sepsis AND sepsis-induced tissue hypoperfusion or organ dysfunction
  - Ex: altered mental status, hypoxemia without overt pulmonary disease, elevated lactate, or oliguria (urine output < 30 mL/hour)

Septic Shock

- Older definition as of 2016 — severe sepsis AND sepsis-induced hypotension despite adequate fluid resuscitation
- New **SOFA** definition — subset of sepsis in which particularly profound circulatory, cellular, and metabolic abnormalities are associated with a greater risk of mortality than with sepsis alone

- ***qSOFA score*** **(Quick Sepsis–related Organ Failure Assessment Score)**
    - Respiratory rate ≥ 22 breaths/minute — 1 point
    - Systolic blood pressure ≤ 100 mm Hg — 1 point
    - Altered level of consciousness (GCS <15) — 1 point
    - < 2 points low risk for sepsis
    - ≥ 2 points high risk for poor outcome in suspected infection
    - Not a diagnostic test to determine sepsis (used for mortality risk assessment)
    - Positive qSOFA score ≥ 2 points should be evaluated for organ dysfunction

Multiple organ dysfunction syndrome (MODS)

- Progressive organ dysfunction in a severely ill patient
- Failure to maintain homeostasis without intervention
- End stage in infectious conditions (sepsis, septic shock) and noninfectious conditions (e.g., SIRS due to pancreatitis)
- The greater the number of organ failures, the higher the mortality risk, with the greatest risk associated with respiratory failure requiring mechanical ventilation
- MODS can be classified as primary or secondary
    - **Primary MODS** is the direct result of identifiable injury or insult with early organ dysfunction
        - Such as renal failure due to a nephrotoxic agent or liver failure due to a hepatotoxic agent
    - **Secondary MODS** is organ failure that has no attributable cause and is a consequence of the host's response
        - Such as acute respiratory distress syndrome in individuals with pancreatitis

Sepsis definition comment

- There is ongoing defining and redefining over time of sepsis categories with different specialty groups disagreeing to varying degrees

Differential diagnosis

- Anaphylactic shock
- Adrenal crisis and shock
- Cardiogenic shock
- Hypovolemic shock
- Hemorrhagic shock
- DKA
- Neuroleptic malignant syndrome
- Toxic shock syndrome
- Heatstroke
- Cardiac tamponade
- Massive pulmonary embolism
- Adult respiratory distress syndrome (ARDS)
- Other forms of shock

Considerations

- Culture positive bacteremia occurs in 30–50%
- Not all patients with bacteremia have signs of sepsis
- Serious bacterial infections with or without bacteremia may be associated with changes in all organ systems
    - Change in organ function mediated by host immune system mechanisms against infection
- The continuum of severity is from sepsis to septic shock to multiple organ dysfunction syndrome
- ARDS occurs in 20–40% of septic shock
- Hyperoxia may impair oxygen delivery in patients with sepsis, and hyperoxia decreases whole-body oxygen consumption in critically ill patients. Patients should be weaned to the lowest necessary FiO_2.
- No relationship between the CVP and intravascular volume and between the CVP and fluid responsiveness
- Pseudosepsis is defined as fever, leukocytosis, and hypotension due to causes other than sepsis
- Lactic acidosis in sepsis commonly caused by high sympathetic (adrenergic) state and not always from hypoperfusion

Sepsis Therapy

(Meeting treatment goals is associated with improved survival in patients with severe sepsis and septic shock)

Treatment goals

- Maintain MAP ≥ 65 mm Hg
- Target a central venous O_2 ($ScvO_2$) saturation ≥ 70%
- Target serum lactate ≤ 2 mmol/L
- Maintain urine output ≥ 0.5 ml/kg/hour
- Correcting peripheral capillary refill delay

Monitoring

- Vital signs every 5 minutes until stabilized
- Maintain an O_2 saturation ≥ 90%
- Central line placement for possible vasopressors and CVP measurement
- Foley catheter placement

Testing

- ABG
- Lactic acid (lactate) level
- CBC
- BMP
- LFTs
- PT/PTT/INR
- Blood cultures X 2 using different sites
- Sputum culture & sensitivity and gram stain
- U/A and urine culture
- Chest x-ray
- EKG
- Troponin and BNP
- Type and screen
- Cortisol level
- Accucheck for glucose

Treatment

IV fluid and pressor treatment

- Current recommendations from various entities including Medicare for severe sepsis or septic shock
    - 30 ml/kg bolus with NS or LR (may use ideal body weight if patient obese)
- Bolus crystalloids IV 500–1,000 ml every 30 minutes and re-assess response of HR, MAP, CVP
    - Goal is to achieve MAP ≥ 65 and CVP 8–12 mm Hg
    - Give at least 30 ml/kg of fluid, but often patients need ≥ 4 L to achieve adequate volume resuscitation
    - Fluid overload is associated with increased mortality so too aggressive IV fluid hydration may be deleterious to the patient
        - Caution in heart failure patients that demonstrate high CVP or pulmonary edema
    - End stage renal failure patients frequently to not receive enough IVF in septic shock
- MAP is < 65 mm Hg then start norepinephrine (Levophed) IV if not responsive to IV NS or LR
    - Norepinephrine start at 2–4 mcg/minute IV — usual dosage range 8–12 mcg/minute (may need up to 30 mcg/minute in refractory shock)
    - Add vasopressin 0.03 units/min when an additional agent is needed to maintain MAP
- For patients with refractory shock and an $ScvO_2$ < 70%, consider the following
    - Consider using dobutamine IV up to 20 mcg/kg/minute especially if there is evidence of myocardial dysfunction
    - If hematocrit < 25% — transfuse packed red blood cells to raise hematocrit > 25%
- Give methylprednisolone 100 mg IV if adrenal sufficiency present or suspected
    - 50 mg IV q6hr until shock resolved

Empiric antibiotic treatment

- Administer antibiotics within one hour of recognition of severe sepsis or septic shock, and after collection of blood cultures when feasible.
- Attempt to achieve source control as soon as the site of infection is identified This may include, but is not limited to, removing indwelling catheters, draining abscesses, or relieving a source of obstruction (ureteral stone, biliary stone blocking the biliary tree, etc.).

Suggested empiric regimens

- Vancomycin 1 gm IV q12hr (adjust for renal insufficiency)

PLUS one of the following

- Piperacillin/tazobactam (Zosyn) 3.375–4.5 gms IV q6hr

OR

- Meropenem (Merrem) 1 gm IV q8hr

OR

- Imipenem (Primaxin) 0.5–1 gm IV q8hr

OR

- Cefepime (Maxipime) 2 gm IV q12hr

OR

- Ceftazidime (Fortaz) 2 gm IV q8–12hr

Consider the addition of an aminoglycoside or fluoroquinolone in patients with:

- Neutropenia
- Pneumonia causing respiratory failure
- Proven resistant infections such as pseudomonas or Acinetobacter

Special considerations

- In addition to the empiric coverage above, patients with suspected or proven intra-abdominal sepsis should receive anaerobic coverage with piperacillin/tazobactam, a carbapenem, clindamycin, or metronidazole.
- A macrolide antibiotic (i.e. azithromycin) should be added to patients with bacteremia from Streptococcus pneumonia.

- Dose adjustments need to be considered in patients with renal or hepatic dysfunction.

Protective lung strategy in ARDS for intubated ventilated patients

Given the high incidence of ARDS in patients with severe sepsis or septic shock, consider

- Tidal volumes of 6 ml/kg of ideal body weight
- Plateau pressure < 30 cm H_2O

Consult recommendations

- Close management of patient care with a physician
- Patients with severe sepsis or septic shock should be cared for in an intensive care unit setting

Notes

References:

Rossi P, et al. *Clin Physiol Funct Imaging* 2007, 27:180–184

Cornet AD, et al. *Crit Care* 2013 Apr 18;17:313

Rivers E et al. *New Engl J Med* 2001; 345:1368–1377

Raghunathan K et al. Crit Care Med. Mar 26 2014. [Epub ahead of print]

The Surviving Sepsis Campaign Guidelines: 2012 – published in Crit Care Med 2013; 41:580–637

Caironi P et al. *New Engl J Med* 2014; 370:1412–1421

The ProCESS Investigators. *New Engl J Med* 2014; 370: 1683–1693

CHEST, June, 2014; pg.1407

ACEP NOW: New Sepsis Definitions Spark Debate on Twitter
Jeremy Samuel Faust, MD, MS, MA on March 16, 2016

Assessment of Clinical Criteria for Sepsis For the Third International Consensus Definitions for Sepsis and Septic Shock (Sepsis-3) *JAMA.* 2016;315(8):762-774. doi:10.1001/jama.2016.0288

Bacterial Sepsis Updated: Feb 05, 2019 Author: Amber Mahmood Bokhari, MBBS; Chief Editor: Michael Stuart Bronze, MD

Am J EM. 2017;35:1946

TETANUS PROTOCOL

When using any protocol, always follow the Guidelines of Proper Use (page 18).

Tetanus infection

Definition

- Anaerobic infection caused by Clostridium tetani producing a toxin that causes muscle spasms and pain

Differential diagnosis

- Conversion disorder
- Meningitis
- Encephalitis
- Dystonic drug reaction
- Mandible dislocation
- Hypocalcemia
- Black widow spider bite
- Subarachnoid hemorrhage
- Peritonsillar abscess
- Retropharyngeal abscess
- Rabies

Considerations

- Found in soil, feces, house dust and is ubiquitous
- Tetanus spores can remain in normal tissue for months to years
- Tetanus infection may occur without apparent wound
- Incidence of tetanus infection has decreased markedly secondary to childhood immunizations and current tetanus prophylaxis recommendations
- Medium incubation period is 7 days, but can be less than 4 days or greater than 14 days
- Tetanus booster does not prevent acute tetanus disease occurrence
    - It prevents future infections
    - Tetanus immune globulin prevents acute infections in under-immunized patients

- Elderly are frequently under-immunized

Signs and symptoms

- 75% have generalized muscle rigidity – "lockjaw"
- Dysphagia
- Fever
- Tachycardia
- Sweating
- Laryngospasms – can cause asphyxia
- Acute abdominal pain mimicking surgical abdomen

Evaluation

- History and physical examination
- No specific lab tests available
- Diagnosis is clinical
- Spatula test
    - Touching tongue with tongue blade causes masseter spasm and biting of the blade
    - Sensitivity 94%
    - Specificity 100%
    - No complications from procedure

Treatment

- Tetanus immune globulin 3,000–5,000 units IM with part of dose injected around infection site
- Rapid sequence intubation per physician if needed acutely
    - Needed in 2/3 of patients
- Wound debridement out to 2 cm from wound edges
- Incision and drainage of any abscesses

Medications

- Valium
    - Adult
        - Mild spasms 5–10 mg PO
        - Moderate spasms 5–10 mg IV
        - Severe spasms 40 mg/hour IV infusion
    - Pediatric

        - Mild spasms 0.1–0.8 mg/kg PO divided tid–qid (NMT 10 mg)
        - Moderate to severe spasms 0.1–0.3 mg/kg IV q4–8h (NMT 10 mg)
    - Antibiotics
        - Efficacy not proven
        - May try penicillin, Flagyl (metronidazole) or doxycycline
    - Vecuronium per physician (if intubated)

Consult criteria

- Immediate physician notification

Tetanus prophylaxis

- Tetanus prophylaxis
    - High risk = every 5 years
    - Low risk = every 10 years
    - Tetanus IG 250–500 units IM at different site from wound if high risk and less than 3 tetanus or unknown history of immunizations previously in life — usually with the elderly

High risk wound

- More than 6 hours old
- Greater than 1 cm deep
- Exposed to saliva or feces
- Stellate wounds
- Crush wounds
- Puncture wounds
- Ischemic appearance

Tdap

- Recommended by CDC for adults (Boostrix)
    - Recommended for adults age ≥ 65 years who have not previously received it
    - For adults having close contacts with infants < 12 months of age who have not previously received it
    - Healthcare workers who have not previously received it
- ACIP recommends a single Tdap dose for persons aged 11 through 18 years who have completed the recommended childhood diphtheria and tetanus toxoids and

pertussis/diphtheria and tetanus toxoids and acellular pertussis (DTP/DTaP) vaccination series and for adults aged 19 through 64 years who have not previously received Tdap

- A substitute for Td once only
- Contains pertussis in addition to tetanus toxoid and diphtheria toxoid
- Boostrix are formulations recommended for adults age ≥ 65 years who have not received it
    - Pediatric Td and Tdap contain 3–4 times more diphtheria toxoid than adult formulation (do not give to adults)
- Use only once, then use regular Td from then on in patients needing a tetanus booster
- Recommended in pregnancy after 20 weeks gestation (ideally between 27 and 36 weeks of gestation) regardless of vaccination history and time since prior Td or Tdap

Discharge instructions

- Wound aftercare instructions
- Refer to health department or primary care provider to complete tetanus primary vaccination series if < 2 vaccines given in past

Notes

References:

Tetanus Author: Patrick B Hinfey, MD; Chief Editor: John L Brusch, MD, FACP emedicine.medscape.com/article/229594

reference.medscape.com/drug/adacel-boostrix-tetanus-reduced-diphtheria-toxoids-acellular-pertussis-vaccine-999568

Updated Recommendations for Use of Tetanus Toxoid, Reduced Diphtheria Toxoid and Acellular Pertussis Vaccine (Tdap) in Pregnant Women and Persons Who Have or Anticipate Having Close Contact with an Infant Aged <12 Months --- Advisory Committee on Immunization Practices (ACIP), 2011

Weekly October 21, 2011 / 60(41);1424-1426

Dermatology

Section Contents

When using any protocol, always follow the Guidelines of Proper Use (page 18).

Human and Animal Bite Protocol

When using any protocol, always follow the Guidelines of Proper Use (page 18).

Human Bites

- 15–20% infection rate
- Staph aureus most common
- Usually hand wounds from fist fight

Evaluation

- Wound exploration
- X-ray
- Assess bone, joint, muscle and tendon for injury

Treatment options

- Consider closure only if all 4 criteria present:
    - Cosmetically significant (face wound)
    - Uninfected wound
    - Less than 12 hours old (< 24 hours on face)
    - Not on hand or foot
- Do not close puncture wounds
- Flush with > 250 cc of 1% betadine solution using 18 gauge angiocath (mix 1 cc of 10% betadine with 9 cc of NS)
- May rinse with NS
- Remove devitalized tissue
- ADT 0.5 cc IM if more than 5 years from last immunization (or Tdap if have not had in past)
- Tetanus immune globulin 250–500 units IM different site if < 3 tetanus immunizations in the past
- Refer to health department or primary care provider to complete tetanus primary vaccination series if < 2 vaccines given in past
    - See Tetanus Protocol (page 756)
- Antibiotics prophylaxis
    - Superficial: none

Deeper wound antibiotic treatment options

- Augmentin (amoxicillin/clavulanate) 875 mg PO bid × 5 days for prophylaxis (adults > 40kg)
- Augmentin (amoxicillin/clavulanate) 15 mg/kg PO bid × 5 days for prophylaxis (pediatrics < 40 kg)
- Doxycycline 100 mg PO bid × 5 days if allergic to penicillin
- Doxycycline 1.5–2 mg/kg PO bid × 5 days if allergic to penicillin (age > 8 years and < 45 kg)
- May refer to Sanford Guide or other drug databases

Discharge criteria

- Superficial wounds without infection
- No bone, joint or tendon involvement

Discharge instructions

- Human bite aftercare instructions
- Return if infection occurs in bite
- Return if pain increases

Consult criteria

- Infected wounds
- Closed fist wounds penetrating to joint, tendon or bone
- Significant bites to hand
- Fever
- Toxicity

Dog Bites

- 15–20% infection rate
- Most common pathogens
  - Aerobes: staph aureus, Pasteurella multocida, streptococcus
  - Anaerobes: enterobacter, pseudomonas, bacillus
- Infection occurring < 24 hours — Pasteurella multocida
- Infection occurring > 24 hours — staph or strep

Evaluation

- Wound exploration
- X-ray
- Assess bone, joint, muscle and tendon for injury
- Assess for foreign body (tooth, etc.)

Treatment

- Flush with > 250 cc of 1% betadine solution (mix 1 cc of 10% betadine with 9 cc of NS using 18 gauge angiocath)
- Rinse with NS
- ADT 0.5 cc IM if more than 5 years from last (or Tdap if have not had in past)
- Tetanus immune globulin 250–500 units IM different site if < 3 tetanus immunizations in the past
- Refer to health department or primary care provider to complete tetanus primary vaccination series if < 2 vaccines given in past
    - See Tetanus Protocol (page 756)
- Add viricidal 1% benzalkonium chloride if risk of rabies
- Remove devitalized tissue
- Consider closure
    - Bite < 8 hours old
    - Bite < 12 hours old on face
    - Do not close puncture wounds
- Antibiotic prophylaxis
    - Usually not needed
    - Use in high risk wounds; facial wounds
    - Use in immunocompromised or asplenic patients
    - Same antibiotic regimen as for human bites
- Consider rabies prophylaxis
- Notify rabies control

Discharge criteria

- Same as human bites

Discharge instructions

- Dog bite aftercare instructions
- Return if infection occurs in bite
- Return if pain increases

Consult criteria

- Severely infected wounds
- Wounds penetrating to joint, tendon, or bone
- Neurovascular deficit or injury
- Significant bites to hand
- Fever
- Toxicity

Cat Bites

- High infection risk
- 25–50% infection rate
- Pasteurella multocida up to 80% of infections
- Infection > 24 hours usually streptococcus — can progress rapidly
- May cause
    - Osteomyelitis
    - Septic arthritis
    - Abscess
    - Sepsis

Evaluation

- Wound exploration
- X-ray
- Assess bone, joint, muscle and tendon for injury
- Assess for foreign body (tooth, etc.)

Treatment

- Flush with > 250 cc of 1% betadine solution using 18 gauge angiocath (mix 1 cc of 10% betadine with 9 cc of NS)
- May rinse with NS
- ADT 0.5 cc IM if more than 5 years from last dose (or Tdap if have not had in past)
- Tetanus immune globulin 250−500 units IM different site if < 3 tetanus immunizations in the past
- Refer to health department or primary care provider to complete tetanus primary vaccination series if < 2 vaccines given in past
    - See Tetanus Protocol (page 756)
- Add viricidal 1% benzalkonium chloride if risk of rabies

- Remove devitalized tissue (not puncture wounds)
- Closure not recommended on
  - Puncture wounds or deep bites
  - Infected wounds
  - Wounds > 24 hours

Antibiotics prophylaxis options

- Augmentin (amoxicillin/clavulanate) 875 mg PO bid-tid × 5 days for prophylaxis (adults > 40 kg)
- Augmentin (amoxicillin/clavulanate) 15 mg/kg PO bid-tid × 5 days for prophylaxis (pediatrics < 40 kg)
- Doxycycline 100 mg PO bid × 5 days if allergic to penicillin
- Doxycycline 1.5–2 mg/kg PO bid × 5 days if allergic to penicillin (age > 8 years and < 45 kg)

Mild infections options

- Augmentin (amoxicillin/clavulanate) 875 mg PO bid × 10–14 days (adults > 40 kg)
- Augmentin (amoxicillin/clavulanate) 15 mg/kg PO bid × 10–14 days (pediatrics < 40 kg)
- Doxycycline 100 mg PO bid × 10–14 days if allergic to penicillin
- Doxycycline 1.5–2 mg/kg PO bid × 10–14 days if allergic to penicillin (age > 8 years and < 45 kg)

Moderate infections options

- Augmentin (amoxicillin/clavulanate) 875 mg PO bid × 10–14 days (adults > 40 kg)
- Augmentin (amoxicillin/clavulanate) 15 mg/kg PO bid × 10–14 days (pediatrics < 40 kg)
- Doxycycline 100 mg PO bid × 10–14 days if allergic to penicillin
- Doxycycline 1.5–2 mg/kg PO bid × 10–14 days if allergic to penicillin (age > 8 years and < 45 kg

    - Rocephin (ceftriaxone) 1–2 gms IM qday × 10–14 days
    - Rocephin (ceftriaxone) 50 mg/kg IM qday × 10–14 days not to exceed adult dose for children
- Consider rabies prophylaxis
- Notify rabies control

Discharge criteria

- Superficial wounds
- Mild to moderate infected wounds

Discharge instructions

- Cat bite aftercare instructions
- Return if infection occurs in bite
- Return if pain increases

Consult criteria

- Severely infected wounds
- Wounds penetrating to joint, tendon, or bone
- Neurovascular deficit or injury
- Significant bites to hand
- Fever
- Toxicity

Wild Animal Bites

- Similar evaluation, treatment and disposition as Dog Bites Protocol
- Notify rabies control

Notes

References:

Human Bites Author: Jeffrey Barrett, MD; Chief Editor: John L Brusch, MD, FACP
emedicine.medscape.com/article/218901

Animal Bites in Emergency Medicine
Author: Alisha Perkins Garth, MD; Chief Editor: Joe Alcock, MD, MS emedicine.medscape.com/article/768875

SPIDER BITE AND INSECT STING PROTOCOL

When using any protocol, always follow the Guidelines of Proper Use (page 18).

Brown Recluse Spider Bite

- Found in dark areas
- Envenomation can be mild if spider has recently fed
- Symptoms develop 4–8 hours after bite
- Symptoms and findings that may occur are
  - Local reaction only
  - Tissue necrosis
  - Severe pain
  - Pruritus
  - Fever
  - Nausea/vomiting
  - Headache
  - Myalgias
  - Initial papule which develops central dark area of necrosis over 48–72 hours

Evaluation

- History of bite
- Exam of lesion area

Systemic symptoms

- CBC to check for thrombocytopenia and anemia
- BMP to check for renal involvement
- PT/PTT/INR and DIC panel if DIC suspected
- U/A to check on dipstick for blood for hemolytic anemia

Treatment options

- Clean wound
- Benadryl (diphenhydramine) or other antihistamines for pruritus and rash
- ADT 0.5 cc IM if more than 5 years from last dose (or Tdap if have not had in past) — see Tetanus Protocol

- Antibiotics if secondary infection present
  - Doxycycline 100 mg PO bid × 10–14 days if allergic to penicillin
  - Doxycycline 1.5–2 mg/kg PO bid × 10–14 days if allergic to penicillin (age > 8 years and < 45 kg) — NMT 100 mg per dose
  - Septra DS (trimethoprim/sulfamethoxazole) bid x 10–14 days
  - Septra (trimethoprim/sulfamethoxazole) 8-12 mg TMP/kg/dose or 0.5 cc/LB bid PO for PO q12hr for 10–14 days for children
    - Contraindicated in ages < 2 months
  - Clindamycin 300 mg PO tid for 10–14 days
  - Pediatric — clindamycin 20-30 mg/kg/day PO divided tid × 10–14 days (NMT 300 mg/dose usually)
- Follow up with primary care provider or surgeon within 7 days if wound necrotic

Discharge criteria

- Nontoxic patient
- No systemic symptoms

Discharge instructions

- Brown recluse spider bite aftercare instructions
- Return if pain worsens
- Return if fever occurs
- Return for occurrence of systemic symptoms

Consult criteria

- Toxic patient
- Systemic symptoms
- Anemia
- Thrombocytopenia
- Acute renal insufficiency
- Significant cellulitis
- Necrotic area > 2 cm

Black Widow Spider Bites

- Red hourglass on abdomen

Grade 1 (mild envenomation)

- Immediate pain at site
- Normal vital signs

Grade 2 (moderate envenomation)

- Muscle pain in bitten extremity
- Muscle pain may extend to abdomen if lower extremity bitten
- Muscle pain may extend to chest if upper extremities bitten
- Diaphoresis at bite site
- Normal vital signs

Grade 3 (severe envenomation)

- Generalized muscular pain
- Generalized diaphoresis
- Nausea/vomiting
- Headache
- Hypertension
- Tachycardia

Evaluation

- U/A for hematuria
- CPK
- Labs and other testing to rule out other acute abdominal process if suspected

Treatment options

- IV NS
- Tetanus prophylaxis (see Tetanus Practice Guide)
- Cool compresses to site
- Benadryl (diphenhydramine) IV 50 mg or weight adjusted for pediatrics if antivenin to be given
- Pain control with narcotics
- Black widow antivenin (consult physician before using)

Consult criteria

- All black widow spider bites
- Before any antivenin given

Bees, Wasps, and Fire Ants

- Refer to Allergy Practice Guide if needed

- Remove stinger
- Cool compresses
- Can make a Adolph Meat Tenderizer paste with water and apply for 1 hour to break down proteins in venom
- NSAID's prn for pain
- Topical hydrocortisone cream may be used
- Tetanus prophylaxis if > 10 years (see Tetanus Practice Guide)
- Respective aftercare instructions

Local Reactions from Insect Bites or Stings

- 1–5 cm of nontender induration usually
- Light pink or red color
- Antihistamine OTC prn
- Cool compresses prn
- Steroids 1–3 day course can be considered — usually not needed (avoid in diabetes)
- If cellulitis present, refer to Cellulitis Practice Guide
- Local reaction aftercare instructions

Notes

References:

Brown Recluse Spider Envenomation

Author: Thomas C Arnold, MD, FAAEM, FACMT; Chief Editor: Joe Alcock, MD,MS emedicine.medscape.com/article/772295

Clark RF, Wethern-Kestner S, Vance MV, Gerkin R. Clinical presentation and treatment of black widow spider envenomation: a review of 163 cases. *Ann Emerg Med*. Jul 1992;21(7):782–787

Widow Spider Envenomation Author: Sean P Bush, MD, FACEP; Chief Editor: Joe Alcock, MD, MS emedicine.medscape.com/article/772196

SNAKE BITE PROTOCOL

When using any protocol, always follow the Guidelines of Proper Use (page 18).

Considerations

- 2,000 venomous snake bites per year
- Alcohol intoxication frequently a contributing factor
- Mortality < 0.5% with advent of antivenin
- Venomous snake bites involve pit vipers (Crotalids) or coral snakes
- Eastern coral snake considered deadly
- Arizona coral snake not deadly
- Oozing at fang bite site reliable predictor of envenomation

Pit vipers (are responsible for majority of venomous bites)

- Rattlesnakes
- Cottonmouths
- Copperheads
- Water moccasins

Identification

Pit vipers

- Depressions or pits between eyes and nostrils
- Triangular head
- Elliptical eyes
- 2 fangs
- Subcaudal plates

Coral snake

- Black nose
- Colored rings
- Confused with King snake
    - "Red on yellow, kill a fellow; red on black, venom lack" denoting color rings of Coral and King snakes respectively
- Venom usually either hemotoxic or neurotoxic

Pit vipers symptoms and findings

- Local injury (swelling starts in 15–30 minutes)
- Systemic vascular damage
- Hemolysis; hematuria; hematemesis
- Fibrinolysis and coagulopathy
- Neuromuscular dysfunction
- Compartment syndrome
- Airway edema

Coral snake symptoms and findings

- No significant local injury
- Respiratory failure
- Cranial nerve dysfunction
- Tremors
- Salivation
- Seizures

Crotalid (Pit Viper) Envenomation Grading

No envenomation

- Snakebite suspected
- Minimal pain
- No systemic symptoms or lab abnormalities in first 12 hours after bite

Mild envenomation

- Local redness, swelling, ecchymosis limited to bite site

Moderate envenomation

- Local redness, swelling, and ecchymosis that extends beyond bite site
- Nausea
- Paresthesias
- Metallic taste in mouth
- Mild hypotension
- Mild tachycardia
- Mild tachypnea
- Coagulation factors normal and no active bleeding signs

Severe envenomation

- Rapidly spreading swelling, redness, and ecchymosis to involve entire limb
- Altered mentation
- Respiratory compromise
- Severe hypotension (7%)
- Extreme tachycardia
- Coagulopathy
- Active bleeding

Coral Snake Envenomation

- Coral snake bite symptoms can be delayed up to 12 hours
- Ptosis early sign
- Muscle weakness
- Salivation
- Slurred speech
- Dizziness
- Respiratory failure
- Other neurologic abnormalities

Diagnosis of Snake Bites

- Fang marks (pit vipers)
- History of snake exposure
- Local tissue injury
- Coral snake may have tiny punctures and minimal local tissue changes

Evaluation of Snake Bites

- History and physical exam
- Mark edematous area with a pen every 15 minutes — 30 minutes to assess progression
- CBC
- CMP
- PT/PTT/INR
- U/A

Moderate to severe envenomation

- EKG
- Chest x-ray

- ABG
- Troponin
- DIC panel

Treatment Options

- Clean wound with antiseptic or soap/water
- No arterial constrictive banding, no wound excisions, no ice
- Venous banding can be considered if there is a large snake bite and prolonged delay reaching hospital
- Keep limb immobilized at heart level
- Tetanus toxoid (ADT) 0.5 cc IM if > 5 years since last dose (or Tdap in never had in past)
- Tetanus immune globulin 250–500 units IM at different site if < 3 tetanus doses in life
- Refer to health department or primary care provider to complete tetanus primary vaccination series if < 2 vaccines given in past
    - See Tetanus Protocol
- Antibiotics choices if infected — usually not needed otherwise
    - Rocephin, dicloxicillin, septra or doxycycline

Pain and nausea control options prn

- Dilaudid (hydromorphone) 0.5–1 mg IV (double if IM) prn — may repeat prn
- Morphine 2–5 mg IV prn — may repeat prn
- Stadol (butorphanol) 0.5–1 mg IV (double if IM) — may repeat prn
- Phenergan (promethazine) 6.25 mg IV or 25–50 mg IM prn
- Zofran (ondansetron) 4–8 mg IV prn

Pit viper antivenin (mainstay of treatment) — notify physician

Crofab (less allergic reactions than horse serum)

- Read package insert
- Mild or no envenomation does not require antivenin for pit vipers
- 4–6 vials IV for moderate to severe envenomation initially — give slowly for first

10 minutes at 25–50 cc/hr to observe for allergic reaction

- 2 vials IV q6hr up to 3 doses if further doses needed after initial dosing

Coral snake (eastern) antivenin

- Read package insert
- Pretreat with Benadryl (diphenhydramine) and Pepcid (famotidine) IV
- Keep epinephrine at bedside
- 3–6 vials IV over 1–2 hours if definitely bitten
- 10 vials IV initially if systemic manifestations present

Complications of antivenin

Acute allergic reaction – see Allergy Protocol Anaphylaxis sections

- Benadryl (diphenhydramine) 50 mg adult; 1.25 mg/kg pediatrics not to exceed 50 mg
- Pepcid (famotidine) 20–40 mg IV adult
- Pepcid (famotidine) 0.25 mg/kg up to 20 mg for children
- Solumedrol (methylprednisolone) 125 mg IV for adults
- Solumedrol (methylprednisolone) 1 mg/kg IV for children not to exceed 125 mg
- If reaction is severe notify physician immediately
    - Epinephrine 0.3–0.5 SQ/IM/IV for adults depending on severity; pediatrics 0.1 mg/kg SQ/IM/IV depending on severity not to exceed 0.5 mg
- It is preferable to consult on venomous snake bite patients

Serum sickness

- Fever
- Arthralgias
- Rash (usually occurs 7–10 days after antivenin; can occur earlier)

Treatment

- Antihistamines prn
- Steroids for 7–10 days PO

Discharge Criteria

- Pit viper bite is dry, and is asymptomatic after 8 hours of observation
- Sonoran and Arizona coral snake bite: can be discharged

Discharge instructions

- Snake bite aftercare instructions
- Refer to primary care provider or surgeon

Consult Criteria

- Notify physician promptly for all snake bites
- All eastern coral snake or suspected eastern coral snake bites (need admission)
- Pit vipers with any envenomation (usually need admission)
- Abnormal vital signs
- Abnormal lab; chest x-ray; EKG
- Neurologic abnormalities
- Suspected compartment syndrome

Notes

References:

Snakebite Author: Brian James Daley, MD, MBA, FACS, FCCP, CNSC; Chief Editor: Joe Alcock, MD, MS emedicine.medscape.com/article/168828

Coral Snake Envenomation

Author: Robert L Norris, MD; Chief Editor: Joe Alcock, MD, MS emedicine.medscape.com/article/771701

Dart RC. Sequelae of pit viper nvenomations. In: Campbel JA, Brodie ED Jr, eds. Biology of the pit vipers. Tyler, Texas.: Selva Publishing, 1992:395–404

Kitchens CS, Van Mierop LHS. Envenomation by the eastern coral snake (Micrurus fulvius fulvius): a study of 39 victims. JAMA 1987; 258:1615–8

CELLULITIS PROTOCOL

When using any protocol, always follow the Guidelines of Proper Use (page 18).

Definition

- Local inflammatory reaction of the skin and subcutaneous tissue secondary to bacterial infection

Differential Diagnosis

- Erysipelas
- Osteomyelitis
- Septic arthritis
- Lymphadenitis
- Abscess
- Deep vein thrombosis
- Necrotizing fasciitis

Considerations

- Pain, tenderness, redness, swelling and warmth
- Abscess frequently co-exists
- Associated with outpatient treatment failure
    - Fever 100.4° F or 38°C
    - Chronic leg ulcers
    - Chronic edema
    - Prior cellulitis in the same area
    - Cellulitis at a wound site
    - Cellulitis of the hand
    - **Subacute spread or redness and edema may extend beyond drawn margins during the first 48 hrs. without representing treatment failure**
        - Decreasing intensity of the erythema is often a more important variable of improvement

Caused by

- S. aureus (MRSA)
- Group A streptococcus
- H. influenzae
- Pseudomonas

- Anaerobes

Complications

- Bacteremia
- Osteomyelitis
- Septic joint
- Cavernous sinus spread

Higher risk

- Diabetics
- Peripheral vascular disease
- Chronic edema
- IV drug abuse
- Immunocompromised

Necrotizing fasciitis

- Prompt diagnosis and treatment reduces mortality and amputations
- Early diagnosis missed in almost 75% of cases
    - Misdiagnosed as cellulitis or abscess
- Pain out of proportion to swelling and erythema most consistent finding
- Other potential findings
    - Tenderness extending beyond the erythema and swelling due to toxins and enzymes spreading along fascia
    - Indistinct margins
    - Lymphangitis rarely seen due to depth of infection
    - Rapidly progressive despite antibiotic treatment

Evaluation

- Complete history and physical examination
- Assess for tissue gas
- Palpate for tenderness

No tests needed

- For small area of involvement
- No fever or systemic signs
- No high risk factors

Testing considerations

- CBC, BMP for high risk factors
- Blood cultures if toxic or septic appearance
- Ultrasound useful to evaluate for possible abscess if suspected
- X-ray if crepitus noted or tissue gas suspected

Treatment Options

Uncomplicated purulent cellulitis (select one)

- Septra (trimethoprim /sulfamethoxazole), doxycycline (age > 8 years) or clindamycin for community acquired MRSA
  - Clindamycin 20-30 mg/kg/day PO/IV divided q6hr–q8hr × 10 days; not to exceed 450 mg/dose
  - Doxycycline 1.5–2 mg/kg PO bid × 10 days (age > 8 years and < 45 kg) not to exceed 100 mg bid

Uncomplicated non–purulent cellulitis (select one)

- Dicloxicilln 500 mg q6hr PO x 5–10 days
  - <40 kg —12.5 –100 mg/kg/day PO depending on severity divided q6hr
- Cephalexin 500 mg q6hr PO x 5–10 days (or other cephalosporins PO/IV)
  - Pediatric 25–50 mg/kg/day PO divided q6hr not to exceed 500 mg/dose
- Cefazolin 1–2 gms IV q8hr x 10 days
  - Pediatric 25-100 mg/kg divided q6hr–q8hr
  - Clindamycin 300–450 mg q6–8hr PO/IV x 10 days
    - Pediatric 20-30 mg/kg/day PO/IV divided q6hr–q8hr × 5– 10 days not to exceed 450 mg/dose

Human, dog or cat bite

- Augmentin x 10 days (amoxicillin/clavulanate) or Sanford guide or antibiotic databases
  - See Cat and Dog bite sections

Preseptal ocular cellulitis

- Augmentin x 10 days (amoxicillin/clavulanate) or Sanford guide or antibiotic database

    - See Preseptal cellulitis section
- Drain associated abscesses and pack as needed
    - Leave pack in usually 2 days
    - Bedside ultrasound frequently changes therapy if abscess found with cellulitis (see examples below)

Waterborne cellulitis

Fresh water

- Commonly aeromonas hydrophilia (or others)
- Treatment
    - Doxycycline (age ≥ 8 years) plus IV gentamicin etc.)
    - Bactrim
    - Ceftriaxone
    - Quinolone such as ciprofloxacin or levofloxacin (caution in children due to possible arthropathy complications)

Salt water

- Commonly vibrio species
    - May progress rapidly to necrotizing infection, even if initially a superficial infection
- Treatment
    - Third generation cephalosporin such as cefepime, ceftriaxone plus doxycycline (age ≥ 8 years)
    - Quinolone such as ciprofloxacin or levofloxacin (caution in children due to possible arthropathy complications)

Bedside ultrasound can change therapy (see below)

Brown recluse spider bite causing both cellulitis and abscess of proximal anterior thigh

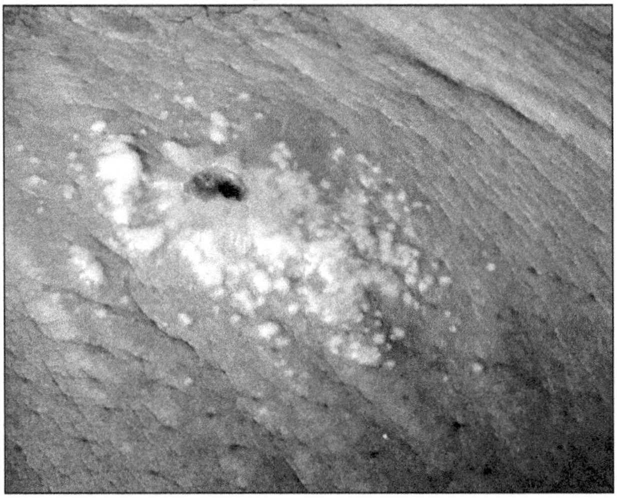

In performing bedside ultrasound for skin soft tissue exams, use the linear high frequency probe

Cobblestone appearance ultrasound image of cellulitis (fat globules with surrounding edema)

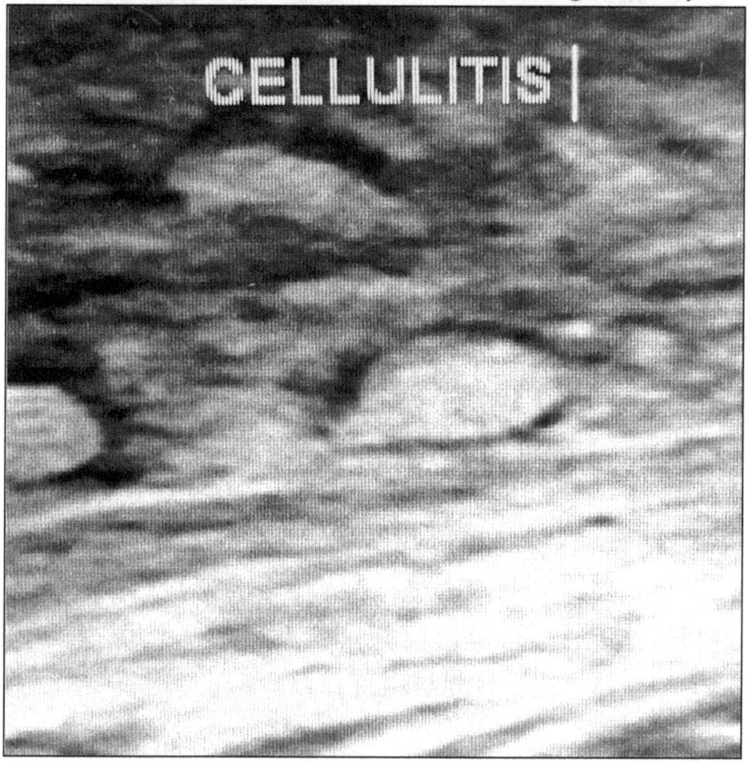

Abscess associated with the cellulitis

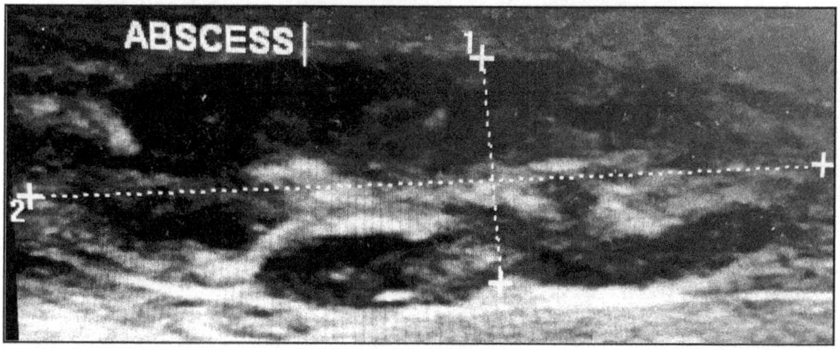

Discharge Criteria

- Mild cellulitis without systemic toxicity
- Available follow up

Discharge instructions

- Cellulitis aftercare instructions
- Follow up with PCP within 3–5 days if not improving
- Return if fever develops or pain increases
- Return for progressive increase in cellulitis

Consult Criteria

- Any documented fever
- Rapidly spreading
- Pain out of proportion to exam
- Crepitus or gas in tissues
- Systemic toxic appearance
- Necrotizing fasciitis or gas gangrene
- Large abscess
- Facial cellulitis
- Orbital cellulitis
- Suspected bony involvement
- Poorly controlled diabetic patients
- Failure of outpatient antibiotics
- Waterborne cellulitis

Higher risk comorbidities

- Diabetics with poor control
- Peripheral vascular disease
- Chronic edema
- IV drug abuse
- Immunocompromised

Vital signs and age consult criteria

- Age < 6 months
- Hypotension
- Any fever

Lab consult criteria

- WBC ≥ 15,000 or < 3,000
- Bandemia ≥ 15%
- Acute thrombocytopenia
- Significant electrolyte abnormally
- Glucose ≥ 350 mg/dL in diabetic patient
- Glucose ≥ 200 mg/dL in non-diabetic patient

- Hyperglycemia with metabolic acidosis (decreased serum CO2 or elevated anion gap)
- Metabolic acidosis

Notes

References:

Goh T, et al. *Br J Surgery* January 2014, Vol. 101, Issue 1, pages e119-e125

Hsiao C, et al. *Am J Emerg Med* 2008; 26: 170-175

Huang KF, et al. *J Trauma* 2011; 71: 467-473

Majeski J, Majeski E. *South Med J* 1997; 90: 1065-1068

Peterson D, et al. *Acad Emerg Med* 2014 May;21(5):526-531

Volz KA, et al. *Am J Emerg Med* 2013 Feb;31(2):360-4

Sabbaj A, et al. *Acad Emerg Med* 2009 Dec;16(12):1290-7

JEM,53(4):485

SOFT TISSUE ABSCESS PROTOCOL

When using any protocol, always follow the Guidelines of Proper Use (page 18).

Definition

- Collection of purulent material in the soft tissues

Differential Diagnosis

- Cellulitis
- Erysipelas
- Osteomyelitis
- Septic arthritis
- Lymphadenitis
- Deep vein thrombosis
- Necrotizing fasciitis

Considerations

- Incision and drainage usually curative without antibiotics
- MRSA most common cause
- Cellulitis frequently surrounds abscess
- May be in deep areas like the buttocks
- Ultrasound useful when in doubt of an abscess being present
- Recurrent groin and axillary abscesses suggest hidradenitis suppurativa

Higher risk comorbidities

- Diabetics
- Peripheral vascular disease
- Chronic edema
- IV drug abuse
- Elderly
- Immunocompromised

Evaluation

- Assess for systemic toxicity
- Bedside ultrasound frequently changes therapy
- Examine for deeper structure involvement

- Culture Bartholin cysts for GC and Chlamydia
    - Usually from E coli or vaginal flora more than STD
- Consider abscess culture
- CBC, BMP for high risk factors
- Blood cultures if toxic or septic appearance

In performing bedside ultrasound for skin soft tissue exams, use the linear high frequency probe

Bedside ultrasound of abscess

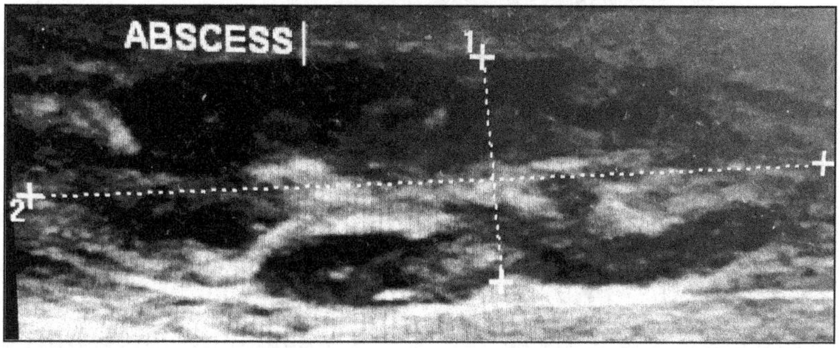

Treatment Options

- Skin prep with betadine
- Local anesthesia with ethyl chloride and/or lidocaine
- May use 18–20 gauge needle to aspirate to confirm an abscess
- Incise with #11 scalpel maximum area of swelling and/or tenderness
- Break any deeper adhesions
- Drain pus
- Pack with gauze if large abscess present for 24–48 hours — patient can remove at home or return to see a Provider
- Do not pack facial abscesses
- NSAID's, Tylenol or narcotics short course prn

Loop drainage technique

- Very useful in pediatrics (also use in adults)
- After local anesthesia and skin prep with betadine, incise lateral edge of abscess 3-5 mm with #11 scalpel
- Introduce small curved hemostat in cavity and break up loculations
- With tip of hemostat find other edge of abscess and tent skin and incise down to hemostat bringing tip through skin

    - Usually 4 cm or less should separate incised openings. If more distance needed then consider additional loops
- Irrigate pus out
- Draw a vessel loop, sterile rubber band or Penrose drain back through the abscess from second opening
- Tie loop loosely with enough space to get a finger under the loop
- Keep area clean with gauze
- Can shower or bathe
- Remove loop when drainage had stopped and cellulitis improved, usually within 7–10 days

Has superior results and decreased pain than conventional I&D

Antibiotic choices

- All abscesses > 2cm by ultrasound treated with MRSA antibiotics 5–10 days (beneficial in smaller abscesses also)
    - Septra DS (trimethoprim/sulfamethoxazole)
        - Pediatric 0.5 ml/kg bid (max dose 20 ml)
    - Doxycycline (age ≥ 8 years)
    - Clindamycin
- Severe infection
    - Patients who have failed I&D plus oral antibiotics
    - Meet SIRS criteria
    - Immunocompromised patients
    - Vancomycin or Daptomycin or Linezolid or Televancin or Ceftaroline
- Consider antibiotics for higher risk patients

Discharge Criteria

- Uncomplicated abscess without toxicity
- No high risk co-morbidity
- Outpatient follow up available

Discharge instructions

- Abscess aftercare instructions
- Return if pain worsens or involved area increases in size
- Return if fever develops or worsens

Consult Criteria

- Rapidly spreading
- Pain out of proportion to exam
- Crepitus or gas in tissues
- Systemic toxic appearance
- Hypotension
- Necrotizing fasciitis
- Gas gangrene
- Vital signs significantly abnormal
- Facial abscess
- Large abscess
- Perirectal or pilonidal abscess
- Suspected bony or muscle involvement
- Poorly controlled diabetic patient
- Failure of recent I&D treatment

Higher risk comorbidities

- Diabetics with poor control
- Peripheral vascular disease
- Chronic edema
- IV drug abuse
- Elderly
- Immunocompromised

Vital signs and age consult criteria

- Age < 6 months or ≥ 70 years old
- Hypotension or relative hypotension SBP < 105 in patient with hypertension history
- Fever > 101°F (38.3°C)

Lab consult criteria

- WBC ≥ 15,000 or < 3,000
- Bandemia ≥ 15%
- Acute thrombocytopenia
- Significant electrolyte abnormally
- Glucose ≥ 350 mg/dL in diabetic patient
- Glucose ≥ 200 mg/dL in non-diabetic patient
- Hyperglycemia with metabolic acidosis (decreased serum CO_2 or elevated anion gap)
- Worsening anemia
- Metabolic acidosis

Notes

Reference:

Stevens DL, et al. Clin Infect DisÂ July 15, 2014; 59(2): 147–159.

Talan DA, et al. Ann of Emerg Med. October 5, 2017.

Aprahamian CJ1, Nashad HH2, DiSomma NM3, Elger BM4, Esparaz JR5, McMorrow TJ4, Shadid AM4, Kao AM3, Holterman MJ1, Kanard RC4, Pearl RH6. Treatment of subcutaneous abscesses in children with incision and loop drainage: A simplified method of care. J Pediatr Surg. 2016 Dec 30. PMID:

Henoch-Schonlein Purpura Protocol

When using any protocol, always follow the Guidelines of Proper Use (page 18).

Definition

- Henoch-Schonlein purpura (HSP) is an inflammatory disorder characterized by a generalized vasculitis involving the small vessels of the skin, kidneys, GI tract, joints, and rarely the lungs and central nervous system

Differential Diagnosis

- Disseminated intravascular coagulation
- Meningitis
- Idiopathic Thrombocytopenic Purpura
- Mononucleosis
- Rocky Mountain spotted fever
- Septic shock
- Acute renal failure
- Intussusception
- Hand-Foot-Mouth disease
- Kawasaki disease
- Acute Glomerulonephritis
- Chicken pox
- Thrombocytopenic Purpura
- Systemic Lupus Erythematosus

Considerations

- Disease of children and young adults
- Diffuse vasculitis of unknown etiology
- Often an antecedent infection history present
- Peak incidence is 4 years of age
- Typical age range 2–11 years of age
- Spring peak
- Renal involvement most serious sequelae
    - Develops within 3 months of rash

  - Renal failure can develop up to 10 years after rash
  - More common in adults
- Generally a benign self-limited condition
- 40% have reoccurrence usually with rash and abdominal pain
- Normal platelet count, PT, and PTT

Signs and Symptoms

- Palpable purpura
- Rash of erythematous papules followed by nonthrombocytopenic purpura
  - Typically on buttocks; lower extremities; can be elsewhere
- Abdominal pain — 2/3 of patients; can mimic acute abdomen
- Low grade fever
- Vomiting
- Diarrhea — can be bloody
- Arthritis — 70% of patients; transient and no permanent deformity
- Nephritis
- End stage renal disease develops in 5% of cases
- Hematuria
- Intussusception
- Intracranial hemorrhage

Evaluation

- CBC
- BMP
- U/A
- PT/PTT/INR
- CT abdomen/pelvis scan if severe abdominal pain or bleeding present

Treatment

- IV NS for signs of hypovolemia
- Ibuprofen per weight
- Prednisone 1 mg/kg qday × 5–7 days if renal or severe GI involvement

    - Long term kidney disease may not be prevented
- Discontinue any known precipitants

Discharge Criteria

- Normal platelet count
- Normal renal function
- Minimal or no abdominal pain
- Discuss with physician prior to discharge

Discharge instructions

- Henoch-Schonlein Purpura aftercare instructions
- Follow up within 24 hours if discharged on prednisone

Consult Criteria

- Severe abdominal pain
- Neurologic abnormalities
- Gastrointestinal bleeding
- Intussusception
- Renal involvement

Notes

References:

Henoch-Schonlein Purpura Author: Noah S Scheinfeld, MD, JD, FAAD; Chief Editor: Craig B Langman, MD emedicine.medscape.com/article/984105

Chartapisak W, Opastirakul S, Hodson EM, Willis NS, Craig JC. Interventions for preventing and treating kidney disease in Henoch-Schönlein Purpura (HSP). Cochrane Database of Systematic Reviews 2009, Issue 3. Art. No.: CD005128. DOI: 10.1002/14651858.CD005128.pub2

ERYTHEMA MULTIFORME PROTOCOL

When using any protocol, always follow the Guidelines of Proper Use (page 18).

Definition

- Erythema multiforme (EM) is an acute, self-limited, and occasionally recurring skin condition thought to be a type IV hypersensitivity reaction associated with certain infections, medications, and other various triggers

Differential Diagnosis

- Urticaria
- Herpes simples
- Pityriasis rosea
- Secondary syphilis
- Viral exanthems
- Septicemia
- Drug eruptions
- Collagen vascular disease
- Serum sickness

Considerations

Erythema multiforme (EM) minor

- Target lesions or raised red papules
- No mortality

Erythema multiforme major

- Similar to EM minor with mucous membrane involvement
- Epidermal detachment < 10% total body surface area
- No mortality

Stevens Johnson Syndrome (SJS)

- Widespread blisters/bullae on trunk and face
- Mucous membrane involvement

- SJS — epidermal detachment < 10% BSA (body surface area)
- Mortality approximately 5%

Toxic Epidermal Necrolysis (TEN)

- Widespread blisters/bullae on trunk and face
- Mucous membrane involvement
- TEN — epidermal detachment > 30% BSA
- Mortality approximately 30%

Symptoms and Findings

Erythema multiforme: minor and major

- Burning sensation of rash
- Pruritus usually absent
- Eye involvement up to 10%; bilateral purulent conjunctivitis
- Any mucous membrane involvement is mild
- Viral type prodrome in 50%

Rash

- Target or iris lesions (red papules and macules with central clearing)
- Vesiculobullous lesions can develop in existing rash
- Sudden onset and symmetrical
- Centripetal spread
- Favors palms and soles
- Dorsal hands
- Extensor limb surfaces
- Face

SJS/TEN

- Generalized cutaneous and/or mucocutaneous vesiculobullous lesions
- Hemorrhagic bullae
- Fever
- Vomiting and diarrhea can occur
- Oral pain may be severe
- Eye pain and discharge
- Dyspnea may occur
- Dysuria

- Oral involvement may appear similar to aphthous ulcers
- Nasal pharynx, respiratory tract, GI and GU systems can be involved

Causes

- No identifiable cause in 50%
- Viral
  - Herpes simplex (10%)
  - Chicken pox
  - Various other viruses
- Bacterial
  - Mycoplasma
  - Salmonella
  - Gonorrhea
  - Various others
- Fungal
- Postvaccination
- Drugs
  - Sulfonamides
  - Hypoglycemics
  - NSAID's
  - Anticonvulsants
  - Various antibiotics
  - Malignancy
  - Hormonal
  - Autoimmune disorders

Evaluation

- Erythema multiforme
  - Testing driven by history and physical exam
  - May not need testing
- SJS/TEN
  - CBC
  - BMP
  - LFT's
  - Chest x-ray
  - Cultures prn

Treatment Options

- Remove offending agents if identified
- Erythema multiforme
    - Symptomatic treatments
    - Narcotics short course prn
    - NSAID's prn
    - Cool compresses with saline or Burrow's solution
    - Saline or Benadryl (diphenhydramine) elixir gargles prn for oral findings/symptoms
    - No oral steroids
    - Acyclovir for herpes associated erythema multiforme
- SJS/TEN
    - IV NS for hydration
    - Cultures prn
    - Burn unit treatment

Discharge Criteria

- Uncomplicated erythema multiforme

Discharge instructions

- Erythema multiforme aftercare instructions
- Return immediately if signs of SJS/TEN develops

Consult Criteria

- Refer to General Patient Criteria Protocol (page 22)
- All suspected SJS/TEN

Notes

References: Erythema Multiforme Author: Jose A Plaza, MD; Chief Editor: William D James, MD
emedicine.medscape.com/article/1122915

Sokumbi O, Wetter DA. Clinical features, diagnosis, and treatment of erythema multiforme: a review for the practicing dermatologist. *Int J Dermatol*. Aug 2012;51(8):889–902

Ann of EM, 8/14, pg. 119

Erythema Nodosum Protocol

When using any protocol, always follow the Guidelines of Proper Use (page 18).

Definition

- Erythema nodosum (EN) is an acute, nodular, erythematous eruption that usually is limited to the extensor aspects of the lower legs, thought to be a hypersensitivity reaction

Differential Diagnosis

- Urticaria
- Nodular vasculitis
- Insect bites
- Erysipelas
- Superficial thrombophlebitis

Considerations

- Delayed hypersensitivity reaction
- Painful red tender 2–6 cm nodules on extensor lower extremities
- Usually acute and self-limited
- May last weeks to years
- More common in females age 30–50 years
- Idiopathic 50% of the time
- Often a marker for systemic disease

Causes

- Idiopathic 50% of the time
- Most commonly secondary to strep infections; sarcoidosis
- Drug reactions
  - Sulfa
  - Penicillin
  - Oral contraceptives
- Systemic infections
  - Tuberculosis
  - Fungal
- Ulcerative colitis

- Malignancy
  - Leukemia
  - Lymphoma

Evaluation

- Strep test of pharynx
- ESR or C-reactive protein (may be very high)

Treatment

- NSAID's prn
- Treat underlying infection or causes if found
- Cool compresses prn
- Elevation of legs
- Bed rest

Discharge Criteria

- All uncomplicated cases

Discharge instructions

- Erythema nodosum aftercare instructions

Consult Criteria

- Refer to General Patient Criteria Protocol (page 22)
- Serious associated comorbidities

Notes

Reference:

Erythema Nodosum Author: Jeanette L Hebel, MD; Chief Editor: Dirk M Elston, MD
emedicine.medscape.com/article/1081633

DYSHIDROTIC ECZEMA PROTOCOL

When using any protocol, always follow the Guidelines of Proper Use (page 18).

Definition

- Vesicular eruption with pruritic deep-seated vesicles of the fingers, hands and feet of unknown etiology

Differential Diagnosis

- Scabies
- Contact dermatitis
- Irritant dermatitis
- Erythema multiforme
- Herpes simplex

Considerations

- Related to stress; drugs; illness
- "Id" reaction from variety of stimuli; distant fungal infections
- Last approximately 3 weeks
- Is a chronic relapsing palmoplantar dermatitis
- Spring and summer prevalence
- Warm climates
- 50% have childhood atopic dermatitis, asthma or similar conditions
- Symmetric distribution

Treatment Options

- Moisturizing lotions (Eucerin)
- Topical steroids
- Oral steroids such as prednisone 20–40 mg or dexamethasone 4–6 mg daily for a short course up to 7–10 days with taper
- Tacrolimus ointment
- Ultraviolet A light
- Oral antihistamines prn itching
- Ointments beneficial where increased moisture is needed

- Creams preferred in scalp and moist areas
- Avoid precipitating agents

Discharge Criteria

- Uncomplicated process

Discharge instructions

- Dyshidrotic eczema aftercare instructions

Consult Criteria

- Moderate to severe superinfection

Notes

References:

National Institute for Clinical Excellence. *Frequency of application of topical corticosteroids for atopic eczema*. London, England: National Institute for Clinical Excellence (NICE); 2004:34

Dyshidrotic Eczema Author: Sadegh Amini, MD; Chief Editor: Dirk M Elston, MD medicine.medscape.com/article/1122527

Dyshidrotic Eczema Author: Sadegh Amini, MD; Chief Editor: Dirk M Elston, MD medicine.medscape.com/article/1122527

Dyshidrotic Eczema emedicine medscape

Updated: Jun 29, 2018 Author: Sadegh Amini, MD; Chief Editor: William D James, MD

ATOPIC DERMATITIS/ECZEMA PROTOCOL

When using any protocol, always follow the Guidelines of Proper Use (page 18).

Definition

- Poorly defined red patchy plaque-like rash with edema acutely and skin thickening chronically, mostly on flexor surfaces
- Also known as Eczema

Differential Diagnosis

- Seborrheic dermatitis
- Discoid eczema
- Contact dermatitis
- Scabies
- Insect bites
- Psoriasis

Considerations

- Can be acute or subacute
- Chronic relapsing most common
- Pruritic inflammation of epidermis or dermis
- Family history of asthma, hay fever, allergic rhinitis, allergic dermatitis
- Immune modulated
- More frequent in formula fed babies
- Manifests in infancy or early childhood usually and persists into adolescence
- Relationship to food allergies: milk, soy, eggs, wheat
- More frequent in winter
- Increased humidity contribution
- Bathing with hot water removes moisture from skin — worsening the rash

Symptoms

- Dry skin

- Erythematous patches and plaques
- Surrounding erythema and scaling may occur
- Skin excoriations frequent
- Often in skin flexures — antecubital and popliteal fossa
- May be generalized

Treatment Options

- Tacrolimus or pimcrolimus ointment
- Antihistamines
- Topical steroids
- May need oral steroids
- Avoid soap and hot water on rash as much as possible
- Topical or oral antibiotic for staph superinfection
- Eucerin
- Tar containing shampoo for scalp seborrheic dermatitis
- Avoid wool clothing

Discharge Criteria

- Uncomplicated process

Discharge instructions

- Atopic dermatitis or eczema aftercare instructions

Consult Criteria

- Moderate to severe superinfection

Notes

References:

Margolis JS, Abuabara K, Bilker W, Hoffstad O, Margolis DJ. Persistence of Mild to Moderate Atopic Dermatitis.*JAMA Dermatol*. Apr 2 2014

Atopic Dermatitis Author: Brian S Kim, MD; Chief Editor: William D James, MD
emedicine.medscape.com/article/1049085

Hanifin JM, Cooper KD, Ho VC, Kang S, Krafchik BR, Margolis DJ, Schachner LA, Sidbury R, Whitmore SE, Sieck CK, Van Voorhees AS. Guidelines of care for atopic dermatitis. J Am Acad Dermatol. 2004 Mar;50(3):391–404

PSORIASIS PROTOCOL

When using any Protocol, always follow the Guidelines of Proper Use (page 18).

Definition

- A chronic, relapsing, multisystem inflammatory condition manifested most commonly with skin rash and arthritis, with a familial predisposition

Differential diagnosis

- Seborrheic dermatitis
- Atopic dermatitis
- Tinea corporis, pedis or capitis
- Contact dermatitis
- Blepharitis
- Syphilis
- Squamous cell carcinoma
- Diaper dermatitis
- Pustular eruptions
- Various skin malignancies

Considerations

- Rash most commonly on elbows, knees, scalp, lumbosacral region, intergluteal clefts and glans penis
- Arthritis occurs in up to 30% of patients
- Plaque-type most common rash
    - Plaques are raised, red, inflamed with silvery white scaly appearance
- Ocular involvement occurs in up to 10% of patients
- Flares may be secondary to recent strep throat or viral infection, immunization or trauma

Guidelines on psoriasis biologic therapy from the British Association of Dermatologists

- Offer biologic therapy to people with psoriasis who require systemic therapy if methotrexate and cyclosporine have failed
- If methotrexate and cyclosporine are not tolerated or are contraindicated

- If psoriasis has a large impact on physical, psychological, or social functioning

Guidelines on the management and treatment of psoriasis with biologics by the American Academy of Dermatology and the National Psoriasis Foundation

- Offer monotherapy with TNF-alpha Inhibitors
- Offer monotherapy Interleukin-17 Inhibitors

Symptoms and Findings

- Scaling red macules, papules and plaques that are frequently pruritic
- Guttate psoriasis are small pink 1–10 mm macules commonly on upper trunk frequently 2–3 weeks after strep throat
- Rash may be pustular
- Fever, chills, hypothermia and dehydration may occur when most of the body is covered with psoriasis rash
- Pits on the nails
- Arthritis is usually of hands and feet, though may include large joints
- White oral lesions and/or cheilosis
- Geographic tongue
- Blepharitis
- Uveitis
- Conjunctivitis

Evaluation options

- Usually a clinically diagnosis
- Joint x-rays may help with determining type of arthritis
- If immunologic therapy started, obtain baseline CBC, BMP, LFT's and TB screening

Treatment options

- Systemic steroids not effective and may worsen the psoriasis when discontinued
- Minimize soap exposure to rash as much as is practical
- Moisturizing lotions

- Sunlight exposure
- Sea bathing
- Topical corticosteroids for rash (avoid very potent steroids in children)
    - Triamcinolone 0.025–0.1% cream is drug of choice for new treatment (have a break from treatment every 4 weeks for potent steroids)
    - Betamethasone 0.025–0.1% for disease resistant to triamcinolone or hydrocortisone creams (have a break from treatment every 4 weeks for potent steroids)
- Ocular corticosteroids for eye involvement
    - Prednisolone 1% (Pred Forte) bid
    - Dexamethasone 1% ophthalmic
- Coal tar 0.5–33% (DHS Tar, Doctar, Theraplex T)
    - Shampoo for scalp lesions
    - Topical corticosteroid in addition to coal tar preparation increases effectiveness
- Salicylic acid preparations help to remove scales
- Calcipotriene (vitamin D analogue)
- Combination therapy with tazarotene (a retinoid) or calcipotriene with a topical corticosteroid more effective than either alone
- Oatmeal baths may help symptoms

Severe cases may need treatment from some of the following

- Systemic retinoids, cyclosporine, methotrexate, azathioprine, a Biologic, or hydroxyurea — **consult dermatologist prior to using and read PDR**
    - Methotrexate monitor patients closely for bone marrow, liver, lung and kidney toxicities
    - Biologics are infliximab (Remicade), etanercept (Enbrel), adalimumab (Humira), and alefacept (Amevive) — **consult dermatologist prior to using and read PDR**
    - Psoralen with ultraviolet A light retinoids PUVA (do not in skin cancer prone patients or if 150 PUVA treatments already given)
    - Ultraviolet B

- Anthralin preparations 0.1–1% (Drithocreme, Anthra-Derm)

Phosphodiesterase-4 inhibitors

- Apremilast (Otezla)

Interleukin inhibitors —Monotherapy treatment option for adults with moderate-to-severe plaque psoriasis

- Ustekinumab (Stelara)
- Secukinumab (Cosentyx)
- Ixekizumab (Taltz)
- Brodalumab (Siliq)

Disease–modifying antirheumatic drugs (DMARD's) methotrexate and azathioprine

Considerations

- Check CBC, creatinine, LFT's and investigate abnormalities before DMARD or Biologics medications used
- Document negative pregnancy test and discussion of contraception in fertile females before treatment
- Consider pneumovax vaccination
- Document PPD results before Biologics therapy
- Be familiar with effects and side effects of medications as listed in the Physician Desk Reference (PDR)

Biologics (tumor necrosis factor inhibitors)

- Infliximab (Remicade)
    - Reserve infliximab for use in people with very severe disease or people in whom other available biologic agents have failed or cannot be used
    - Monotherapy treatment option for adults with moderate-to-severe plaque psoriasis
    - British Association of Dermatologists recommendation
- Etanercept (Enbrel)
    - Monotherapy treatment option for adults with moderate-to-severe plaque psoriasis

- Adalimumab (Humira)
  - Offer adalimumab as a first-line biologic agent to adults with psoriasis, particularly when psoriatic arthropathy is a consideration
- **Avoid TNF antagonist therapy in people with severe cardiac failure**
  - Stop in the event of new or worsening preexisting heart failure and seek specialist advice

Cautions

- Severe infection risk exists
- Stop all DMARDs and Biologics if infection identified or suspected until treated and resolved
- Malignancy risks may be increased
- Do not use in optic neuritis or multiple sclerosis patients or in a first degree relative of these patients
- Do not use in patients with significant heart failure
- Avoid live vaccines
- Biologics may be used with or without DMARDs
- Be familiar with effects and side effects of medications as listed in the Physician Desk Reference (PDR)

Discharge criteria

- Uncomplicated psoriasis

Discharge instructions

- Psoriasis aftercare instructions
- Referral to PCP or dermatologist

Consult criteria

- Systemic symptoms or findings
- Fever
- Systemic treatment needed for severe disease
- Prescribing Biologics or DMARDs

Notes

References:

National Institute for Health and Clinical Excellence (NICE). Psoriasis: the assessment and management of psoriasis. London (UK): National Institute for Health and Clinical Excellence (NICE); 2012 Oct. 61 p. (NICE clinical guideline; no. 153)

Mason AR, Mason J, Cork M, Dooley G, Hancock H. Topical treatments for chronic plaque psoriasis. Cochrane Database of Systematic Reviews 2013, Issue 3. Art. No.: CD005028. DOI: 10.1002/14651858.CD005028.pub3

Psoriasis Author: Jeffrey Meffert, MD; Chief Editor: Robert E O'Connor, MD, MPH
emedicine.medscape.com/article/1943419

[Guideline] Smith CH, Jabbar-Lopez ZK, Yiu ZZ, Bale T, Burden AD, Coates LC, et al. British Association of Dermatologists guidelines for biologic therapy for psoriasis 2017. *Br J Dermatol*. 2017 Sep. 177 (3):628-636

[Guideline] Menter A, Strober BE, Kaplan DH, et al. Joint AAD-NPF guidelines of care for the management and treatment of psoriasis with biologics. *J Am Acad Dermatol*. 2019 Feb 13

Psoriasis Updated: Feb 28, 2019 Author: Jacquiline Habashy, DO, MSc; Chief Editor: William D James, MD
Emedicine medscape

CONTACT DERMATITIS PROTOCOL

When using any protocol, always follow the Guidelines of Proper Use (page 18).

Definition

- Hypersensitivity reaction manifested by acute or chronic inflammatory reactions to substances that contact the skin

Differential Diagnosis

- Cellulitis
- Scabies
- Atopic dermatitis/eczema
- Psoriasis
- Herpes simplex
- Erythema multiforme

Considerations

- Comprises 90% of workman's compensation dermatologic claims
- Rash limited to exposure area with sharp margins or linear excoriations

Some causes

- Rhus dermatitis (toxicodendron)
    - Poison ivy, poison oak, poison sumac
- Metals: nickel common
- Chemical
    - Hair dyes; paraphenylenediamine

Treatment Options

- Identify and limit exposure
- Soothing moist dressings
- Topical steroids
- Systemic steroids with severe cases up to 10 days
- Toxicodendron or Rhus dermatitis (poison ivy, etc.) use soap and water, especially under nails
- Zanfel over the counter can be used for Rhus dermatitis acutely

- Psoralen plus UVA, azathioprine and cyclosporine are used for steroid-resistant chronic hand dermatitis
  - Azathioprine — chronic immunosuppression with this purine antimetabolite increases neoplasia risk, mutagenic risk, and hematologic toxicities

Discharge Criteria

- Uncomplicated process

Discharge instructions

- Contact dermatitis aftercare instructions

Consult Criteria

- Severe superinfection

Notes

References:

Allergic Contact Dermatitis Author: Daniel J Hogan, MD; Chief Editor: William D James, MD
emedicine.medscape.com/article/1049216

Bourke J, Coulson I, English J, British Association of Dermatologists Therapy Guidelines and Audit Subcommittee. Guidelines for the management of contact dermatitis: an update. Br J Dermatol. 2009 May;160(5):946–54

IMPETIGO PROTOCOL

When using any protocol, always follow the Guidelines of Proper Use (page 18).

Definition

- Impetigo is a highly contagious gram-positive bacterial infection of the superficial layers of the epidermis that exists in 2 forms which are bullous impetigo and non-bullous impetigo

Differential Diagnosis

- Erythema multiforme
- Fixed drug eruption
- Bullous pemphigoid
- Herpes simplex
- Herpes zoster
- Insect bites
- Stevens-Johnson syndrome
- Toxic Epidermal Necrolysis
- Varicella (Chicken pox)
- Atopic dermatitis
- Scabies

Considerations

- Contagious superficial bacterial infection of epidermis
- Crusted erosions or ulcers
- Most common in children ages 2–5 years
- Clinical diagnosis
- Predisposing factors
- Close contact with infected person
- Warm/humid climates
- Poor hygiene
- Crowding
- Poverty
- Non-bullous form most common
- MRSA most prevalent
- GABHS still occurs

Treatment Options

- Gentle washing of crusts with soap and washcloth
- Mupirocin topical for 5–10 days or until lesions gone for 2 days (as effective as cephalexin)
- Retapamulin bid for 5 days
    - Superior to mupirocin and oral antibiotics
    - Not for mucosal membranes
- More widespread and severe cases can give systemic antibiotics — choices
    - Septra (trimethoprim/sulfamethoxazole)
    - Doxycycline
    - Clindamycin
    - Beta-lactams if strep infection suspected

Discharge Criteria

- Uncomplicated infection

Discharge instructions

- Impetigo aftercare instructions
- Return if fever develops
- Follow up with PCP if rash persists > 10 days

Consult Criteria

- Systemic symptoms
- Immunocompromised

Notes

References:

Scheinfeld N. A Primer In Topical Antibiotics For The Skin And Eyes. *J Drugs Dermatol*. 2008;7(4):409–415

Impetigo Author: Lisa S Lewis, MD; Chief Editor: Russell W Steele, MD emedicine.medscape.com/article/965254

Koning S, van der Sande R, Verhagen AP, van Suijlekom-Smit LWA, Morris AD, Butler CC, Berger M, van der Wouden JC. Interventions for impetigo. Cochrane Database of Systematic Reviews 2012, Issue 1. Art. No.: CD003261. DOI: 10.1002/14651858.CD003261

SCABIES PROTOCOL

When using any protocol, always follow the Guidelines of Proper Use (page 18).

Definition

- Dermatitis secondary to the mite Sarcoptes scabiei, spread by direct contact with hosts or fomites

Differential Diagnosis

- Insect bites
- Atopic dermatitis
- Contact dermatitis
- Urticaria
- Psoriasis
- Lice
- Secondary syphilis
- Bedbug bites
- Dyshidrotic eczema
- Chicken pox
- Folliculitis

Considerations

- Excruciating pruritus especially at night
- Transmission primarily from skin to skin
- Transmission can occur from infected linens or clothing
- Eggs hatch in 3 days
- Mite viable 2–5 days
- Lesions are small excoriations with erythematous papules
- Burrow not always present, but pathognomonic
- Burrow is grey to red to brown thin line 2–15 mm in length
- Does not affect scalp in adults
- Can affect scalp in infants
- Diagnosis is clinical
- Can be confirmed with microscopic visualization of mite

- Itching can last 4 weeks after treatment due to hypersensitivity reaction to dead mite
- Itching lasting > 4 weeks search for another cause of the itching

Distribution

- Intertriginous areas
- Sides and webs of fingers
- Axillary folds
- Flexor wrists
- Extensor elbows
- Waist
- Genital folds
- Buttocks
- Thighs
- Extensor knees
- Posterior feet

Evaluation options if desired

Burrow ink test

- Washable felt tip marker across suspected burrow and ink removed with alcohol
- Remaining ink outlines the burrow

Skin scraping

Treatment

- Permethrin cream 5%
    - Massage cream in from neck to soles of feet
    - Leave on 8–14 hours
    - Second application one week later
- Lindane (Kwell lotion)
    - Massage cream from neck to soles of feet
    - Leave on 8–14 hours
    - Second application one week later
- Oral ivermectin 200 mcg/kg × 1 dose
    - Not recommended in pregnant or lactating women
    - Not recommended in children < 15 kg
    - Repeat in 2 weeks
- Benadryl (diphenhydramine) prn itching

- Topical steroids prn once mite eradicated
- Treat all family members or close contacts
- Infected linens and clothing washed in hot water and dried with heat or ironing
- Crusted scabies should be removed (warm soaks and then 5% salicylic acid in petrolatum and then scraped off (avoid salicylic acid in large surface areas due to toxicity)
    - Crusted scabies have heavy mite burden and may need repeated treatments

Discharge Criteria

- Nontoxic patient with routine symptoms

Discharge instructions

- Scabies aftercare instructions
- Follow up with PCP as needed

Consult Criteria

- Moderate to severe topical or systemic superinfection

Notes

References:

Scabies Author: Megan Barry, MD; Chief Editor: William D James, MD emedicine.medscape.com/article/1109204

Strong M, Johnstone P. Interventions for treating scabies. Cochrane Database of Systematic Reviews 2007, Issue 3. Art. No.: CD000320. DOI: 10.1002/14651858.CD000320.pub2

Centers for Disease Control and Prevention (CDC). Ectoparasitic infections. In: Sexually transmitted diseases treatment guidelines, 2010. MMWR Recomm Rep. 2010 Dec 17;59(RR-12):88–90

CUTANEOUS CANDIDIASIS PROTOCOL

When using any Practice Guide, always follow the Guidelines of Proper Use (page 18).

Definition

- Infections of the skin caused by the yeast *Candida albicans* or other *Candida* species

Considerations

- Present in normal flora in GI tract and vagina
- May colonize skin but not normal flora
- Disease caused by overgrowth
- Tissue damage resulting from trauma, xerostomia, radiation-induced mucositis, ulcerations, skin maceration, or occlusion
- Predisposed in endocrine conditions such as diabetes mellitus, Cushing syndrome, corticosteroid use
- Predisposition in immunocompromised states
- Candida auris is an emerging fungus that presents a global health care threat with severe illness in hospitalized patient and is often resistant to multiple medications

Differential diagnosis

- Intertrigo
- Mucosal candidiasis
- Onychomycosis
- Seborrheic dermatitis

Presentation

- Red moist, occasionally macerated rash, commonly see in skin folds (**Intertrigo**)
- Itching and pain/soreness
- White papules or plaques
- May be present in nails

Diagnosis

- Usually a clinical diagnosis
- KOH prep is easiest lab test for yeast and pseudohyphae

Treatment

Candidal vulvovaginitis

- Topical antifungal agents including miconazole nitrate (Micatin, Monistat-Derm) or clotrimazole (Lotrimin, Mycelex) creams
- Fluconazole (150 mg) PO x 1
- Itraconazole (600 mg) PO x 1

Oral candidiasis in infant

- Nystatin oral suspension 1 mL (100,000 U) to each side of the mouth 4 times daily for 10–14 days or until symptoms gone for 48–72 hours
    - Preterm infants is half the mg dose with same frequency and length of treatment

Oral candidiasis in adults

- Nystatin (1:100,000 U/mL, 5 mL oral rinse and swallow qid)

Candidal diaper dermatitis

- Air drying
- Frequent diaper changes
- Baby powders and zinc oxide paste are adequate preventive measures

Intertrigo

- Keep skin dry
- Topical nystatin powder, clotrimazole, or miconazole bid for 10–14 days (may need longer term treatment)
- Fluconazole 100 mg PO qd for 1-2 wk. (may need longer term treatment)
- Itraconazole 100 mg PO qd for 1-2 wk.
- May add low potency steroid cream short term treatment for inflammatory relief
- Ketoconazole shampoo with showers or bathing to rash 10–14 days (may need long term treatment)

- Ketoconazole cream bid to rash x 10–14 days or longer
- Ketoconazole 200 mg PO qd for if other treatment unsuccessful 1-2 wk.
    - **Black box warning** for liver toxicity and QT .prolongation
    - **Tinea versicolor** may use off label ketoconazole 400 mg PO x 1 every several months as needed

Disposition

Admission or consult criteria

- Severe inflammatory disease
- Immunocompromised state
- Systemic symptoms

Discharge criteria

- Most patients with localized disease

Notes

References:

Cutaneous Candidiasis Author: Noah S Scheinfeld, JD, MD, FAAD; Chief Editor: Dirk M Elston, MD

May 22, 2018 emedicine.medscape.com/article/1090632-overview

www.cdc.gov/fungal/diseases/candidiasis

TINEA CAPITIS PROTOCOL

When using any protocol, always follow the Guidelines of Proper Use (page 18).

Definition

- A disease caused by superficial fungal infection of the skin of the scalp

Differential Diagnosis

- Alopecia areata
- Psoriasis
- Drug eruptions
- "Id" reaction
- Contact dermatitis
- Seborrheic dermatitis
- Secondary syphilis
- Impetigo
- Systemic lupus erythematosus

Considerations

- Is a fungal superficial infection of the scalp
- Most common in younger pediatric population
- Spread by person to person contact
- Spread by shared objects such as combs and hair brushes
- Erythematous patch increasing over time
- Alopecia can occur
- May develop painful lymphadenopathy
- Kerion can develop — multiple boggy nodules of pus with associated hair loss
- Diagnosis can be clinical or confirmed with KOH prep

Treatment Options

- Adult
    - Oral griseofulvin 500 mg to 1 gm microsize PO qday for 6–8 weeks, may need 8–12 weeks
    - Sporanox 200 mg PO qday for 2 weeks
    - Terbinafine 250 mg PO qday for 4–6 weeks

- Pediatric
    - Oral griseofulvin 20–25 mg/kg microsize PO qday for 6–8 weeks (do not exceed adult doses)
    - Sporanox 3–5 mg/kg PO qday for 2 weeks (do not exceed adult doses)
- Monitor LFT's due to possible liver toxicity of griseofulvin
- Six weeks or more may be needed for treatment

Discharge Criteria

- Uncomplicated rash
- Children may return to school once appropriate treatment has started

Discharge instructions

- Tinea capitis aftercare instructions
- Follow up within 14 days if no improvement in rash
- Follow up in 3–4 weeks if rash persists

Consult Criteria

- Moderate to severe superinfection
- Systemic symptoms
- Immunocompromised

Notes

References:

Shemer A, Plotnik IB, Davidovici B, Grunwald MH, Magun R, Amichai B. Treatment of tinea capitis - griseofulvin versus fluconazole - a comparative study. *J Dtsch Dermatol Ges*. Apr 10 2013

González U, Seaton T, Bergus G, Jacobson J, Martínez-Monzón C. Systemic antifungal therapy for tinea capitis in children. Cochrane Database of Systematic Reviews 2007, Issue 4. Art. No.: CD004685. DOI: 10.1002/14651858.CD004685

Tinea Capitis Author: Grace F Kao, MD; Chief Editor: Dirk M Elston, MD emedicine.medscape.com/article/1091351

TINEA CORPORIS PROTOCOL

When using any protocol, always follow the Guidelines of Proper Use (page 18).

Definition

- Superficial fungal infection of the body

Differential Diagnosis

- Tinea versicolor
- Cutaneous candidiasis
- Seborrheic dermatitis
- Psoriasis
- Impetigo
- Pityriasis rosea
- Secondary syphilis

Considerations

- Commonly called "ring worm"
- Erythematous lesion with central clearing
- Diagnosis usually clinical
- KOH prep will show the fungal hyphae

Treatment Options

- Luliconazole 1% cream qday for 1 week (recent FDA approval)
- Topical Lamisil qday for 1–4 weeks (apply on rash and 2 cm out from rash)
- Lotrimin bid for 2–6 weeks (apply on rash and 2 cm out from rash)
- Treat until no rash visible for 2 days
- Oral griseofulvin or ketoconazole for more severe infection (monitor LFT's)
    - May combine with topical treatment
    - May use in immunosuppressed patients
    - Use in tinea unguium (nails) or tinea Capitis
- Fluconazole at 50–100 mg/day or 150 mg once weekly for 2–4 weeks for more severe infection

- Oral itraconazole in doses of 100 mg/d for 2 weeks for more severe infection
- Avoid sharing infected objects
- Launder all possible infected linens and clothing separately
- Good hand washing
- Topical steroids can be used for initial 1–4 days to relieve symptoms

Tinea unguium treatment options

- Menthal ointment OTC daily for many months (Vicks VapoRub)
- Oral itraconazole 200 mg PO qday for 12 weeks
- Terbinafine 250 mg PO qday for toenail for 12 weeks, for fingernail for 6 weeks

Discharge Criteria

- Uncomplicated rash
- Children may return to school once appropriate treatment has started

Discharge instructions

- Tinea corporis aftercare instructions
- Follow up within 14 days if no improvement in rash
- Follow up in 3–4 weeks if rash persists

Consult Criteria

- Moderate to severe superinfection
- Systemic symptoms
- Immunocompromised

Notes

References:

Brooks M. FDA Approves New Topical Antifungal Luliconazole 1%. Medscape Medical News. Nov 15 2013

Tinea Corporis Author: Jack L Lesher Jr, MD; Chief Editor: Dirk M Elston, MD
emedicine.medscape.com/article/1091473

Crawford F, Hollis S. Topical treatments for fungal infections of the skin and nails of the foot. Cochrane Database of Systematic Reviews 2007, Issue 3. Art. No.: CD001434. DOI: 10.1002/14651858.CD001434.pub2

Tinea Pedis Author: Courtney M Robbins, MD; Chief Editor: Dirk M Elston, MD
emedicine.medscape.com/article/1091684

TINEA PEDIS (ATHLETE'S FOOT) PROTOCOL

When using any protocol, always follow the Guidelines of Proper Use (page 18).

Definition

- Superficial fungal infection of the foot

Differential Diagnosis

- Cutaneous candidiasis
- Erythema multiforme
- Psoriasis
- Secondary syphilis
- Dyshidrotic eczema
- Pustular psoriasis

Considerations

- Most common superficial dermatophyte fungal infection
- Commonly called "athletes foot"
- Excessive sweating and occlusive footwear predispose to infection
- Acute and chronic states occur
- Inflammatory vesicles and bullae
- Located in toe webs — most common 4th and 5th
- Clinical diagnosis usually
- Can confirm with KOH prep if desired
- Can lead to cellulitis

Treatment Options

- Luliconazole for the treatment of interdigital tinea pedis in adults that requires a 2-week treatment period
- Topical Lamisil qday 1-4 weeks or until rash gone for 2-4 days
- Oral terbinofine, itraconazole or ketoconazole for more severe infection

    - May combine with topical treatment
- Avoid sharing infected objects
- Launder all possible infected linens and clothing separately
- Good hand washing
- Avoid tight fitting shoes
- Keep feet dry
- May use topical steroid initial 2–4 days of treatment to relieve symptoms

Discharge Criteria

- Uncomplicated rash
- Children may return to school once appropriate treatment has started

Discharge instructions

- Tinea pedis aftercare instructions
- Follow up with PCP within 14 days if no improvement in rash
- Follow up with PCP in 3–4 weeks if rash persists

Consult Criteria

- Moderate to severe superinfection
- Systemic symptoms
- Immunocompromised

Notes

References:

Tinea Pedis Author: Courtney M Robbins, MD; Chief Editor: Dirk M Elston, MD medicine.medscape.com/article/1091684

Crawford F, Hollis S. Topical treatments for fungal infections of the skin and nails of the foot.. Cochrane Database of Systematic Reviews 2007, Issue 3. Art. No.: CD001434. DOI: 10.1002/14651858.CD001434

URTICARIA PROTOCOL

When using any protocol, always follow the Guidelines of Proper Use (page 18).

Definition

- Vascular reaction of the skin with transient wheals, soft papules and plaques usually with pruritus

Differential Diagnosis

- Erythema multiforme
- Angioedema
- Serum sickness
- Cutaneous vasculitis
- Toxic epidermal necrolysis
- Leprosy
- Juvenile rheumatoid arthritis
- Thrombophlebitis
- Cellulitis
- Pityriasis rosea
- Drug eruptions

Considerations

- Transient wheals — soft papules and plagues
- Is pruritic
- Acute reaction lasting < 30 days — usually allergic
- Chronic reaction lasting > 30 days — often idiopathic
- Angioedema can occur with chronic urticaria
- Ask about precipitants as in Causes

Causes

- Idiopathic
- Food allergies
- Infections
- Medications
- Insect bites or stings
- Sunlight
- Physical and emotional stressors
- Autoimmune diseases

- Hashimoto's thyroiditis
- Systemic diseases
- Serum sickness
- Transfusion reaction

Treatment Options

Benadryl (diphenhydramine)

- Adult: 25–50 mg PO, IM or IV
- Pediatrics: 1–2 mg/kg PO or IM (NMT 50 mg)
- May continue for 5–7 days PO

Pepcid (famotidine) with diphenhydramine

- Adult: 20 mg IV or 40 mg PO
- Pediatric: 0.25 mg/kg IV or 0.5 mg/kg PO (not to exceed maximum adult dose)

Epinephrine

- Adult 0.3 mg SQ/IM if urticaria part of anaphylaxis reaction (see Allergy Protocol)

Consider steroids (caution if diabetic)

- Prednisone 40–60 mg PO qday for 5–10 days (> 40 kg)
- Prednisone/prednisolone 1 mg/kg PO qday for 5–10 days (< 40 kg)
- Dexamethasone 4–6 mg qday for 5–10 days

- Avoid offending agent if known

Discharge Criteria

- Good resolution of rash and itching

Discharge instructions

- Urticaria aftercare instructions
- Return if rash persists or worsens
- Follow up with primary care provider within 7 days

Consult Criteria

- Systemic symptoms
- Hypotension
- See General Patient Criteria Protocol (page 22)

Notes

References:

Fedorowicz Z, van Zuuren EJ, Hu N. Histamine H2–receptor antagonists for urticaria. Cochrane Database of Systematic Reviews 2012, Issue 3. Art. No.: CD008596. DOI: 10.1002/14651858.CD008596.pub2

Acute Urticaria Author: Henry K Wong, MD, PhD; Chief Editor: Michael A Kaliner, MD emedicine.medscape.com/article/137362

Urticaria (Hives) Updated: Jun 13, 2018
Author: Henry K Wong, MD, PhD; Chief Editor: Dirk M Elston, MD

PITYRIASIS ROSEA PROTOCOL

When using any protocol, always follow the Guidelines of Proper Use (page 18).

Definition

- Common skin disorder observed in otherwise healthy people, more frequently in children and young adults which manifests as an acute, bilateral, self-limiting, papulosquamous eruption with a 6–week to 8–week duration

Differential Diagnosis

- Viral exanthem
- Tinea corporis
- Erythema multiforme
- Secondary syphilis
- Drug eruption
- Tinea versicolor
- Seborrheic dermatitis

Considerations

- More common in late childhood to early adulthood
- Spring and fall prevalence
- Etiology unknown
- Not contagious
- Self-limited
- Resolves in 6–12 weeks
- Differential diagnosis considerations are secondary syphilis or drug eruption

Appearance

- Herald patch — single oval slightly raised plaque 2–5 cm, red color, on trunk usually
- Generalized eruption 1–2 weeks after herald patch
  - Fine scaling plaques and papules
  - Dark pink "Christmas tree" pattern along cleavage lines
  - Most noticeable on back

Treatment Options

- Benadryl (diphenhydramine) prn
- Aveeno or calamine prn
- UV exposure may hasten resolution
- Topical steroids

Discharge Criteria

- Self-limited disease so no consultation usually needed

Discharge criteria

- Pityriasis rosea aftercare instructions
- Follow up within 7–10 days as needed

Consult Criteria

- See General Patient Criteria Protocol as needed (page 22)

Notes

References:

Pityriasis Rosea Author: Robert A Schwartz, MD, MPH; Chief Editor: Dirk M Elston, MD
emedicine.medscape.com/article/1107532

Chuh AAT, Dofitas BL, Comisel G, Reveiz L, Sharma V, Garner SE, Chu FKM. Interventions for pityriasis rosea. Cochrane Database of Systematic Reviews 2007, Issue 2. Art. No.: CD005068. DOI: 10.1002/14651858.CD005068.pub2

HERPES SIMPLEX GINGIVOSTOMATITIS PROTOCOL

When using any protocol, always follow the Guidelines of Proper Use (page 18).

Definition

- Grouped vesicles on erythematous base of the skin or mucous membranes usually causes by herpes simplex–1

Differential Diagnosis

- Aphthous stomatitis
- Hand-Foot-Mouth disease
- Candidiasis
- Chanchroid
- Pharyngitis
- Secondary syphilis
- Urethritis

Considerations

- Regional lymphadenopathy can occur
- Oral lesions are HSV-1 type usually
- HSV-1 type can cause genital herpes
- Recurrent outbreaks in one-third of patients; decreases over time
- Prodrome of tingling, itching or pain approximately 24 hours preceding rash
- Diagnosis clinical
- Can be confirmed with Tzanck smear

Triggers

- Skin infections
- Stress
- UV radiation

Treatment Options

- Avoid contact with infected individuals

- Antiviral treatment within 48–72 hours of onset of lesions

Antiviral choices

- Acyclovir ointment 5% 5 times a day for 5 days
- Acyclovir 400 mg PO qid × 7 days for severe infection
- Pediatric acyclovir oral dosing 15 mg/kg 5 times a day for 7 days (do not exceed adult doses)
- Valtrex (valacyclovir) 2000 mg PO q12h × 1 day
- Abreva cream 10% OTC may help

Aphthous stomatitis

- Unknown etiology
- Many triggers
- May last weeks to months
- Recurrent

Treatment

- Local treatment with lidocaine 2% solution 5 ml swish and swallow qid prn (caution pediatric patients)
- Chlorhexidine, salt water or dilute hydrogen peroxide rinse
- Dexamethasone elixir 0.5mg/5 ml swish and spit qid — NPO 30 minutes after
- Aphthasol (amlexanox) 0.5 cm to affected area qid after brushing teeth

Discharge Criteria

- Benign local disease

Discharge instructions

- Herpes simplex–1 aftercare instructions
- Follow up with PCP within 7–10 days as needed
- Return if rash increases or spreads

Consult Criteria

- Encephalitis
- Altered mental status
- Disseminated infection
- Severity of symptoms enough to cause dehydration

- Immunocompromised
- Ocular involvement
- Refer to General Patient Criteria Protocol (page 22) as needed

Notes

References:

Nasser M, Fedorowicz Z, Khoshnevisan MH, Shahiri Tabarestani M. Acyclovir for treating primary herpetic gingivostomatitis. Cochrane Database of Systematic Reviews 2008, Issue 4. Art. No.: CD006700. DOI: 10.1002/14651858.CD006700.pub2

Herpes Simplex Author: Michelle R Salvaggio, MD, FACP; Chief Editor: Burke A Cunha, MD emedicine.medscape.com/article/218580

HERPETIC WHITLOW PROTOCOL

When using any protocol, always follow the Guidelines of Proper Use (page 18).

Definition

- Herpes simplex infection of the digits manifested as painful grouped vesicles

Differential Diagnosis

- Felon
- Paronychia
- Cellulitis

Considerations

- Patients usually less than 20 years of age
- Usually caused by HSV-1 (60%)
- From autoinoculation
- Incision not recommended
- Lesions crust over in 10–14 days and viral shedding stops at this point (heals in another 5–7 days after that)
- May have prodrome of fever and malaise
- Herpetic gingivostomatitis is almost pathognomonic in children
- Process is self-limited

Treatment Options

- Avoid skin contact with uninfected individuals
- Antiviral treatment within 48–72 hours of rash onset
- **Do not incise**

Antiviral choices

- Acyclovir ointment 5% 5 times a day for 5 days
- Acyclovir 400 mg PO qid × 7 days for severe infection
- Pediatric acyclovir oral dosing 15 mg/kg 5 times a day for 7 days (do not exceed adults doses)
- Valtrex (valacyclovir) 500–1000 mg PO bid × 7 days for adults

Discharge Criteria

- Most patients without severe superinfection

Discharge instructions

- Herpetic whitlow aftercare instructions
- Follow up with PCP within 7–10 days

Consult Criteria

- Moderate to severe superinfection
- Immunocompromised

Notes

References:

Herpetic Whitlow Author: Michael S Omori, MD; Chief Editor: Steven C Dronen, MD, FAAEM
emedicine.medscape.com/article/788056

Nasser M, Fedorowicz Z, Khoshnevisan MH, Shahiri Tabarestani M. Acyclovir for treating primary herpetic gingivostomatitis. Cochrane Database of Systematic Reviews 2008, Issue 4. Art. No.: CD006700. DOI: 10.1002/14651858.CD006700.pub2

GENITAL HERPES PROTOCOL

When using any protocol, always follow the Guidelines of Proper Use (page 18).

Definition

- Sexual transmitted disease by skin to skin contact caused by herpes simplex type 2 usually and occasionally by herpes simplex type 1 virus

Differential Diagnosis

- Candidiasis
- Syphilis
- Chanchroid
- Herpes zoster

Considerations

- May be transmitted during asymptomatic periods
- Recurrent outbreaks less frequent over time
- May cause systemic complaints
- Grouped vesicles crusting over in 4–15 days
  - New lesions appears 75% of time forming in 4–10 days
- Viral shedding lasts about 12 days
- Reactivation recurs in 90% of patients in the first year, sometimes multiple times
- May be asymptomatic

Treatment Options

- Avoid sexual contact with infected individuals
- Antiviral treatment within 48–72 hours of rash onset
- Analgesics prn

Antiviral choices

- Acyclovir ointment 5% 5 times a day for 5 days
- Acyclovir 400 mg PO tid × 7–10 days for severe infection
- Acyclovir 200 mg orally five times a day for 7–10 days

- Pediatric acyclovir oral dosing 15 mg/kg 5 times a day for 7 days (do not exceed adults doses)
- Valacyclovir 1 g orally twice a day for 7–10 days for adults
- Famciclovir 250 mg orally three times a day for 7–10 days
- Treatment can be extended if healing is incomplete after 10 days of therapy

Discharge Criteria

- Immunocompetent patient without systemic symptoms

Discharge instructions

- Genital herpes aftercare instructions
- No sexual relations during prodrome and until lesions healed
- Follow up within 7–10 days
- Return if unable to void
- Return if rash worsens

Consult Criteria

- Systemic symptoms
- CNS infection
- Severe local symptoms
- Immunocompromised
- Urinary retention secondary to severe pain or sacral nerve involvement
- Refer to General Patient Criteria Protocol (page 22) as needed

Notes

References:

Herpes Simplex Author: Michelle R Salvaggio, MD, FACP; Chief Editor: Burke A Cunha, MD
emedicine.medscape.com/article/218580

Centers for Disease Control and Prevention (CDC). Diseases characterized by genital, anal, or perianal ulcers. In: Sexually transmitted diseases treatment guidelines, 2010. MMWR Recomm Rep. 2010 Dec 17;59(RR-12):18–39

HERPES ZOSTER (SHINGLES) PROTOCOL

When using any protocol, always follow the Guidelines of Proper Use (page 18).

Definition

- Acute dermatomal reactivation of varicella virus (chickenpox) in dorsal nerve roots ganglia

Differential Diagnosis

- Herpes simplex virus infection
- Varicella (chickenpox)
- Impetigo
- Cellulitis
- Folliculitis
- Contact dermatitis
- Prodromal pain thought to be
    - Biliary colic
    - Appendicitis
    - Angina

Considerations

- Seen with increasing age and decreasing immunocompetence
- Many patients have normal immune systems
- 10–20% of the general population will eventually develop herpes zoster
- Can have mild symptoms
- Immunosuppression increases risk of occurrence
- Prodrome of pain 3–5 days before rash occurs in 75% of cases
- Rash may be pruritic
- Rash crusts over in 7–10 days
- Complete healing may take more than 4 weeks
- Prodrome frequently causes medical evaluation for unrelated diseases
- Pain duration is usually < 1 month

- Recurrence is rare
- Herpes zoster can cause varicella (chickenpox) in exposed non-immunized patients
- Increased incidence of stroke and acute MI

Findings

- Initially a vesicular patchy dermatomal rash on a red base that may involve 1 or more adjacent dermatomes
- Usually no more than 2–3 adjacent dermatomes involved with normal hosts
- Thoracic dermatomes followed by lumbar dermatomes are the most commonly involved areas
- Fever, malaise, headache and fatigue occur in < 20% of patients
- Can involve cranial nerves and visceral organs
- Pain is usually described as burning, stabbing or throbbing

Post-herpetic neuralgia (PHN)

- Pain > 1 month is defined as post-herpetic neuralgia
- Increases with increasing age, rash severity and severity of pain
- Occurs in 10–15% of cases
- Most debilitating symptom of disease
- May be difficult to control pain
- Antiviral therapy early in disease may help prevent PHN

Postherpetic Neuralgia Treatment Guidelines (American Academy of Neurology 2008)

- Tricyclic antidepressants (TCAs)
    - Amitriptyline
    - Nortriptyline
    - Desipramine
    - Maprotiline(tetracyclic)
- Gabapentin
- Pregabalin
- Opioids
- Topical lidocaine patches are effective in the treatment of PHN

    - Topical lidocaine may be considered first line in elderly patients, especially if there are concerns regarding the adverse CNS effects with oral medications
  - Strong opioids and capsaicin cream are second-line choices
    - Capsaicin patches show promise but the long-term effects of repeated applications, particularly on sensation, are unclear
  - SSRI's limited usefulness

Treatment Options

- Antiviral treatment started within 72 hours of rash
  - Many experts recommend that if new skin lesions are still appearing or complications of herpes zoster are present, treatment should be started even if the rash began more than 3 days ago
- Valtrex (valacyclovir) 1,000 mg PO tid × 7 days
- Oral antiviral therapy should be considered for patients younger than 50 years with mild pain and rash and truncal involvement to decrease PHN
  - Brivudin, famciclovir, and valacyclovir show greater efficacy than acyclovir
- Topical antiviral therapy is not recommended
- Consider varicella immune globulin in elderly or pediatric patients
- Shingrix (zoster vaccine recombinant, adjuvanted) for the prevention of shingles in adults aged 50 years and older
- Steroids may help quality of life in patients at risk for PHN — controversial
  - Prednisone 40–60 mg qday × 1 week; taper over following week
- The treatment of choice is high-dose intravenous acyclovir for immunocompromised patients
- Pain management approaches should be individualized based on pain severity, underlying conditions, and prior response to specific medications
- Acetaminophen and/or NSAIDs
  - For mild to moderate pain
    - Alone or in combination with weak opioids such as codeine or tramadol

- For moderate to severe pain, strong opioids such as oxycodone or morphine may be used
- Moderate to severe pain not rapidly reponsive to treatment with an opioid analgesic or unable to tolerate opioids
    - Add or use one or some of following
        - Gabapentin or pregabalin
        - Tricyclic antidepressants (TCAs) (especially nortriptyline)
        - Corticosteroids (e.g., prednisone) may be considered
- For patients with pain that is inadequately controlled, refer to a pain specialist to evaluate eligibility for neural blockade

Discharge Criteria

- Uncomplicated infection

Discharge instructions

- Herpes zoster aftercare instructions
- Return for systemic symptom develop
- Follow up within 7–10 days

Consult Criteria

- Immunosuppression
- Severe or disseminated disease
- 3 or more dermatomes affected
- Ophthalmic disease or ophthalmic dermatomal involvement
- Involvement of trigeminal nerve
- Visceral involvement
- Intractable pain
- Ramsey Hunt syndrome (7–8th cranial nerve involvement)
- Acute altered mental status
- Meningitis or encephalitis

Notes

References:

Gagliardi AMZ, Gomes Silva BN, Torloni MR, Soares BGO. Vaccines for preventing herpes zoster in older adults. Cochrane Database of Systematic Reviews 2012, Issue 10. Art. No.: CD008858. DOI: 10.1002/14651858.CD008858.pub2

Sampathkumar P, et al. Herpes Zoster (Shingles) and Postherpetic Neuralgia *Mayo Clin Proc*2009;84:274–280

Yawn BP, et al. A population-based study of the incidence and complication rates of herpes zoster before zoster vaccine introduction *Mayo Clin Proc* 2007; 82: 1341–1349.

Herpes Zoster Author: Camila K Janniger, MD; Chief Editor: Dirk M Elston,MD emedicine.medscape.com/article/1132465

NEJM, Vol. 369, pg. 255

Mayo Clin Proc, Vol. 84, pg. 274

[Guideline] Dworkin RH, Johnson RW, Breuer J, Gnann JW, et al. Recommendations for the management of herpes zoster. *Clin Infect Dis*. 2007 Jan 1. 44 Suppl 1:S1-26

[Guideline] Fashner J, Bell AL. Herpes zoster and postherpetic neuralgia: prevention and management. Am Fam Physician. 2011 Jun 15. 83 (12):1432-7

[Guideline] Stevens DL, Bisno AL, Chambers HF, Dellinger EP, Goldstein EJ, Gorbach SL, et al. Practice guidelines for the diagnosis and management of skin and soft tissue infections: 2014 update by the infectious diseases society of America. *Clin Infect Dis*. 2014 Jul 15. 59 (2):147-59.

Herpes Zoster (Shingles) Updated: Jan 25, 2019
Author: Camila K Janniger, MD; Chief Editor: Dirk M Elston, MD; emedicine medscape

Tick Bite Protocol

When using any protocol, always follow the Guidelines of Proper Use (page 18).

Definition

- Various disease processes transmitted by tick bites

Differential Diagnosis

- Lyme disease
- Rocky Mountain spotted fever
- Babesiosis
- Ehrlichiosis
- Measles
- Meningococcemia
- Rubella
- Varicella
- Mononucleosis
- Disseminated gonorrhea
- Typhus
- Kawasaki disease
- Toxic shock syndrome
- Secondary syphilis
- Gastroenteritis
- Allergic vasculitis
- Collagen vascular disease
- Juvenile rheumatoid arthritis
- Heat illness

Considerations

- Many patients with tick borne disease do not recall a tick bite
- Degree of tick engorgement is a marker for length of attachment
- Most tick borne illness occurs after attachment for 24–48 hours
    - Low risk of infection within 36 hours of tick attachment
- Hard body ticks cause most disease

- Ticks are found in brushy or wooded areas usually
- Lifecycle over 2–3 years
- Have to brush against where tick is (they do not jump, fly, or drop on to people)
- Spring and summer time when most tick borne diseases are transmitted
- "Summer fever" or "summer virus" check CBC for thrombocytopenia
- Can cause DIC (disseminated intravascular coagulation)
- Can cause acute renal failure
- Beef and pork allergy thought to occur from Lone Star tick among others

Tick removal

- Grasp head and mouth parts at skin and pull with gentle pressure for several minutes until tick is removed
- Can inject skin at site with lidocaine 1% to see if tick will release on its own
- Any mouth parts left in skin are not infectious

Tick types

Deer tick

- Lyme
- Ehrlichiosis
- Babesiosis

Dog tick

- Rocky Mountain spotted fever (RMSF)

Lone Star tick

- Lyme
- RMSF
- Ehrlichiosis
- Tularemia

Tick-borne diseases

- Lyme disease
- Rocky Mountain spotted fever (RMSF)
- Babesiosis
- Relapsing fever
- Tularemia

- Ehrlichiosis
- Q-fever
- Colorado Tick fever
- Tick paralysis

Lyme Disease

- See Lyme Disease Protocol

Rocky Mountain Spotted Fever

Symptoms and findings

- Fever and chills
- Up to 30–40% of patients report no tick bite within the past 14 days
- Headache
- Photosensitivity
- Nausea and vomiting
- Diarrhea
- Myalgias
- Maculopapular rash on extremities 3–5 days after fever onset spreading to rest of body
    - 10–20% do not get rash
    - 40–60% gets petechial rash 6 days after illness onset

Lab testing for

- Leukopenia
- Anemia
- Thrombocytopenia
- Elevated LFT's and creatinine
- Single titer of 1:64 supportive; 4 fold rise diagnostic
- PCR can be ordered

Treatment

- Adult: doxycycline 100 mg PO bid for 7 days continuing until afebrile for 2 days
- Children > 45 kg: doxycycline 100 mg PO qday for 7 days continuing for 2 days until afebrile
- Children < 45 kg: doxycycline 2–4 mg/kg PO qday for 7 days continuing until afebrile for 2 days

- Age < 8 consult physician (usually can use doxycycline for the treatment course needed in rickettsial infections)
- Macrolides (erythromycin or Zithromax (azithromycin) do not work

Babesiosis

Malarial like disease

- Diffuse weakness is hallmark of disease
- Fever and chills
- Nausea and vomiting
- Headache
- Cough
- Diarrhea
- Splenomegaly
- Jaundice
- Petechiae

Lab findings

- Hemolytic anemia
- Thrombocytopenia
- Elevated LFT's
- Organisms can be seen on a slide smear prep

Treatment

- Adults — Zithromax (azithromycin) 600 mg qday for 7–10 days plus Atovaquone 750 mg PO bid for 7–10 days
- Children — Zithromax (azithromycin) 12 mg/kg qday for 7–10 days plus Atovaquone 20 mg/kg PO bid for 7–10 days (do not exceed adult doses)

Ehrlichiosis

Considerations

- Transmitted by Lone Star tick

Symptoms and findings

- Appear toxic
- Fever, chills and rigors
- Headache
- Nausea and vomiting

- Rare maculopapular rash 5–10% of patients
- Arthralgias

Lab testing for

- Leukopenia
- Anemia
- Thrombocytopenia
- Elevated LFT's and creatinine

Treatment

- Adult: doxycycline 100 mg PO bid for 14 days
- Children > 45 kg: doxycycline 100 mg PO qday for 14 days
- Children < 45 kg: doxycycline 3 mg/kg PO qday for 14 days
- Age < 8 consult physician (usually can use doxycycline for the treatment course needed in rickettsial infections)

Discharge Criteria

- Mild disease in healthy patient
- Sanford Guide or other drug databases can be used

Discharge instructions

- Tick bite aftercare instructions
- Follow up within 1–2 days
- Return if symptoms worsens or rash develops

Consult Criteria

- Ill appearing patient
- Thrombocytopenia
- Hepatitis
- Splenectomy
- Immunocompromised
- Hemolytic anemia
- Significant comorbidities
- Refer to General Patient Criteria Protocol (page 22)

Notes

References:

Rocky Mountain Spotted Fever Author: Burke A Cunha, MD; Chief Editor: Michael Stuart Bronze, MD
emedicine.medscape.com/article/228042

Ehrlichiosis Author: Burke A Cunha, MD; Chief Editor: Michael Stuart Bronze, MD
emedicine.medscape.com/article/235839

American Academy of Pediatrics. Rocky Mountain Spotted Fever. In: Pickering LK, ed. 2003 Red Book: Report of the Committee on Infectious Disease. Elk Grove Village, IL: American Academy of Pediatrics; 2005:532–533

American Academy of Allergy, Asthma and Immunology (AAAAI) and World Allergy Organization (WAO) 2018 Joint Congress: Abstract 627, presented March 3, 2018; Abstract 721, presented March 5, 2018

LYME DISEASE PROTOCOL

When using any protocol, always follow the Guidelines of Proper Use (page 18).

Definition

- Infection caused by the spirochete Borrelia burgdorferi

Differential Diagnosis

- Rocky Mountain spotted fever (RMSF)
- Babesiosis
- Relapsing fever
- Tularemia
- Ehrlichiosis
- Q-fever
- Colorado Tick fever
- Rheumatic fever
- Viral meningitis
- Septic arthritis
- Juvenile rheumatoid arthritis
- Brown recluse spider bite
- Fibromyalgia
- Reiter syndrome

Considerations

- Transmitted by bite of infected tick
- Most common tick infection in North America
- Peak April and November prevalence
- Transmitted by deer tick most commonly
- 1/3 of patients recall a tick bite
- Can cause hepatitis
- Ocular involvement — keratitis, iritis, optic neuritis
- No person-to-person transmission

Symptoms

Stage 1

Erythema migrans (EM)

- Is initial rash
- "Bull's eye" rash
- Macule with distinct red border that enlarges with central clearing
- Diameter > 5 cm
- Occurs in 90% of patients
- May be multiple in 10–20% of patients
- May have central induration, vesiculation or necrosis

Other symptoms/findings

- Headache
- Regional lymphadenopathy
- Myalgias
- Arthralgias
- Fatigue and malaise

Stage 2

- Days to weeks after tick bite
- Aseptic meningitis
- Cranial neuritis
- Radiculoneuritis
- Bell's palsy most common nerve involvement
- May present without rash
- Prognosis generally good

Cardiac

- Tachycardia
- Bradycardia
- AV block
- Myopericarditis

Stage 3

- Onset > 1 year after tick bite
- Acrodermatitis (resembles scleroderma)
- Arthritis
    - Brief attacks
    - Monoarthritis or oligoarthritis

- Occasionally migratory
- Most common joints: knee, shoulder, elbow

Evaluation

- CBC — leukocytosis, anemia, thrombocytopenia
- ESR > 30 seconds
- BMP
- LFT's
- Serology

Treatment

- Remove tick
- NSAID's prn
- ASA for cardiac involvement
- Vaccine (LYMErix) for prevention
- Doxycycline 100 mg PO within 72 hours of a deer tick bite effective in preventing Lyme disease

Stage 1 choices

- Amoxicillin or doxycycline or cefuroxime for 21 days
- Zithromax (azithromycin) for 14–21 days

Stage 2 choices

- Amoxicillin with probenecid for 30 days
- Doxycycline for 10–21 days
- Consult physician

Stage 3

- Consult physician

Discharge Criteria

- Patients treated with oral therapy

Discharge instructions

- Tick bite aftercare instructions
- Follow up within 3–7 days
- Return if symptoms worsens

Consult Criteria

- Stage 2 or 3

- Immunocompromised
- Systemic symptoms
- Meningeal signs

Notes

References:

Nadelman RB, et. al. Prophylaxis with single-dose doxycycline for the prevention of Lyme disease after an *Ixodes Scapularis* tick bite *NEJM*July 12, 2001

Mayo Clin Proc, 4/10,e13

Final Report of the Lyme Disease Review Panel of the Infectious Diseases Society of America April 22, 2010

emedicine.medscape.com/article/330178

VARICELLA (CHICKEN POX) PROTOCOL

When using any protocol, always follow the Guidelines of Proper Use (page 18).

Definition

- Successive crops of pruritic vesicles evolving to pustules and crusts caused by varicella zoster virus primarily in childhood

Differential Diagnosis

- Herpes simplex infection
- Herpes zoster
- Impetigo
- Hand-Foot-Mouth disease
- Henoch-Schonlein Purpura
- Erythema multiforme
- Stevens-Johnson syndrome
- Toxic Epidermal Necrolysis
- Scabies
- Toxic shock syndrome

Considerations

- Fever and malaise may occur
- Primarily childhood disease
- Older patients may have more severe disease — pneumonia or encephalitis
- Transmission by airborne droplets or direct contact
- Infectious period is from 2 days before first vesicle to when all vesicles are crusted
- Epidemics occur in winter and early spring in 3–4 year cycles
- Diagnosis is clinical
- "Dew drop" vesicle is initial finding
- New lesions usually stop appearing by day 5
- Palms and soles spared
- Self-limiting

Treatment and Prevention

- Supportive
- Vaccination
- Antivirals may decrease duration of infection (acyclovir and valacyclovir)
  - Especially useful in adults and immunocompromised
- No aspirin (can cause Reyes syndrome)
- Antibiotic choices for secondary bacterial infection
  - Mupirocin topical for 5–10 days
  - Retapamulin topical bid for 5 days
  - Septra (trimethoprim/sulfamethoxazole)
  - Doxycycline
  - Clindamycin
  - Beta-lactams
- Varicella zoster immune globulin for post-exposure up to 10 days in high risk individuals (pregnancy, immunocompromised)

Discharge Criteria

- Uncomplicated infection in children
- Trim nails

Discharge instructions

- Varicella aftercare instructions
- Return if systemic symptoms worse

Consult Criteria

- Encephalitis
- Altered mental status acutely
- Pregnancy
- Immunocompromised
- Systemic symptoms
- Moderate to severe secondary superinfection
- Adult infection

Notes

References:

Klassen TP, Hartling L. Acyclovir for treating varicella in otherwise healthy children and adolescents. Cochrane Database of Systematic Reviews 2005, Issue 4. Art. No.: CD002980. DOI: 10.1002/14651858.CD002980

Chickenpox Author: Anthony J Papadopoulos, MD; Chief Editor: Dirk M Elston, MD
emedicine.medscape.com/article/1131785

HAND INFECTION PROTOCOL

When using any protocol, always follow the Guidelines of Proper Use (page 18).

Definition

- Local inflammatory reaction of the skin and/or subcutaneous tissue of the hand secondary to bacteria or viral infection

Paronychia

Definition

- Cellulitis or abscess of nail margins and/or nail bed

Differential diagnosis

- Felon
- Draining osteomyelitis
- Herpetic whitlow
- Neoplasm

Considerations

- Secondary to trauma, nail biting, chemicals, incorrect nail trimming or chronic moist environment (dishwashers, bartenders, etc.)
- Acute infection: staph or strep
- Chronic infection: C. albicans or other fungi
- Vesicles suggest herpes infection
- Do not incise herpes infection (herpetic whitlow)

Evaluation

- CBC, BMP if signs of systemic infection present
- X-ray if chronic or recurrent to check for osteomyelitis

Treatment

No abscess

- Warm soaks and antibiotics

Subcuticular Abscess

- Local 1% plain lidocaine digital block (without epinephrine); may add 5% Marcaine (bupivacaine)
- Elevate eponychial fold at the nail plate
- Incise at maximal swelling and tenderness to allow drainage
- If pus extends below nail, remove lateral ¼ – ½ of nail
- Give antibiotics for any associated cellulitis — MRSA coverage (see Soft Tissue Abscess Protocol) or antibiotic database

Discharge criteria

- Noncomplicated paronychia without systemic symptoms/findings or bony involvement

Discharge instructions

- Paronychia aftercare instructions
- Refer to primary care provider or hand surgeon within 7–10 days as needed

Consult criteria

- Osteomyelitis
- Systemic symptoms/findings
- Associated proximal hand or tendon infection

Felon

Definition

- Infection/abscess of the pulp space of the distal finger

Differential diagnosis

- Paronychia
- Draining osteomyelitis
- Herpetic whitlow

Considerations

- Wooden splinters, minor cuts or diabetic testing methods are the common causes
- Paronychia spreading to pulp
- Staph aureus most common infection
- Can lead to osteomyelitis

Evaluation

- X-ray if osteomyelitis is suspected
- Neurovascular and tendon examination

Treatment

- Discuss with physician unless experienced
- Digital block with 1% plain lidocaine ± Marcaine (bupivacaine)

Longitudinal incision in the midline is effective without serious complications that are observed with other recommended incisions (incise skin only)

OR

- Lateral incision 5 mm distal to DIP joint on the dorsal 1/3 avoiding the neurovascular bundle, extending not past the distal nail corner (incise skin only)
    - Avoid incising the ulnar thumb side, and the radial side of index or middle finger to avoid a scar that interferes with pinching
- Lateral incision 5 mm distal to DIP joint on the dorsal 1/3 avoiding the neurovascular bundle, extending not past the distal nail corner
- Avoid incising the ulnar thumb side, and the radial side of index or middle finger to avoid a scar that interferes with pinching
- Pack with gauze
- Splint and elevate finger

Antibiotics choices

- Cefazolin IV, then cephalexin or dicloxicillin PO × 10 days
- Septra DS bid × 10 days
- Clindamycin 300 mg tid × 10 days

Discharge instructions

- Felon aftercare instructions
- Follow up in 24 hours
- NSAID's or narcotic short course

Consult criteria

- Osteomyelitis
- Flexor tenosynovitis
- Systemic symptoms or findings

Herpetic Whitlow Protocol

Definition

- Herpes simplex infection of the digits manifested as painful grouped vesicles

Differential diagnosis

- Felon
- Paronychia
- Cellulitis

Considerations

- Patients usually less than 20 years of age
- Usually caused by HSV-1
- Do not incise

Treatment options

- Avoid contact with infected individuals
- Antiviral treatment within 48–72 hours

Antiviral medication choices

- Acyclovir ointment 5% 5 times a day for 5 days
- Acyclovir 400 mg PO qid × 7 days for severe infection
- Pediatric acyclovir oral dosing 15 mg/kg 5 times a day for 7 days (do not exceed adult doses)
- Valtrex (valacyclovir) 500–1000 mg PO bid × 7 days for adults

Discharge criteria

- Most patients without severe superinfection

Discharge instructions

- Herpetic whitlow aftercare instructions
- Follow up with PCP within 7–10 days

Consult criteria

- Moderate to severe superinfection
- Immunocompromised

Closed (Clenched) Fist Infection or Injury

Definition

- Laceration or skin injury from a clenched fist striking human teeth

Differential diagnosis

- Cellulitis
- Osteomyelitis
- Abscess

Considerations

- Assumed to be from human teeth
- High risk for infection
- All bite wounds with evidence of infection require physician consultation
- Usually over the MP dorsal joint

Evaluation

- Neurovascular and tendon examination
- X-ray
- CBC if fever present
- Assess for infection

Treatment

- No suturing of wound
- Irrigate with > 250 cc of 0.1% betadine with 18 gauge angiocath (1% betadine: mix 1 cc of 10% betadine with 99 cc NS)
- May use tap water mixed with soap initially, then flushed with tap water (ok to use faucet)
- If no infection present, and no neurovascular or tendon acute deficits or injuries, then prescribe Augmentin (amoxicillin/clavulanate) or follow Sanford Guide or other drug databases for prophylaxis treatment
- Pain treatment prn
- See Human and Animal Bite Protocol

Discharge criteria

- Noninfected wound
- No bony, tendon or neurovascular acute abnormality
- Reliable follow up

Discharge instructions

- Human bite aftercare instructions
- Return if infection occurs in bite
- Return if pain increases

Consult criteria

- Infected wound
- Bony, tendon or neurovascular acute abnormality
- Hand surgeon preferred if available

Deep Space Infection

- Consult physician

Flexor Tenosynovitis

Definition

- Infection or inflammation of the flexor tendon sheath

Differential diagnosis

- Noninfectious flexor tenosynovitis
- Fracture
- Septic joint
- Tendon rupture
- Gout
- Rheumatoid arthritis
- Endocarditis

Considerations

- Usually penetrating injury history to volar surface; frequently cat bites
- Kanavel's signs
    - Pain on passive extension
    - Finger held in flexed position
    - SEVERE tenderness along tendon sheath
    - Symmetric swelling (sausage finger)
    - May see with ultrasound using linear probe in water bath as dark fluid collections around tendon

Consult criteria

- All patients
- Admission

- Surgical treatment
- IV antibiotics

Notes

References:

Herpetic Whitlow Author: Michael S Omori, MD; Chief Editor: Steven C Dronen, MD, FAAEM emedicine.medscape.com/article/788056

Nasser M, Fedorowicz Z, Khoshnevisan MH, Shahiri Tabarestani M. Acyclovir for treating primary herpetic gingivostomatitis. Cochrane Database of Systematic Reviews 2008, Issue 4. Art. No.: CD006700. DOI: 10.1002/14651858.CD006700.pub2

Felon Author: Glen Vaughn, MD; Chief Editor: Steven C Dronen, MD, FAAEM emedicine.medscape.com/article/782537

Common Acute Hand Infections
Dwayne C. Clark, CDR, MC, USN, Naval Hospital Jacksonville, Jacksonville, Florida
Am Fam Physician. 2003 Dec 1;68(11):2167–2176

Hand Infections Author: Rohini J Haar, MD; Chief Editor: Rick Kulkarni, MD emedicine.medscape.com/article/783011

Hematology and Oncology

Section Contents — one protocol

When using any protocol, always follow the Guidelines of Proper Use (page 18).

VENOUS THROMBOEMBOLIC DISEASE PROTOCOL

When using any protocol, always follow the Guidelines of Proper Use (page 18).

Definition

- Formation of thrombus within veins that may or may not propagate toward the central circulation

Differential diagnosis

- Cellulitis
- Hematoma
- Superficial thrombophlebitis
- Varicose veins
- Contusion or muscle strain/tear
- Arterial insufficiency
- Postphlebitic syndrome
- Dependent edema
- Lymphedema
- Baker's cyst

Considerations

- Deep vein thrombosis (DVT) and pulmonary embolism (PE) are manifestations of the same disease process
- DVT involves the legs most commonly, followed by the arms
- Early recognition and treatment are very important in decreasing morbidity and mortality
- Thrombus damages vein valves causing reflux of blood and postphlebitic syndrome — chronic edema and venous stasis ulcers
- Most DVT's develop complete or partial recanalization and collaterals over time
  - More than half of patients with proximal DVT have residual vein thrombosis on ultrasound 6 months - 1 year after completion of therapy
  - Presence of residual DVT has been shown to be a risk factor for recurrent VTE

- Proximal large vein thrombosis can cause pulmonary embolism
- PE occurs in ~ 10% of DVT
- Calf DVT may produce 1/3 of PE
- Most DVT is occult and resolves spontaneously
- Up to 40% of DVT patients when diagnosed have a silent PE
- CTA should only be performed in the context of clinical suspicion and in patients with an appropriate pre-test probability
- Thrombophilia screening should only be performed if the results alter therapeutic management
    - Almost exclusively the case in young female first-degree relatives of patients with venous thromboembolism contemplating estrogen medications or pregnancy
    - Tests should never be performed in the acute setting: both anticoagulatory therapy and the inflammatory state accompanying any thromboembolic event falsify the results and preclude any conclusions
- Paradoxical emboli may pass through an atrial septal defect and cause a CVA or distal arterial occlusion
- D-dimers remain elevated for 3 days after symptomatic thrombus

Risk factors

- Cancer
- Advanced age
- Immobilization > 3 days
- Major surgery in the prior 4 weeks
- Clotting disorders are common risk factors for venous thromboembolism (VTE)
    - 5–10% of VTE is from protein C, protein S or antithrombin III disorders
    - Factor V Leiden mutation
- Most common risk factor is prior VTE
- CHF
- AMI
- CVA
- Sepsis
- Estrogens

- IV drug abuse
- Pregnancy and postpartum period
- Thrombocytosis and polycythemia vera

Virchow triad for formation of thrombus

- Venous stasis
- Activation of the coagulation system
- Vein damage

Goals of DVT treatment

- Reduce morbidity
- Prevent postphlebitic syndrome
- Prevent pulmonary embolism

Signs and symptoms

DVT

- Extremity pain
- Involved area red and swollen
- May be asymptomatic

Severe DVT

Phlegmasia alba dolens

- Blanched leg appearance
- Massive iliofemoral thrombotic occlusion

Phlegmasia cerulea dolens

- Follows phlegmasia alba dolens
- Associated with arterial spasm
- Risk of gangrene
- Shock may occur
- Mortality 20–40% if venous gangrene develops
- Notify or consult promptly a physician for phlegmasia of any type
- May be treated conservatively with heparin and elevation if no ischemia present

Pulmonary embolism (see section in Dyspnea Protocol and below)

- Hypoxemia
- Chest pain

- Shock or hypotension
- May have no symptoms or findings

EKG

- Sinus tachycardia most common
- Nonspecific STT wave changes or with ischemic appearing biphasic T waves in V2 and V3
- New right bundle branch block
- S1Q3T3 pattern in 19%
- Right axis deviation in 5%
- Left axis deviation in 10%
- New onset atrial fibrillation
- EKG may be normal in 13%

Evaluation options

- Chest x-ray
- CBC if fever or tachycardia present
- BMP if diabetic or tachycardia present
- D-dimer (if negative with Well's criteria 0–1 makes PE unlikely)
- CT chest (see below)
- Apply Well's pulmonary embolism and DVT criteria and chart Well's score as indicated
- Extremity venous ultrasound for moderate to high probability Well's criteria as indicated
    - CT abdominal/pelvis scan for suspected intra-abdominal or pelvic DVT
- Record positive or negative calf tenderness and Homan's sign (for malpractice considerations)

Evaluation with D-dimer

D-dimer (LIA method) — some methods currently in use not reliable

- Useful if negative at cutoff value to rule out DVT or PE
    - Rare exception is cancer (especially hematological cancer) patients with PE may have negative d–dimer in small percentage (0.4%)

- Negative D-dimer with low to moderate probability Well's DVT or PE score largely excludes venous thromboembolic disease
- Well's DVT criteria high probability: order ultrasound scan regardless of D-dimer result
- If positive — not as useful as a negative result which usually rules out VTE (venous thromboembolic) disease
- Frequently positive with
    - Hospitalization in past month
    - Chronic bedridden or low activity state
    - Increasingly positive with age without significant acute disease process
        - D-dimer increases 10 mcg/L for every year over 50 years of age if the upper cutoff is 500 mcg/L (80 year old with d-dimer 700 mcg/L would be in the normal range)
        - If another assay used, then 2% increase/year over age 50 may be used to adjust upper limit for age
        - D–dimer age adjusted calculators
    - CHF
    - Chronic disease processes
    - Edematous states

Well's DVT criteria

- One point each:
    - Active cancer
    - Paralysis/recent cast immobilization
    - Recently bedridden > 3 days or surgery < 4 weeks
    - Deep vein tenderness
    - Entire leg edema
    - Calf swelling > 3 cm over other leg
    - Pitting edema > other calf
    - Collateral superficial veins
- Two points — alternative diagnosis less likely

High probability: ≥ 3 points

Moderate probability: 1–2 points

Low probability: 0 points

Well's PE criteria score 3 or greater consider D-dimer and CT chest PE protocol

- Suspected DVT = 3
- Alternative diagnosis less likely than PE = 3
- Heart rate > 100 = 1.5
- Immobilization/surgery past 4 wks. = 1.5
- Previous DVT/PE = 1.5
- Hemoptysis = 1
- Cancer past 6 months = 1

Well's score ≥ 6: order CTA chest PE protocol

Document positive or negative Homan's sign or calf tenderness regardless of Well's scores

Document PERC and/or Well's scores when appropriate

Pulmonary Embolism (PE)

Definition

- Blockage of pulmonary artery usually by a migrating blood clot from legs (most commonly) or pelvic veins

Differential diagnosis

- Acute coronary syndrome
- Acute pericarditis
- ARDS
- Panic disorder
- Aortic stenosis
- Atrial fibrillation
- Cardiogenic shock
- Cor pulmonale
- Cardiomyopathy
- COPD
- Fat embolism
- Mitral stenosis

- Acute MI
- Pneumothorax
- Pulmonary hypertension
- Sudden cardiac death
- Superior vena cava syndrome
- Syncope or near syncope

Considerations

- Can be either minimally asymptomatic or catastrophic
- Occurs 1 person per 1,000/year
- Clinical assessment performed by experienced physicians has proven non-inferior to standardized prediction scores and has an important place in everyday clinical practice
- CTA should only be performed in the context of clinical suspicion and in patients with an appropriate pre-test probability
- Commonly a missed diagnosis on initial evaluation
- PE are increasingly observed as incidental findings, i.e., without clinical correlate
- Reliability of detection of PE via CTA decreases significantly in peripheral clots with small filling defects (<6mm) and, overall, the incidence is overestimated
- Present in 60–80% of DVT patients even though one half have on PE symptoms
- More common cause of hospitalized patient death
- One year mortality is 24%
    - Mainly due to cardiac disease, recurrent PE, infection or cancer
- NT-proBNP >500 ng/L associated with central PE and possible predictor of increased death risk (pre–existing conditions such renal failure and atrial fibrillation that have chronic increased NT-proBNP would make this assumption not as useful)
- Elevated troponin is an increased severity risk marker — 19% probability of death during hospitalization
- Massive PE second only to sudden cardiac death as a cause of sudden death
- Majority of deaths from PE occur in the first 1–2 hours of care

- Nonmassive PE defined as a systolic BP ≥ 90 mmHG and accounts for 95.5–96% of patients
- See Well's Pulmonary Embolism Criteria in above section

Pulmonary Embolism Rule-out Criteria (PERC Rule)

(Reportedly decreases significantly the likelihood of pulmonary embolism if all 8 criteria met — not superior to clinical gestalt)

- Age < 50
- Pulse oximetry > 94%
- Heart rate < 100
- No history of DVT or VTE
- No hemoptysis
- No estrogen use
- No unilateral leg swelling
- No recent surgery or trauma hospitalization past 4 weeks

American College of Physicians (ACP) 2015

- Plasma D-dimer tests are more appropriate for those at intermediate risk for a PE, and no testing may be necessary for some patients at low risk
- Use either the Wells or Geneva rules to choose tests based on a patient's risk for PE
- Low risk patients clinicians should use the 8 Pulmonary Embolism Rule-Out Criteria (PERC) and if negative for all 8 criteria then no testing is needed
- Intermediate risk patients or for those at low risk who do not meet all of the rule-out criteria, use a high-sensitivity plasma D-dimer test initially
- In patients >50 years use an age-adjusted threshold age × 10 ng/mL
    - Normal D-dimer levels increase with age
- D-dimer level below the age-adjusted cutoff should not receive any imaging studies
    - Patients with elevated D-dimer levels should receive imaging
- Patients at high risk skip the D-dimer test and proceed to CT pulmonary angiography
    - Negative D-dimer test does not eliminate the need for imaging in these patients

- Obtain ventilation-perfusion scans in patients with a contraindication to CT pulmonary angiography or if CT pulmonary angiography is unavailable
- Use validated clinical prediction rules to estimate pretest probability in patients in whom acute PE is being considered

American College of Emergency Physicians (ACEP) 2011

- Negative quantitative D-dimer assay results can be used to exclude PE in patients with a **low** pretest probability for PE
- Negative quantitative D-dimer assay results may be used to exclude PE in patients with an **intermediate** pretest probability for PE
- Low or PE unlikely patients (Wells score 4) pretest probability for PE who require additional diagnostic testing (positive D-dimer result or highly sensitive D–dimer not available), a negative multidetector CT pulmonary angiogram alone can be used to exclude PE
- Intermediate or high pretest probability for PE and a negative CT pulmonary angiogram result in whom a clinical concern for PE still exists and CT venogram has not already been performed, consider additional diagnostic testing (e.g., D-dimer, lower extremity imaging, VQ scanning, traditional pulmonary arteriography) prior to exclusion of VTE disease
- Venous ultrasound
    - May be considered as initial imaging in patients with obvious signs of DVT for whom venous ultrasound is readily available
    - Patients with relative contraindications for CT scan (e.g., borderline renal insufficiency, CT contrast agent allergy)
    - Pregnant patients
    - A positive finding in a patient with symptoms consistent with PE can be considered evidence for diagnosis of VTE disease and may preclude the need for additional diagnostic imaging

Risk factors

Virchow triad

- Endothelial injury
- Stasis or turbulence of blood flow
- Blood hypercoagulability

- Immobilization
- Malignancy
- Inherited or acquired thrombophilia states (hypercoagulable states)
- Acute medical illness
- Surgery past 3 months
- Trauma (mostly lower extremities or pelvis) past 3 months
- Oral contraceptives or estrogen
- Pregnancy
- Prior pulmonary embolism
- COPD
- Heart failure
- Stroke, hemiplegia or paralysis
- Central venous lines within past 3 months

Signs and symptoms

- Tachypnea (respiratory rate >16/min) — 96%
- Rales — 58%
- Accentuated second heart sound — 53%
- Tachycardia (heart rate >100/min) — 44%
- Fever>37.8°C (100.04°F) — 43%
- Diaphoresis — 36%
- S_3 or S_4 gallop — 34%
- Clinical signs and symptoms suggesting thrombophlebitis — 32%
- Lower extremity edema: 24%
- Cardiac murmur — 23%
- Cyanosis — 19%

Presenting complaints and findings

- Dyspnea — 73%
- Pleuritic chest pain — 66%
- Cough — 37%
- Hemoptysis — 13%

- Hypoxia
- Delirium in elderly
- Wheezing
- Productive cough
- Syncope or near syncope
- Hypotension or relative hypotension (for the patient with hypertension history)
- Lung infarction
- New onset atrial fibrillation
- Ventricular arrhythmia
- Pleural effusion
- Pulseless electrical activity

Testing options

- Chest x–ray (may be normal or nonspecific)
    - Westermark sign — decreased vascularity
    - Hampton hump — pleural based triangular density from pulmonary infarction (rare)
- CBC
- EKG
    - Sinus tachycardia most common
    - Nonspecific STT wave changes or with ischemic appearing biphasic T waves in V2 and V3
    - New right bundle branch block
    - S1Q3T3 pattern in 20%
    - Right axis deviation in 5%
    - Left axis deviation in 10%
    - New onset atrial fibrillation
- D–dimer (do not use in high clinical PE probability — scan instead)
    - More useful in eliminating younger healthy patients if negative
- ABG (may be normal or have increased A–a gradient or hypoxemia)
- BNP or NT-proBNP
- Troponin
- Echocardiogram RV strain have 10% mortality, 0% mortality with normal RV function
- Chemistries
- CTA chest pulmonary embolism protocol

- V/Q lung scan if CTA chest not available or contraindicated
    - May be performed in healthy low risk patients (if normal then very useful)
    - Low probability scans can have PE from 4–20% depending whether clinical suspicion is low or high
- Leg venous ultrasound

Treatment guidelines

American College of Chest Physicians (ACCP)

- Dabigatran, rivaroxaban, apixaban, or edoxaban are preferred over vitamin K antagonist (VKA) therapy as long-term (first 3 months) anticoagulant therapy for noncancer patients
- Low-molecular-weight heparin (LMWH) is recommended over VKA therapy, dabigatran, rivaroxaban, apixaban, or edoxaban as long-term (first 3 months) anticoagulant therapy for patients with cancer-associated thrombosis
- Aspirin is recommended over no aspirin to prevent recurrent venous thromboembolism (VTE) in patients who are stopping anticoagulant therapy and do not have a contraindication to aspirin
- In most patients with acute PE not associated with hypotension, systemically administered thrombolytic therapy is not recommended
- Selected patients with acute PE who deteriorate after starting anticoagulant therapy but have yet to develop hypotension and who have a low bleeding risk, systemically administered thrombolytic therapy is preferred over no such therapy
- Thrombolytic therapy is suggested in select patients with acute PE not associated with hypotension and with a low bleeding risk whose initial clinical presentation or clinical course after starting anticoagulation suggests a high risk of developing hypotension

- Thrombolytic therapy is not recommended for most patients with acute PE not associated with hypotension
- First episode of VTE and with a low or moderate risk of bleeding should have extended anticoagulant therapy
- First episode of VTE with a high bleeding risk should have therapy limited to 3 months
- Patients who have PE and preexisting irreversible risk factors, such as deficiency of antithrombin III, proteins S and C, factor V Leiden mutation, or the presence of antiphospholipid antibodies, should be placed on long-term anticoagulation

Treatments

- IV NS 250–500 ml bolus if hypotensive and notify physician promptly **(severe PE patients may decompensate with IVF bolus due to acute very high right ventricular pressure and strain from PE — exercise caution and consider norepinephrine drip instead)**
- **Embolectomy** in very unstable patients in centers with CV surgery available and thrombolytics thought not to be adequate therapy or contraindicated
  - Nitric oxide 10ppm inhalation may be tried to temporize condition prior to surgery or thrombolytics

Anticoagulation

- Is a passive anticoagulation—prevents new thrombus formation while body breaks down existing thrombus
- **Enoxaparin** (LMWH) 1mg/kg q12hour SQ or 1.5 mg/kg q24hours SQ
  - Do not use with creatinine clearance <30
  - Do not use with history of heparin induced thrombocytopenia (HIT)
  - No PTT monitoring
- **Heparin** (unfractionated) load 80units/kg IV and 18 units/kg/hour IV
  - Goal is PTT 1.5–2.5 times normal
  - Creatinine clearance <30 increased bleeding risk

Do not use with history of heparin induced thrombocytopenia Stop all heparins if platelet count drops to 100,000, or a 50% decrease in baseline platelet count occurs, or 30% decrease in platelet count with new thrombus formation development (heparin induced thrombocytopenia) — a life threatening immune process

- **Warfarin** 15 mg PO load
    - Overlap with heparin until INR 2–3
    - 2–10mg PO daily (start >6 hours after LMWH)
    - **Contraindicated in pregnancy**

Direct oral anticoagulants (DOACs)

- **Apixaban (Eliquis)** 10 mg PO BID x 7 days, then 5 mg BID
    - Not recommended in severe liver disease
- **Rivaroxaban (Xarelto)** 15 mg PO q12hr for 21 days with food, then 20 mg PO qday

Thrombolytics

- **TPA** 100mg IV over 2 hours
- May give 100mg IVP during CPR in PE or suspected PE coding patients
- Heparin bolus and drip near end to TPA infusion or immediately following

Disposition

Consult criteria

- Discuss all patients with a physician

Admission

- Unstable or severe PE admit to ICU
- Patients not meeting Hestia criteria
- New elevation of troponin and/or NT-proBNP
- Clinical judgment that overrides Hestia criteria

Discharge

Hestia criteria for outpatient PE therapy — A "No" answer to all questions needed to treat outpatient

- Hemodynamically unstable
- Clot busting necessary

    - Bleeding issues
    - Oxygen required
    - Ongoing anticoagulation
    - Severe pain
    - Inpatient status needed
    - Renal failure
    - Liver disease
    - Pregnancy
    - Documented HIT
- Clinical judgment that outpatient therapy is safe for patient
- No tachycardia

Treatment options

DVT

May be treated as outpatient if none of the following present

- Pulmonary embolism
- Significant cardiopulmonary comorbidities
- Pregnancy
- Morbid obesity
- Homeless
- Creatinine > 2 mg/dL
- No follow up
- Inherited bleeding disorder
- Iliofemoral DVT
- Contraindications to anticoagulation
- Disorder of coagulation
- Patient does not want to be discharged

- Enoxaparin (Lovenox) 1 mg/kg SQ q12hr (1 mg/kg SQ q24hr if creatinine clearance<30 ml/minute)

OR

- Heparin (unfractionated) 80–100 U/kg IV loading dose and 15–18 U/kg/hour IV (keep PTT 2–2.5 times normal

OR

- Fondaparinux (Arixtra) – no INR or PTT monitoring needed

    - < 50 kg: 5 mg SQ qday
    - 50–100 kg: 7.5 mg SQ qday
    - > 100 kg: 10 mg SQ qday

  Stop all heparins if platelet count drops to 100,000, or a 50% decrease in baseline platelet count occurs, or 30% decrease in platelet count with new thrombus formation development (heparin induced thrombocytopenia) — a life threatening immune process

- Warfarin (Coumadin)
    - 2–10 mg PO qday to achieve INR 2–3
    - Treatment for 3–6 months
    - Can cause initially a transient hypercoagulable state if started without heparin treatment
    - Has a myriad of drug and other substances interactions
    - Can cause life threatening hemorrhage
    - Read drug information before using to determine interactions and patient risks
- Thrombin inhibitors
    - Argatroban for heparin-induced thrombocytopenia
- Thrombolytics
    - Use under direction of physician
    - For severe iliofemoral DVT (Phlegmasia cerulea dolens) — catheter directed

Direct oral anticoagulants (DOACs)

- **Rivaroxaban** 15 mg PO q12hr for 21 days with food, then 20 mg PO qday for 6 months
- **Dabigatran** for prophylaxis and if patient on parenteral anticoagulant 5–10 days already
- **Apixaban (Eliquis)** 10 mg PO BID x 7 days, then 5 mg BID
    - Not recommended in severe liver disease

- Mechanical extraction
    - Consult vascular surgeon or interventional physician with appropriate skill set

Pulmonary embolism (see Pulmonary Embolism section above)

- Same medication treatment as DVT
- Oxygen
- IV NS 250–500 ml bolus if hypotensive and notify physician promptly **(severe PE patients may decompensate with IVF bolus due to acute very high right ventricular pressure and strain from PE — exercise caution and consider norepinephrine drip instead)**
    - Thrombolytics may be considered if PE caused hypotension is present
    - Improves mortality but with increased bleeding

DVT prophylaxis

- Enoxaparin (Lovenox) 40 mg SQ q24hr

  OR
- Heparin (unfractionated) 5,000 units SQ q8–12h

For admitted patients with any of the following

- Age > 60 years
- CHF
- Systemic infection
- History of DVT or PE
- Inflammatory disorders
- Cancer
- ICU admission
- Hypercoagulable state
- Immobilization ≥ 3 days or severely compromised ambulation

Discharge criteria

- DVT not meeting exclusionary criteria above
    - Discuss with physician

Consult criteria

- All DVT and PE patients, or suspected DVT/PE diagnosis
    - Tachycardia
    - Hypotension or relative hypotension (SBP < 105 with history of hypertension)

- Dyspnea

Notes

References:

Deep Venous Thrombosis Author: Kaushal (Kevin) Patel, MD; Chief Editor: Barry E Brenner, MD, PhD, FACEP emedicine.medscape.com/article/1911303

Büller HR, Prins MH, Lensin AW, Decousus H, Jacobson BF, Minar E, et al. Oral rivaroxaban for the treatment of symptomatic pulmonary embolism. *N Engl J Med*. Apr 5 2012;366(14):1287–97

Boyles S. Thrombolysis aids PE survival, but ups bleeding risk. *MedPage Today* [serial online]. June 17, 2014; Updated June 18, 2014;Accessed June 22, 2014

Pulmonary Embolism Author: Daniel R Ouellette, MD, FCCP; Chief Editor: Zab Mosenifar, MD emedicine.medscape.com/article/300901

Age-Adjusted D-Dimer Cutoff Levels to Rule Out Pulmonary Embolism: The ADJUST-PE Study *JAMA.* 2014;311(11):1117-1124. doi:10.1001/jama.2014.2135

Circulation;129:917

J Emerg Med. 2017;52:184

Clin Chest Med. 2018;39:539

Myths in the Evaluation of Acute Pulmonary Embolism; emedhome.com clinical pearl

Stussi-Helbling M, et al. *Am J Med.* 2019

SICKLE CELL ANEMIA PROTOCOL

When using any protocol, always follow the Guidelines of Proper Use (page 18).

Definition

- Inherited disorder of hemoglobin synthesis causing sickling and destruction of RBC's with resulting vascular obstruction and tissue ischemia

Differential Diagnosis

- Appendicitis
- Cholecystitis
- Pneumonia
- Pulmonary embolism
- Acute myocardial infarction
- Priapism
- Anemia from other causes
- Hemorrhage
- Pancreatitis
- Osteomyelitis
- CVA
- Meningitis
- Hepatitis

Considerations

- Has increased incidence of life threatening infections
- Functional asplenia
- Chronic hemolysis
- Hand-foot syndrome — ages 6–24 months
- Aseptic necrosis of bone and osteomyelitis may occur
- Vascular occlusion pain most common presentation
- Stroke common
- Pulmonary embolism increased risk
- Mean survival: females 48 years; males 42 years from SS disease
- WBC elevated; platelet count elevated; reticulocyte count averages > 2–3%
- Precipitants

- Infection
- Cold exposure
- Dehydration

Crises types

Vaso–occlusive crises

- Bones
- Lungs (acute chest syndrome)
- Musculoskeletal pain most common complaint
- Abdominal pain 2nd most common complaint

Acute chest syndrome (ACS)

- Pulmonary infiltrates with one of the following:
    - Chest pain
    - Cough
    - Fever
    - Tachypnea
    - Wheezing
- Leading cause of death
- 50% of ACS cases develop in patients admitted for other sickle cell disease diagnoses

Aplastic Crises

- Severe anemia from cessation of erythropoiesis; can be related to parvovirus B19V infection
- Low reticulocyte count

Acute splenic sequestration crises

- Sudden hemoglobin decrease ≥ 2 gms
- Syncope
- Abdominal distension

Priapism

- Sickle cell patients may need exchange transfusion
- Consult physician and urologist immediately
- See Male Genitalia Protocol

Pediatric sickle cell disease (SCD) and fever

Admission criteria

- Age < 2 years with hemoglobin SS (HbSS) disease or hemoglobin S–β° (HbS–β°)
  - HbSC or HbS–β+ less likely to have bacteremia and age alone not an admission criteria
- Temperature > 104°F (40°C)
- WBC > 30,000 or < 5,000
  - Both associated with increased bacteremia risk
  - Bandemia > 1,000 with bacterial infection
- Hemoglobin ≥ 2 gms below baseline in HbSS or HbS–β°
- Hemoglobin ≤ 5 gms
- Previous bacteremia or invasion infection
- Indwelling vascular lines
- Signs of systemic toxicity, vital sign instability or serious infection
- Previously treated with clindamycin or vancomycin instead of ceftriaxone
- Presence of SCD manifestations that require inpatient management
  - Acute chest syndrome
  - Painful crisis
  - Aplastic crisis
  - Splenic sequestration
- Concerns about family not able to recognize changes in patient's condition or inability/difficulty for follow–up (Need clear method to contact family if cultures are positive)

Outpatient management

- Patient that do not meet admission criteria can be considered for discharge (discuss with physician)
- Clinically stable
- Specific plan for follow–up the next day
- Recorded working telephone number recorded in chart

- Ceftriaxone 50–75 mg/kg IM or IV daily unless discontinued by medical provider
    - 100 mg/kg if meningitis present or suspected
- Stress oral hydration
- If vomiting occurs then return for further evaluation
- Adequate PO pain medications

Evaluation of sickle cell anemia

- Complete physical exam
- CBC
- BMP
- U/A
- Reticulocyte count (should be elevated)
- Chest x-ray
- ABG if significant dyspnea
- LFT's for abdominal pain
- Blood cultures if febrile
- O_2 saturation measurement

History for

- Prior episodes
- Transfusion history
- Dyspnea
- Fever
- Cough
- Headache
- Neurologic deficits
- Previous hemoglobin level

Treatment Options

- D5½NS at maintenance rate if not hypotensive or hypovolemic — otherwise IV NS as needed for hypovolemia or hypotension
- Pain control
- Toradol (ketorolac) 10 mg PO or 30 mg IV prn (avoid IM)
    - Do not use Toradol (ketorolac) if creatinine is elevated

Narcotics IM or IV options prn

- Dilaudid (hydromorphone) 0.5–1 mg IV or 1–2 mg IM — may repeat × 2 prn
- Morphine 2–5 mg IV or 5–10 mg IM — may repeat × 2 prn
- Phenergan (promethazine) or Zofran (ondansetron) with narcotics
- Hydrocodone or oxycodone PO prn if discharged

- Supplemental oxygen if hypoxic or O_2 saturation < 92%
- Albuterol aerosol if dyspneic without CHF
- IV 1/2NS or NS at 125–150 cc/hour or 150% maintenance
- Folic acid PO as outpatient if not already taking it
- Hydroxyurea outpatient treatment
    - Start: 15 mg/kg PO qd
    - Titrate by 5 mg/kg/d q8–12wk
    - NMT 35 mg/kg/d

Exchange transfusion indicated for

- Significant cardiopulmonary decompensation
- Priapism
- Acute nervous system event

Transfusion indicated for

- Severe anemia (hemoglobin < 6 gms)
- Symptomatic anemia (consult physician)

Discharge Criteria

- Resolution of the painful crises to the satisfaction of provider and patient
- No indications for admission

Discharge instructions

- Sickle cell anemia aftercare instructions
- Return if pain persists or worsens
- Return if fever develops
- Follow up with PCP in 1–2 days
- See Pediatric sickle cell section above

Consult Criteria

- Refractory pain crises
- Signs of bacterial infection
- Fever
- Acute chest syndrome
- Acute splenic sequestration crises
- Aplastic crises (reticulocyte count not elevated)
- CVA or TIA
- Refractory priapism
- Symptomatic anemia

Notes

References:

Sickle Cell Anemia Author: Joseph E Maakaron, MD; Chief Editor: Emmanuel C Besa, MD
emedicine.medscape.com/article/205926

Benjamin LJ, Swinson GI, Nagel RL. Sickle cell anemia day hospital: an approach for the management of uncomplicated painful crises. Blood. 2000;95:1130–1136

Embury SH, Garcia JF, Mohandas N, et al. Effects of oxygen inhalation on endogenous erythropoietin kinetics, erythropoiesis, and properties of blood cells in sickle-cell anemia. N Engl J Med.1984;311:291–295

CANCER EMERGENCY PROTOCOL

When using any protocol, always follow the Guidelines of Proper Use (page 18).

Definition

- Cancer conditions and treatments resulting in urgent and emergent symptoms and findings

Considerations

- There is an increase in the amount of cancer patients surviving longer
- Cancer is the second most common cause of death in the U.S.

3 most common categories of cancer emergencies

- Neutropenic fever (most common)
- Mechanical complications
- Metabolic derangements

Neutropenic fever

Definition

- WBC (white blood count) < 500 cells/μL
- WBC < 1000 cells/μL with anticipation of WBC < 500 cells/μL
- Temperature > 101°F (38.3°C) on one reading or 100.4°F (38.0°C) > 1 hour

Considerations for neutropenic fever

- May have minimal symptoms besides fever
  - Pneumonia patients may have no infiltrates on chest x-ray and or any cough
  - CT chest may be needed to make diagnosis
- UTI patients may not have much frequency, dysuria or pyuria
- Progression of symptoms may be rapid
- Staphylococcus aureus and coagulase negative staphylococcus are the most common pathogens

Evaluation

- CBC

- CMP
- Chest x-ray
- Blood cultures 5 minutes apart x 2
- Blood culture from any central venous catheters
- U/A
- Urine culture and sensitivity
- Lactic acid level if hypotensive or evidence of tissue hypoperfusion

Treatment

- Early empiric antibiotic monotherapy with
  - Ceftazidime 1 gm IV q8–12hr or cefepime 1 gm IV q12hr

    Or
  - Imipenem-cilastatin 500–1000 mg IV q6hr or meropenem 1 gm IV q6hr

Add

- Vancomycin 1 gm IV q12hr for the following
  - Suspected central catheter related infection
  - History of MRSA colonization
  - Preliminary blood culture growth of gram positive bacteria
  - Hypotension or cardiovascular compromise
- Neupogen (filgrastim) may be added per physician or oncologist
- Reverse isolation room if admitted and available

Discharge criteria

- Per physician consultation
- Most patients will be admitted

Consult criteria

- All febrile neutropenic patients
- Notify physician promptly if patient is hypotensive (or recent history of hypotension) or appears toxic, or signs/symptoms of hypoperfusion present

Mechanical cancer emergencies

- Spinal cord compression
- Superior vena cava syndrome
- Neoplastic cardiac tamponade

- Hyperviscosity syndrome
- Leukostasis

Spinal cord compression

Definition

- Compression of the spinal cord by tumor

Considerations

- Back pain with history of cancer is a Red Flag
- Patient outcomes improved with rapid detection
- Very important to consider this as a possible diagnosis

Symptoms and findings

- Back pain worsened by cough, worse at night or in supine position
- Numbness and paresthesia
- Loss of proprioception
- Bowel or bladder incontinence
- Bladder retention with overflow incontinence
- Decreased rectal tone
- New onset radicular pain on occasion may be caused by nerve root compression by tumor
- Back pain and tenderness may or may not be midline

Evaluation

- Complete history and physical exam with detailed neurologic and rectal tone exam
- MRI scan is the preferred imaging modality
- CBC, BMP, U/A as indicated
- Plain spine films for vertebral lesions

Treatment

- Decadron (dexamethasone) 0.1 mg/kg IV when suspected or diagnosed
- Radiation therapy may be needed

Discharge criteria

- Per physician and/or oncologist

Consult criteria

- All suspected or diagnosed spinal cord compression patients to be discussed with physician or oncologist and neurosurgeon

Superior vena cava syndrome

Definition

- Obstruction of the superior vena cava

Considerations

- More of an urgency than emergency unless
    - Cerebral edema or laryngeal edema present

Common causes are

- Lung cancer
- Lymphoma
- Central line related DVT (deep vein thrombosis) of superior vena cava

Symptoms or findings

- May be vague
- Venous distension of neck, chest or upper extremities
- Facial or neck swelling
- Chronic cough
- Hoarseness
- Supine facial cyanosis (rare but pathognomonic)
- Dyspnea
- Fatigue
- Headache

Evaluation options

- Thorough history and physical exam
- CBC and BMP
- Chest x-ray
- CT scanning with contrast may be considered

Treatment options

- Elevate head of bed
- Radiation therapy
- Corticosteroid therapy with dexamethasone 0.1 mg/kg IV or IM (NMT 10 mg)

- Diuretic therapy
- Outpatient management

Discharge criteria

- No cerebral edema or airway impairments/ concerns
- Diagnosis firm

Discharge instructions

- Follow up with PCP or oncologist within 1–2 days
- Return if worsening symptoms

Consult criteria

- Discuss all patients with suspected or diagnosed superior vena cava syndrome with physician

Neoplastic cardiac tamponade

Definition

- Pericardial effusion with impairment of cardiac filling and function

Considerations

- May present with stable vital signs or hypotension
- Beck's triad of hypotension, muffled heart sounds and jugular venous distension may not present

Symptoms and findings (may or may not be present)

- Beck's triad
- Cardiomegaly on chest x-ray
- Low EKG voltage
- Dyspnea
- Pulsus paradoxus present up to 60% of patients (decrease in blood pressure > 10 mm Hg with inspiration — may be seen with COPD and asthma patients also)
- Volume depletion may mask findings
- Associated malignant pleural effusion may occur

Evaluation

- Chest x-ray
- CBC and BMP

- EKG
- Echocardiogram (diastolic collapse diagnostic)

Treatment

- Needle pericardiocentesis per physician
- Pericardial window per cardiothoracic surgeon

Consult criteria

- All suspected or diagnosed cardiac tamponade patients

Hyperviscosity syndrome

Definition

- Elevation of blood viscosity from increase in plasma proteins or blood component cells causing impaired circulation to tissues

Considerations

- Symptoms related to degree of hyperviscosity

Symptoms and findings (variable)

- Mental status changes (may be only manifestation)
- Unexplained dyspnea
- Headache
- Total serum protein minus albumin > 4
- Vision changes
- Somnolence
- Epistaxis
- Vertical nystagmus
- Hearing impairment
- Ataxia
- Retinal hemorrhages
- Paresthesias
- Congestive heart failure
- Low anion gap may be seen with multiple myeloma
    - Low anion gap may also be seen with lithium treatment or low serum albumin

Evaluation

- Serum viscosity measurement
- CBC and BMP

- Other tests as dictated by symptoms or findings

Treatment options

- Per physician
- Phlebotomy of 2–3 units of blood
- IV NS hydration

Consult criteria

- All suspected or diagnosed hyperviscosity syndrome patients

Leukostasis

Definition

- Tissue hypoperfusion secondary to elevated WBC

Considerations

- Seen with acute leukemias
- Typically seen when WBC > 100,000 cells/μL
- Can be seen with monoblastic leukemia of 25,000–50,000 cells/μL
- Watch out for tumor lysis syndrome with leukemia chemotherapy
    - Hyperkalemia
    - Hyperuricemia
    - Hyperphosphatemia
    - Renal failure

Evaluation

- CBC
- BMP
- Chest x-ray
- Uric acid as needed for tumor lysis syndrome

Treatment

- Chemotherapy
- Tumor lysis syndrome treated with
    - Aggressive IV fluid hydration
    - Allopurinol 300 mg PO
    - Amphojel 30–60 cc PO for hyperphosphatemia
    - Hemodialysis

- Blood transfusion can cause hyperviscosity and rapid patient deterioration
- Supplemental oxygen for dyspnea or O_2 saturation < 92%

Consult criteria

- All patients with leukostasis or tumor lysis syndrome

Immune checkpoint inhibitors

- The potential presence of immune-related adverse events necessitates a new approach to the evaluation of cancer patients in the ED if they are on Immune Checkpoint Inhibitors
- Restores immune system function
- Some examples:
  - Pembrolizumab (Keytruda)
  - Nivolumab (Opdivo)
- Patients with dyspnea, in addition to considering pneumonia or pulmonary embolus, consider immune-mediated pneumonitis
- Patients with chest pain, consider myocarditis and pericarditis
- Patients with headache, consider hypophysitis
- Neutropenia is not likely to be present
- Thyroiditis is a common adverse effect
- With potentially serious immune-related adverse effects such as neurologic, pulmonary, and cardiac toxicities, systemic glucocorticoids may need to be initiated expeditiously

Metabolic emergencies

Syndrome of Inappropriate Antidiuretic Hormone Secretion (SIADH)

Definition

- Excess release of ADH (antidiuretic hormone) causing hyponatremia with water retention in euvolemic patient

Considerations

- Less than maximally dilute urine

- Urine sodium > 30
- Normal renal, adrenal and thyroid function
- Absence of diuretic therapy

Symptoms and findings

- Hyponatremia
- As in above **Considerations**
- Frequently chronic and stable
- Anorexia
- Weakness
- Confusion

Evaluation

- CBC
- BMP
- Urine sodium
- Chest x-ray

Treatment options

- Depends on degree of hyponatremia and associated symptoms or findings
- Demeclocycline 250 mg PO q6hr
- See Hyponatremia Protocol
    - Hypertonic saline 3% IV 100 mg/hr. for 2 hours if needed
        - Or 1–2 cc/kg/hour in order to raise the serum sodium by 2.5 mEq/hour
    - Fluid restriction 500–1,000 cc of water per day
    - Be cautious of rapid hyponatremia correction

Consult criteria

- Discuss all suspected or diagnosed SIADH patients with a physician

Notes

References:

Neutropenic Fever Empiric Therapy

Author: Mary Denshaw-Burke, MD, FACP; Chief Editor: Thomas E Herchline, MD

emedicine.medscape.com/article/2012185

Nieto AF, Doty DB. Superior vena cava obstruction: clinical syndrome, etiology, and treatment. Curr Probl Cancer 1986;10:441–484

Hughes WT, Armstrong D, Bodey GP, et al. 2002 Guidelines for the use of antimicrobial agents in neutropenic patients with cancer-IDSA Guidelines. Clin Infect Dis 2002;34:730–751

Kralstein J, Fishman WH. Malignant pericardial disease: Diagnosis and treatment. Cardiol Clin 1987;5:583–589

Gross P, Reimann D, Henschkowski J, et al. Treatment of severe hyponatremia: conventional and novel aspects. J Am Soc Nephrol 2001; 12:S10–14

El Majzoub I, et al. *Ann Emerg Med*. 2019 Jan;73(1):79-87

Bischof JJ, et al. *Ann Emerg Med*. 2019 Jan;73(1):88-90

Psychiatric and Social

Section Contents

When using any protocol, always follow the Guidelines of Proper Use (page 18).

ADULT AND ADOLESCENT PSYCHIATRIC PROTOCOL

When using any protocol, always follow the Guidelines of Proper Use (page 18).

Considerations

- Suicide 9th leading cause of death
- Actively suicidal patient or patient dangerous to others is not competent to refuse evaluation and treatment, and may not depart from the department until psychiatrically and medically cleared by an evaluation to do so
- Patients with depression, substance abuse or schizophrenia are at higher risk of suicide
- Evaluation of medical causes of psychiatric symptoms important
- Evaluation for patient being dangerous to self or others very important

Restraints used when all interventions to reduce patient's dangerous behavior fail

- Placed without discussion or negotiation
- Carries risk of injury and death

Indications

- Prevent harm to patient or staff
- Prevent disruption of treatment
- Decrease stimulation of patient
- Honor patient's request for them to be applied to keep patient from harming themselves

Relative contraindications

- Delirium
- Dementia

General guidelines

- Team of at least 4 persons
- Leather restraints recommended
- Explain to patient need for restraints
- Staff member should be visible to patient at all times

- Placed so an IV is accessible
- Remove potentially dangerous objects from patient
- Raise patient's head to reduce aspiration
- Use verbal or chemical restraints after physical restraints placed if needed
- Check of circulation and limb swelling by nursing staff q15 minutes
- Remove restraints one at a time until 2 left, then last 2 together
- Never leave only one limb restrained
- Place in private area assessable and visible to staff
- Provide bedpan and nursing call light

Contraindications

- Organic brain syndrome
- Sepsis
- Cardiac illness
- Fever or hypothermia
- Metabolic disturbance
- Orthopedic problems

Restraints Time Rules

- Not to exceed 4 hours in adults
- Not to exceed 1 hour children < 9 years of age
- New order needed when time expires
- Restraint protocols change with time and apply new directives as they occur

Evaluation

- Directed by history and physical examination
- Routine lab tests are low yield and need not to be performed frequently unless indicated by history and physical exam
- Routine drug screens in alert, awake, and cooperative need not to be routinely performed
- Consider use of observation period to determine if psychiatric symptoms are from intoxication when substance abuse has occurred

Mental Status Examination

OMI HAT (OMI = organic disease; HAT = psychiatric or functional)

- O – Orientation
- M – Memory
- I – Intellect
- H – Hallucinations
- A – Affect disorder
- T – Thought disorder

Suicidal Ideation or Attempt

- All patients with significant psychiatric symptoms need to be asked about suicidal ideation or attempt
- Need acute psychiatric evaluation
- Cannot leave until cleared of acute suicide risk or a risk of danger to others
- Treat injuries or ingestions as per appropriate protocols

Thought Disorders

- Acute psychosis
- Brief reactive psychosis
- Schizophrenia
- Delusional

Acute psychosis

- Loss of contact with reality
- Hallucinations (usually auditory)
- Fixed delusions (a fixed false belief)
- Rule out organic conditions or drug causes

Treatment

- Treat any organic causes
- No acute treatment besides an outpatient referral if stable, chronic and not dangerous to self or others

Agitation treatment — alone or combination therapy (combination more effective)

- Lorazepam 2–4 mg IM or Versed 3–5 mg IM prn (may be combined with Haldol)

- Haldol 5–10 mg (in elderly use 1–2 mg) IM or Droperidol 5 mg IM (works faster) prn (read droperidol's black box warning about fatal arrhythmias
- Geodon (ziprasidone) 10–20 mg IM (use Haldol if dementia–related psychosis)
- Cooperative patient — Lorazepam 4 mg PO with Risperdal (risperidone) 3 mg PO prn (use Haldol instead of risperidone if dementia–related psychosis)

Brief reactive psychosis

- Acute psychosis caused by a marked stressor
- One day to < 1 month
- Treatment same as acute psychosis

Schizophrenia (present for 6 months)

- Same as acute psychosis
- Disorganized speech and behavior, and a flat affect may be present

Treatment

- No acute medication therapy if not dangerous to self or other
- Outpatient antipsychotics and referral

Delusional disorder

- Non-bizarre delusions (jealousy or persecutory)
- Other schizophrenia symptoms not present
- Assess for organic brain syndrome
- Treatment as outpatient

Mood Disorders

Anxiety disorder

- Evaluate for organic cause
- Benzodiazepines useful if symptoms are severe
- Outpatient referral if not dangerous to self or others

Depression

- Evaluate for organic cause
- Consider antidepressant if symptoms are severe

- Outpatient referral if not dangerous to self or others and can care for self

Personality Disorder

- Outpatient referral if not dangerous to self or others and can care for self

Pain Management in Psychiatric Patients

- Treat with analgesics as indicated in limited amounts prn
- Antidepressants for chronic pain prn
- Pain clinic and psychiatric referral prn
- Refer to primary care provider prn

Discharge Criteria

- Cleared by psychiatric evaluation or provider medical evaluation
- Not dangerous to self or others
- Able to care for self or has support systems to care for self
- No suspected organic cause of psychiatric symptoms
- See General Patient Criteria Protocol (page 22)

Discharge instructions

- Respective psychiatric aftercare instructions
- Return if suicidal or homicidal

Consult Criteria

- Agitated patients requiring chemical or physical restraints
- Dangerous to self or others
- Cannot care for self and no support systems
- Organic causes of symptoms
- Delirium
- See General Patient Criteria Protocol (page 22)

Notes

References:

Chemical Restraint Author: Benjamin B Mattingly, MD; Chief Editor: Rick Kulkarni, MD
emedicine.medscape.com/article/109717

Emergent Treatment of Schizophrenia Author: Paul S Gerstein, MD; Chief Editor: Pamela L Dyne, MD
emedicine.medscape.com/article/805988

Depression Author: Jerry L Halverson, MD; Chief Editor: David Bienenfeld, MD
emedicine.medscape.com/article/286759

ALCOHOL INTOXICATED PATIENT PROTOCOL

When using any protocol, always follow the Guidelines of Proper Use (page 18).

Definition

- Blood level over legal limit by State Statute
- Causing impairment of cognition or function

Differential Diagnosis

- Subdural hematoma
- CVA
- Coexisting intoxicating substances
- Meningitis
- Encephalitis
- Delirium
- Withdrawal syndromes
- Hepatic encephalopathy
- Postictal state

Considerations and comorbidities

- Alcohol metabolized around 20–30 mg% per hour regardless of blood concentration (zero order kinetics)
- Neurologic disorders
    - Altered mental status
    - Nystagmus
    - Pupillary dilation
    - Ataxia
- Minor head trauma from
    - Seizures
    - Falls
    - Altercations
    - Assaults
- Increased traumatic brain injury (coagulopathy common)
    - Intracerebral hemorrhage
    - Subdural hematoma

  - Epidural hematoma
- Embolic stroke
  - Atrial fibrillation
- Hemorrhagic stroke
- Alcohol related seizures
  - Withdrawal seizures
  - Usually single
  - Treat with Ativan (lorazepam) 1–4 mg IV Q15–30 minutes prn
  - Occur within 6–12 hours of withdrawal
  - No other anticonvulsant treatment besides Ativan needed usually
  - May continue any existing seizure medication in addition to Ativan
- Increased infections
  - Altered immune system
  - Fever not uniformly present
  - WBC not necessarily increased
- Hypoglycemia
  - Alcoholic ketoacidosis
  - Mild lactic acidosis
- Thiamine deficiency
- Hypomagnesemia
  - Contributes to withdrawal symptoms
  - Can be present despite normal blood levels
- Rhabdomyolysis
  - Complication of chronic alcoholism and binge drinking
  - Impaired gluconeogenesis
  - Compartment syndrome incidence increased

Evaluation

- Complete history and physical examination
- CMP; Magnesium level prn
- Bedside glucose check if hypoglycemia suspected
- CBC — if infection suspected
- U/A — ketosis, infection or rhabdomyolysis if suspected
- CPK if rhabdomyolysis or compartment syndrome suspected

- Blood alcohol level
- LFT's if chronic alcoholic and mental status worse than expected from blood alcohol level
- CT head scan
  - Evidence of head trauma with:
    - Significant headache
    - Nausea
    - Vomiting
    - Evidence of skull fracture
    - Neurologic acute abnormalities
    - Altered mental status changes worse than expected from degree of alcohol intoxication
    - New onset seizure
- Chest x-ray
  - Fever
  - Respiratory finding or complaints
  - O_2 saturation decreased from patient's baseline or < 94%
- Evaluation for other injuries or comorbidities as indicated

Osmolol gap > 10–20 suspect substance ingestion (Normal < 10)

- Gap = Osmolality measured – Osmolality calculated (calculation equation: 2(Na+K) + glucose/18 + BUN/2.8; normal 280–300mOsm/L)
- Ethanol mg%/4.6 is added to osmolol gap equation if present
- Gap > 50 carries high specificity for toxic alcohol such as methanol, ethylene glycol, or isopropyl alcohol
- Normal gap < 10

Treatment Options

- IV D5NS hydration as indicated
- Ativan IV for seizures
- Feed awake patient without acute neurologic deficits
- Thiamine 100 mg IM or slow IV
- MgSO4 (magnesium sulfate) 2 gms IM or IV unless in renal failure
- Appropriate antibiotic treatment

Discharge Criteria

- Clinically sober or blood alcohol < 300 and decreasing, and patient alert and has a ride home and not driving
- Unlikely to acutely decompensate
- Has support system

Discharge instructions

- Alcohol abuse aftercare instructions
- Follow up with PCP or local alcohol treatment center

Consult Criteria

- Fever
- Significant infectious process
- Acute neurologic deficits
- Acute imaging abnormalities
- Poor support system
- Hypoglycemia
- Acute hepatitis
- Mental status changes not attributable to intoxication
- Osmolol gap > 10 if checked
- Alcoholic ketoacidosis
- Metabolic acidosis
- Pneumonia
- Seizure
- Suicidal or dangerous to others
- Refer to General Patient Criteria Protocol (page 22)

Notes

References:

Rathlev NK, et al. Alcohol-related seizures J of Emerg Med 2006; 31:157–163

Morton WA, et al. A prediction model for identifying alcohol withdrawal seizures Am J Drug Alcohol Abuse 1994;20:75–86

Withdrawal Syndromes Author: Nathanael J McKeown, DO;
Chief Editor: Asim Tarabar, MD
emedicine.medscape.com/article/819502

WITHDRAWAL PROTOCOL

When using any protocol, always follow the Guidelines of Proper Use (page 18).

Definition

- Acute systemic manifestations of withdrawal from a substance to which the patient is addicted

Differential Diagnosis

- Subdural hematoma
- CVA
- Coexisting intoxicating substances
- Meningitis
- Encephalitis
- Delirium
- Withdrawal syndromes
- Hepatic encephalopathy
- Postictal state

Considerations for Ethanol Withdrawal

- Mild ethanol withdrawal resolves in 1–2 days
- Need to determine cause of altered mental status in alcoholic patients
- Determine degree of intoxication
- Seizures have increased occurrence
- Postictal state as a cause of altered mental state
- Infection risk increased
- Head trauma incidence increased
- Wernicke's encephalopathy may occur
- Hepatic encephalopathy from chronic alcoholism can be caused by upper gastrointestinal bleeding if hepatic cirrhosis present
- Fluid and electrolyte abnormalities increased incidence

Ethanol Withdrawal Signs and Symptoms

- Tachycardia
- Fever
- Hypertension

- Diaphoresis
- Tremor
- Anxiety
- Agitation
- Seizures
- Hallucinations
- Delirium tremens
- Each successive withdrawal occurrence can have more severe symptoms

Early withdrawal symptoms

- Occurs within hours after alcohol intake reduction
- Can occur without a total cessation of alcohol intake
- Headache
- Insomnia
- Vivid dreams
- Malaise
- Hand tremor
- Hallucinations

Ethanol related seizures

- Can occur from intoxication
- Can occur from ethanol withdrawal
- Lifetime risk is 5–10%
- Withdrawal seizures progress to delirium tremens 30% of the time
- May occur within 7 hours following decreased ethanol intake
- Ativan (lorazepam) seizure prophylaxis may be given as 1–4 mg IV or IM
- Ativan is seizure treatment of choice: 1–6 mg IV prn (NMT 10 mg)
- Dilantin not effective
- Usually there is a single seizure; not focal usually

Delirium tremens

- Severe autonomic dysfunction plus delirium
- Rarely occurs before 48–72 hours of decreased ethanol intake
- Can start magnesium replacement in withdrawal patients with normal or low serum levels

Comorbidities

- Pneumonia
- Pancreatitis
- Hepatitis
- Hepatic cirrhosis
- Intracranial hemorrhage

Wernicke's encephalopathy

- Thiamine deficiency
- Confusion
- Oculomotor abnormalities
- Ataxia
- Korsakoff's psychosis has long term sequelae

Alcoholic ketoacidosis

- Can occur after binge drinking
- Free fatty acids metabolized from adipose tissue as a starvation ketosis
- Suppressed gluconeogenesis and insulin release occurs
- Usually occurs 24–72
- Beta-hydroxybutyrate is most common ketone which is not measured on ketone routine testing
    - Serum ketones may be minimal or negative
    - Acetone is the ketone that is measured in lab

Symptoms and findings

- Nausea and vomiting
- Abdominal pain
- Dehydration
- Confusion
- Tachycardia and tachypnea
- Arterial pH usually > 7.2

Evaluation Options

- Cardiac monitor and O_2 saturation for moderate to severe withdrawal
- Complete history and physical examination
- CMP; magnesium level
- Bedside glucose check
- CBC
- U/A

- CPK
- Blood alcohol level
- LFT's
- CT head scan for
  - Evidence of head trauma with:
    - Headache
    - Nausea
    - Vomiting
    - Evidence of skull fracture
    - Neurologic acute abnormalities
    - New onset seizure
    - Acute altered mental status not attributed to withdrawal
- Chest x-ray
  - Fever
  - Respiratory finding or complaints
  - O_2 saturation decreased from patient's baseline
- Evaluation for other injuries or comorbidities as indicated

Treatment Options

- IV D5NS hydration as indicated (rate 50–250 cc/hr.) if not hypotensive
- IV NS or LR 500–1000 bolus if hypotensive (notify physician immediately)
- Ativan 1–4 mg IV q 15–30 minutes prn for moderate to severe withdrawal symptoms or findings (monitor for respiratory depression)
- Feed awake patient without acute neurologic deficits besides intoxication
- Thiamine 100 mg IM or slow IV
- MgSO4 (magnesium sulfate) 2 gms IM or IV unless in renal failure
- Potassium as needed PO or IV
- Appropriate antibiotic treatment if infection present
- Avoid antipsychotic medications

Discharge Criteria

- Mild withdrawal
- Good social support

- Next day follow-up preferred
- Consider valium 10 mg qid taper by 25% every 2 days for 7–10 days of treatment

Discharge instructions

  - Withdrawal aftercare instructions
  - Return if withdrawal symptoms worsen
  - Referral to addiction program

Consult Criteria

- Symptoms do not respond to 3 doses of benzodiazepines
- Moderate to severe withdrawal
- Alcoholic ketoacidosis
- Vomiting
- Delirium tremens
- Fever
- Pneumonia
- Significant infectious process
- Acute neurologic deficits
- Acute imaging abnormalities
- Poor acute support system
- Hypoglycemia
- Acute hepatitis
- Mental status changes not attributable to intoxication or withdrawal
- Osmolol gap > 10 if checked
- Metabolic acidosis
- Refer to General Patient Criteria Protocol (page 22)

Opioid Withdrawal

- Symptoms
  - Restlessness
  - Dilated pupils
  - Lacrimation
  - Nausea and vomiting
  - Abdominal cramps
  - Diarrhea
  - Muscle cramps
- Mental status remains normal

- Not life threatening except in neonates

Evaluation

- Complete history and physical examination
- CBC optional
- CMP or BMP optional
- U/A optional
- Other testing as indicated by history, examination or findings

Treatment Options

- Supportive
- Clonidine 0.1 mg q8hr for 3–10 days prn withdrawal if not hypotensive
- Consider lorazepam 1–2 mg PO q4–6h prn for 3–5 days
- Loperamide 2 mg PO tid prn diarrhea (NMT 6 qday)
- Rehydration if needed
- Inpatient treatment program if available and patient agreeable

Discharge Criteria

- Stable patient without significant comorbidities
- Support systems available

Discharge instructions

- Withdrawal aftercare instructions
- Return if withdrawal symptoms worsen
- Referral to addiction program

Consult Criteria

- Refer to General Patient Criteria Protocol (page 22)
- Suicidal ideation
- Significant comorbidities

Notes

References:

Rathlev NK, et al. Alcohol-related seizures J of Emerg Med 2006; 31:157–163

Morton WA, et al. A prediction model for identifying alcohol withdrawal seizures Am J Drug Alcohol Abuse 1994;20:75–86

Withdrawal Syndromes Author: Nathanael J McKeown, DO; Chief Editor: Asim Tarabar, MD emedicine.medscape.com/article/819502

SEXUAL ASSAULT PROTOCOL

When using any protocol, always follow the Guidelines of Proper Use (page 18).

Definition

- Defined as carnal knowledge of victim with force or threat against will of patient and varies state to state

Considerations

- Assess for nonsexual injuries
- 5–6% of victims are male
- Preexisting STD rate of victims are higher than the rate of what is acquired from the sexual assault
- Sexual assault exam and evidence collection is up to 72–96 hours post assault
- Notify police
- HIV PEP is indicated in all HIV-negative patients following significant exposure to a substantial-risk bodily fluid
    - Substantial-risk fluid to vagina, rectum, eye, mouth, nonintact skin (including dermatitis), or percutaneously is considered a significant exposure
        - Blood
        - Semen
        - Vaginal secretions
        - Rectal secretions
        - Breast milk
        - Any fluid visibly contaminated with blood
    - Negligible-risk fluids (if not visibly blood) are as follows:
        - Urine
        - Tears
        - Saliva
        - Nasal secretions
        - Sweat
- HIV PEP is recommended only in patients who present to care 72 hours or sooner since the last exposure

Infection and pregnancy risks

- Gonorrhea: 4%
- Chlamydia: 1.5%
- Trichomonas: 12%
- Syphilis: 0.1%
- HIV: 0.1% if assailant HIV positive
- Pregnancy: 1–5%

Evaluation

- Be compassionate
- Evaluate for other injuries
- UCG or serum pregnancy tests in fertile female patients

HIV testing

- Ag/Ab combination (alternative, Ab only) upon presentation and then at 4-6 weeks and 3 months
- Testing at 6 months indicated if patient recently infected with hepatitis C

Hepatitis B testing

- Hepatitis B surface antigen (HBsAg) upon presentation and then at 6 months, if susceptible
- Hepatitis B surface antibody (HBsAb) upon presentation and then at 6 months, if susceptible
- Hepatitis B core antibody (HBcAb) upon presentation and then at 6 months, if susceptible

Hepatitis C testing

- Surface antibody upon presentation and then at 6 months, if susceptible

Other tests, if applicable

- Syphilis serology upon presentation and then at 4-6 weeks and 6 months
- Gonorrhea (nucleic acid amplification) from all exposed sites (genital, pharyngeal, anal)
- Chlamydia (nucleic acid amplification) from all exposed sites (genital, pharyngeal, anal)

Baseline laboratory tests for PEP medications

- Urine human chorionic gonadotropin (HCG), if applicable, upon presentation and then at 4-6 weeks

- Complete blood cell (CBC) count
- Aspartate transaminase (AST) and alanine transaminase (ALT)

Source testing

- HIV Ab/Ag (and quantitative polymerase chain reaction [PCR], if applicable), hepatitis B, hepatitis C, and STI screening as above.
- Individual state laws on source testing have substantial variability, and legal ramifications should be known for each jurisdiction
    - See cdc.gov/hiv/policies/law/states/

PEP is not 100% effective

History

- Date, time and location of event?
- Areas of body involved?
- Number of assailants?
- Is assailant known to victim?
- Weapons, threats, restraints and foreign bodies used?
- Type of sexual acts?
- Did ejaculation occur?
- Was condom used?
- What clean-up occurred by victim: shower, defecation, or douche?
- Were clothes changed?
- Conception prophylaxis used?
- Last menstrual period?
- Date of last consensual sexual intercourse?

Examination

- Performance of "rape kit" by provider or SANE personnel
- Activate SANE nurse program if available to perform "rape kit" and protocols
- Pelvic exam
- Rectal exam
- GC and chlamydial cultures
- RPR
- Hepatitis B testing
- Offer HIV testing

- X-rays as indicated by comorbid trauma
- Document trauma to genital and rectal areas, along with rest of body

Treatment Options

Sexual transmitted disease (STD) prophylaxis options

Antibiotics

- Ceftriaxone 250 mg IM in a single dose

PLUS

- Metronidazole 2 g orally in a single dose

PLUS

- Azithromycin 1 g orally in a single dose OR doxycycline 100 mg orally twice a day for 7 days

- Offer hepatitis B vaccination if none previously; repeat in 1 and 6 months in no history of prior hepatitis B vaccination

Pregnancy prophylaxis if patient agreeable

- Ovral 2 tablets PO now and 2 tablets PO in 12 hours

OR

- Preven 2 tablets PO now and 2 tablets PO in 12 hours

- Offer sexual assault counseling by trained counselor

CDC Postexposure Assessment 2010

- Assess risk for HIV infection in the assailant
- Evaluate characteristics of the assault event that might increase risk for HIV transmission
- Consult with a specialist in HIV treatment, if PEP is being considered
- If the survivor appears to be at risk for HIV transmission from the assault, discuss antiretroviral prophylaxis, including toxicity and lack of proven benefit
- If the survivor chooses to start antiretroviral PEP, provide enough medication to last until the next return visit; reevaluate the survivor 3–7 days

after initial assessment and assess tolerance of medications

- If PEP is started, perform CBC and serum chemistry at baseline (initiation of PEP should not be delayed, pending results)
- Perform HIV antibody test at original assessment; repeat at 6 weeks, 3 months, and 6 months.

Discharge Criteria

- No comorbid conditions needing admission
- Safe home environment or shelter

Discharge instructions

- Sexual assault aftercare instructions
- Refer to primary care provider and counseling resources
- Notify DHS as indicated

Consult Criteria

- Comorbid conditions needing admission
- Refer to General Patient Criteria Protocol (page 22)

Notes

References:

CDC Sexually Transmitted Disease Guidelines, 2010 Sexual Assault and STDs, updated January 28, 2011

Sexual Assault Author: William Ernoehazy Jr, MD, FACEP; Chief Editor: Pamela L Dyne, MD
emedicine.medscape.com/article/806120

Centers for Disease Control and Prevention, 2015 Sexually Transmitted Diseases Treatment Guidelines

HIV Prophylaxis in Sexual Assault Updated: Dec 04, 2018 Author: Derek T Larson, DO; Chief Editor: Michael Stuart Bronze, MD

DOMESTIC VIOLENCE PROTOCOL

When using any protocol, always follow the Guidelines of Proper Use (page 18).

Definition

- Pattern of assaultive or coercive behaviors including physical, sexual, and/or psychological attacks

Considerations

- Intimate partner abuse (IPV) occurs not infrequently in pregnancy
- Economic coercion occurs
- Barriers exist to leaving a relationship — economic; religious; children
- Reported statistic of 7 attempts to leave before actually leaving
- IPV patients often present with injuries — frequently central body or defensive areas (arms and feet used for protection)
- History can be vague and evasive
- Can present with a STD from abuser
- Increased incidence of depression, anxiety and PTSD
- 60% increase in physical disorders
- 4–6 times increase in depression
- Children frequently abused also
- Most dangerous time for the abused is in disclosure of abuse and in attempting to leave relationship

Evaluation

- Evaluation for injuries
- Establish IPV diagnosis
- For emotional disorders

SAFE questions

S – Stress/safety: Do you feel safe in your relationship? What stress do you experience?

A – Afraid/abused: Have you or your children been abused? Have you ever felt afraid in your relationship?

F – Family: Does your family or friends know of your abuse? Can you tell them? Will they help?

E – Emergency plan: Do you have one? Do you have a safe place to go? Enough money available?

Treatment

- Provide safe environment
- Develop a safety plan
- Referral to abuse counseling and shelter
- Provide community IPV/domestic violence resources and contact numbers
- Do not prescribe sedatives (can interfere with ability to flee)

Discharge instructions

- Domestic abuse aftercare instructions

Consult Criteria

- Patients that need admission for injuries
- Patient that need admission for safety
- Suicidal or homicidal ideation
- Refer to Psychiatric Protocol
- Refer to General Patient Criteria Protocol (page 22)

Notes

References:

Domestic Violence Author: Lynn Barkley Burnett, MD, EdD, LLB(c); Chief Editor: Barry E Brenner, MD, PhD, FACEP emedicine.medscape.com/article/805546

CDC Injury Prevention and Control: Intimate Partner Violence updated June 24, 2014
cdc.gov/violenceprevention/intimatepartnerviolence

CHILD ABUSE PROTOCOL

When using any protocol, always follow the Guidelines of Proper Use (page 18).

Definition

- Physical and/or psychological abuse of children, or neglect of children

Considerations

- Types of child abuse
  - Physical
  - Psychological
  - Sexual
  - Neglect
- Bruises most common abuse finding
- Bruises may be in various stages of healing
- Nonambulatory infants rarely bruise themselves
- Inflicted visceral injury usually is of hollow viscera
- Head injury most common cause of mortality
- More common where mother is also abused
- Mother's boyfriend who is not the father is common suspect
- Injuries with no plausible explanation

Head injury symptoms or finding in abused infants (increasing in seriousness)

- Extreme fussiness
- Inconsolable crying
- Irritability
- Lethargy
- Hypotonia
- Poor feeding
- Vomiting
- Tachypnea
- Bradycardia
- Hypothermia
- Seizures
- Gaze preferences
- Unequal pupils

- Unreactive pupils
- Stupor
- Coma
- Death

Shaken baby syndrome

- Usually < 1 year of age
- Retinal hemorrhages commonly present

Triad — some or all may be present

- Subdural or subarachnoid hemorrhage
- Cerebral edema
- Retinal hemorrhages

CT head scan best diagnostic approach for brain injury

Fractures with higher abuse association

- Posterior rib fractures
- Metaphyseal fractures
- Bilateral or multiple fractures
- Multiple fractures in various stages of healing
- Digit fractures
- Scapular fractures
- Complex skull fractures

Evaluation

- Maintain high index of suspicion
- Is directed toward injuries
- CBC
- U/A
- CMP
- Skeletal survey
- CT head if suspected head or brain injury
- Cervical spine protection until cleared by imaging if altered mental status and suspected head injury

Treatment

- Aimed at injuries
- Child protection actions

Disposition

- Discuss with physician

- Contact Child Protective Services or DHS if abuse diagnosed or suspected
- Do not discharge patient until cleared to do so by physician
- Admission if patient safety is in question
- Report to police if a crime has occurred
- Contact primary care physician to discuss case for similar previous concerns and if discharged to arrange close follow up

Notes

References:

CDC Injury Prevention and Control: Child Maltreatment Prevention updated May 23, 2014

cdc.gov/violenceprevention/childmaltreatment

Child Abuse Author: Julia Magana, MD; Chief Editor: Richard G Bachur, MD emedicine.medscape.com/article/800657

ELDER ABUSE PROTOCOL

When using any protocol, always follow the Guidelines of Proper Use (page 18).

Definition

- Pattern of assaultive or coercive behaviors including physical, sexual, psychological attacks

Considerations

- 3% of elderly have been abused
- Increased incidence of cognitive impairment

Signs may include

- Injuries in various stages of healing
- Unexplained injuries
- Delay in seeking treatment
- Injuries inconsistent with history
- Contradictory explanations given by the patient and caregiver
- Laboratory findings indicating under dosage or over dosage of medications
- Bruises, welts, lacerations, rope marks, burns
- STD's
- Dehydration, malnutrition, decubitus ulcers, poor hygiene
- Signs of withdrawal, depression, agitation, or infantile behavior
- Abuser may not leave medical provider alone with patient
- Abuser more concerned about medical bill
- Abuser displays anger or indifference toward patient

Evaluation

- High index of suspicion
- Complete history and physical exam
- Pelvic exam for STD (may need "rape kit")
- Aimed at injuries and home situation
- CBC prn

- CMP prn
- U/A prn
- Drug levels of medications prn
- UDS (urine drug screen) prn
- Blood alcohol prn
- Relevant x-rays
- CT head, abdomen or chest as indicated

Treatment

- Directed toward injuries and comorbidities
- Protection of patient

Disposition

- Discuss with physician
- Contact DHS if abuse diagnosed or suspected
- Do not discharge patient until cleared to do so by physician
- Admission if patient safety is in question
- Report to police if crime occurred

Notes

References:

CDC Injury Prevention and Control: Elder Abuse
cdc.gov/violenceprevention/elderabuse

Elder Abuse Author: Monique I Sellas, MD; Chief Editor: Barry E Brenner, MD, PhD, FACEP
emedicine.medscape.com/article/805727

Environmental

Section Contents

When using any protocol, always follow the Guidelines of Proper Use (page 18).

HEAT ILLNESS PROTOCOL

When using any protocol, always follow the Guidelines of Proper Use (page 18).

Definition

- Heat induced metabolic derangements with possible tissue injury

Differential Diagnosis

- Meningitis
- Encephalitis
- Serotonin syndrome
- Thyroid storm
- Thyrotoxicosis
- Sepsis and septic shock
- Neuroleptic malignant syndrome
- Tetanus
- Delirium
- Delirium tremens
- Heat stroke
- Infection in elderly without sepsis
- Malignant hyperthermia
- Intracerebral hemorrhage
- CVA
- Drugs

Considerations

- Normal temperature range is 97°F–100.4°F or 36.1°C–38°C
- Prior heat illness increases risk of developing future heat illness

Excessive heat causes damage to multiple organ systems

- Heart
- Liver
- Kidneys
- Lungs

- Muscles
- Central nervous system

Heat regulation mainly by

- Radiation
- Evaporation
- Conduction
- Convection

Risk Factors for Heat illness

Age

- Elderly
- Neonates

Medical Illness

- Alcoholism
- Hyperthyroidism
- Obesity

Medications

- Anticholinergics
- Beta–blockers
- Diuretics
- MOA inhibitors
- Phenothiazines
- Tricyclic antidepressants

Illicit drugs

- Amphetamines
- Cocaine

Social

- Bedridden
- Living alone
- Lack of air conditioning
- Unable to care for self

Mild Forms of Heat illness

Heat edema

- Swollen hands and feet after prolonged sitting/standing in hot temperatures

Heat rash ("prickly heat")

- Sweat glands become blocked

Heat cramps

- Electrolyte imbalance; volume depletion; hyperventilation
- May be hyponatremic and hypochloremic
- No rhabdomyolysis

Heat tetany

- Carpopedal spasm from hyperventilation secondary to hyperthermia

Heat syncope

- Benign syncope from prolonged standing in hot environment

Severe Forms of Heat illness

Heat exhaustion

- Water or salt depletion
- Fatigue
- Weakness
- Hyperventilation
- Headache
- Dizziness
- Vertigo
- Nausea
- Vomiting
- Muscle cramps
- No CNS dysfunction
- Temperature usually < 104°F (40°C)
- Sweating present

Heat stroke

- Hyperthermia with CNS dysfunction:
    - Confusion
    - Delirium
    - Ataxia
    - Seizures
    - Coma
- Temperature usually > 104.5°F (40.5°C)

- May or may not have sweating present
- Mortality 30–80%
- Fatigue
- Weakness
- Hyperventilation
- Headache
- Dizziness
- Vertigo
- Nausea
- Vomiting
- Muscle cramps
- Rhabdomyolysis
- Compartment syndrome
- Multi-organ dysfunction
- Lactic acidosis

Evaluation

Heat illness excluding heat stroke

- CBC prn
- BMP prn
- U/A in elderly; diabetics; immunocompromised

Heat stroke

- CBC
- BMP
- LFT's
- Lactic acid level
- CPK
- Chest x-ray
- EKG

Treatment

Mild forms of heat illness

- Oral or IV rehydration and sodium replacement

Heat exhaustion

- Remove from hot environment
- No antipyretic medication (may impair heat dissipation)

Rapid cooling as needed

- Remove clothing
- Ice packs to axilla, groin and/or behind neck all prn
- Spray with tepid water and fanned prn
- IV NS or LR rehydration prn

Heat stroke

- Remove from hot environment
- No antipyretic medication (may impair heat dissipation)
- Place foley

Rapid cooling

- Remove clothing
- Ice packs to axilla; groin; behind neck
- Spray with tepid water and fanned (lower temperature to 38.3°C (101°F) to avoid overshoot
- Ativan or valium to control shivering, treat seizures and sedate patient prn
- IV NS or LR rehydration
    - NS 500–1000 cc bolus if hypotensive in adults
    - NS 20 cc/kg bolus if hypotensive in children
        - Avoid too rapid IV NS replacement — may cause cerebral edema (free water deficit corrected over 48 hours)
    - Water deficit in liters = Total body water [0.6 × Kg] – Total body water [desired Na^+ / measured Na^+] (For hypernatremia patients)
    - Free water deficit should be replaced slowly over 48 hours

Discharge Criteria

- All heat illness patients without heat stroke or severe heat exhaustion with good response to therapy
- Not hypotensive
- Refer to General Patient Criteria Protocol

Discharge instructions

- Heat illness aftercare instructions
- Return if symptoms worsen

Consult Criteria

- Heat stroke
- Severe heat exhaustion
- Significant electrolyte disturbances
- Refer to General Patient Criteria Protocol (page 22)
- Age ≥ 70 years

Notes

References: Inter-Association Task Force on Exertional Heat Illness. Consensus Statement 2002. (Guidelines)

Heatstroke Author: Robert S Helman, MD; Chief Editor: Joe Alcock, MD, MS emedicine.medscape.com/article/166320

Environmental Emergencies: Heat Illness in Emergency Medicine David A. Townes, MD, MPH, FACEP emedhome.com/features

cdc.gov/niosh/mining/userfiles/work/pdf/2017-125.pdf

HYPOTHERMIA PROTOCOL

When using any protocol, always follow the Guidelines of Proper Use (page 18).

Definition

- Pathologic state in which core body temperature falls below 35°C (95°F)

Differential Diagnosis

- Cerebrovascular accident
- Toxicity
- Alcohols
- Barbiturates
- Benzodiazepines
- Carbon monoxide
- Narcotics
- Ethylene glycol
- Gamma-hydroxybutyrate
- Sedative hypnotics

Considerations

- Core temperature regulated in thermoneutral zone of 36.5°C and 37.5°C (97.7°F and 99.5°F)
- Heat production is a function of metabolism
- Hypothermia affects all organ systems
- Afterdrop in core temperature can occur after rewarming started due to peripheral cold blood return perfusing the body
- Most hypothermia patients will by dehydrated

Heat loss occurs by

- Radiation – most rapid (50% of heat loss)
- Conduction
- Convection
- Evaporation

Hypothermia severity

- Mild = 32–35°C or 89.6–95°F
- Moderate = 28–32°C or 82.4–89.6°F

- Severe = 20–28°C or 68–82.4°F
- Profound < 20°C or 68°F

Risk Factors

- Burns
- Environmental cold exposure or immersion
- Toxicological causes
- Extremes of age
- Hypoadrenalism
- Hypothyroidism
- Hypoglycemia
- Hypopituitarism
- Malnutrition
- Spinal cord injury
- Sepsis
- Uremia

Findings as Temperatures Decrease

Mild hypothermia progression

- Shivering, impaired judgment, confusion
- Tachycardia, tachypnea, cold diuresis
- Bradycardia, respiratory depression, hyperglycemia, ataxia, dysarthria

Moderate hypothermia progression

- Stupor, lethargy, arrest of shivering
- Atrial arrhythmias, Osborn J-waves on EKG (upward deflection of terminal S wave), increased bradycardia
- Insulin ineffective, decreased oxygen utilization
- Progressive decreased level of consciousness, bradycardia, and respiratory rate

Severe hypothermia progression

- Ventricular fibrillation susceptibility increased
- Pulse decreased by 50%
- Oxygen consumption decreased by 50%
- Loss of reflexes and voluntary movement
- Acid-base abnormalities
- No pain response

- Decreased cerebral perfusion by 2/3
- Pulmonary edema
- Apnea
- Hypotension

Profound hypothermia progression

- Lowest level for resumption of cardiac activity, pulse 20% of normal
- Asystole

Evaluation

- Complete history and physical examination (auscultate up to 60 seconds if needed)
- CBC
- BMP
- Chest x-ray
- EKG
- ABG (temperature correction not needed)
- PT/PTT/INR (coagulation panel)
- CPK
- Blood alcohol and toxicology panel as indicated
- Cardiac, oxygen saturation and vital sign monitoring

Treatment Considerations and Options

- IV fluid resuscitation as needed with NS or D5NS (avoid lactated ringer's solution)
    - Do not give D5 IV containing fluids as a bolus (too high tonicity)
- Immunocompromised patients should receive empiric antibiotics
- Intubation as needed
- NG tube if intubated
- Most cardiac dysrhythmias correct with rewarming alone
- Malignant ventricular dysrhythmias use amiodarone (avoid lidocaine and procainamide)
- Defibrillation likely ineffective with core temperature < 30°C (86°F)

Passive rewarming

- Increases temperature 0.3–1.2°C/hour

- For mild hypothermia where shivering is present and patient is healthy
- No external heat added
- Patient covered with blankets
- Remove wet garments
- Cover patient's head except face

Active external rewarming

- Increases temperature 0.3–1.2°C/hour
- For mild hypothermia with impaired thermogenesis due to illness, intoxication, medications or comorbidities
- For moderate hypothermia
- Forced warmed air systems used
- Warmed blankets
- Heat packs
- Heat lamps

Active core rewarming

- Increases temperature approximately 3°C/hour
- For severe hypothermia
- Warmed IV fluids (44°C or 111°F) — warm 1 liter for approximately 2 minutes in microwave
- Warmed humidified air or oxygen in addition to passive and active external rewarming

Extracorporeal rewarming

- Increases temperature approximately 1–18°C/hour
- Indicated for severe or profound hypothermia
- Hypothermia unresponsive to other rewarming methods
- Completely frozen extremities
- For no signs of perfusion
- Hemodialysis (can increase temperature 1–4°C/hour)
- Cardiopulmonary bypass (can increase temperature 18°C/hour)

Discharge Criteria

- Mild hypothermia that responds to passive rewarming in healthy patient

Discharge instructions

- Hypothermia aftercare instructions

Consult Criteria

- Discuss all hypothermia patients with physician

Admission Criteria

- Hypothermia < 32°C or 89.6°F

Notes

References:

N Engl J Med 2012;367(20):1930–8 Accidental Hypothermia Douglas J.A. Brown, M.D., Hermann Brugger, M.D., Jeff Boyd, M.B., B.S., and Peter Paal, M.D.

emedicine.medscape.com/article/770542

Frostbite and Exposure Skin Injury Protocol

When using any protocol, always follow the Guidelines of Proper Use (page 18).

Definition

- Cold related injury or death of tissue from freezing secondary to prolonged cold exposure

Differential Diagnosis

- Hypothermia
- Frostnip
- Trench foot
- Pernio
- Chilblains (3–6 hours of cold moist exposure without freezing)

Frostbite

Considerations

- Extremities, head, and nose most commonly affected
- Initial appearance of injury often fails to predict depth or eventual outcome

Degrees of Injury

First-degree injury

- Erythema, edema, waxy appearance, hard white plaques, and loss of sensation

Second-degree injury

- Erythema, edema, and formation of blisters filled with clear or milky fluid
- Form within 24 hours of injury

Third-degree injury

- Blood-filled blisters
- Progressing to a black eschar in several weeks

Fourth-degree injury

- Full-thickness damage affecting muscles, tendons, and bone, with necrosis of tissue

Evaluation

- Assess for hypothermia
- No lab needed in mild cases
- Assess for severe frostbite
  - CBC
  - CMP
  - U/A for evidence of myoglobin
  - CPK
  - Cultures if infection suspected
  - Technetium-99 scintigraphy 2–7 days after injury is helpful in decision making about amputation

Treatment

- Remove wet clothing
- Ibuprofen 400 mg PO prior to rewarming to improve tissue salvage
- Protect from refreezing
- Rapid rewarming for more severe cases
- Put affected area in warm water (40–42°C or 104–108°F) for 20–30 minutes
- Elevate extremity after rewarming
- Separate damaged digits with dry gauze
- Apply aloe vera (without alcohol, salicylates or other additives) after thawing
  - May be used for debridement also
- Tetanus prophylaxis (see Tetanus Protocol)
- Antibiotics not indicated unless infection present
- Liberal use of analgesics up to 7–10 days
- Leave hemorrhagic blisters intact
- Debride clear fluid filled blisters
- Physical therapy post discharge or admission
- Avoid massaging frostbite area (may increase injury)
- Splinting prn
- Cycloplegia, artificial tears and eyelid closure with dressing for corneal cold injury

Discharge Criteria

- First degree injury

Discharge instructions

  - Frostbite aftercare instructions

Consult Criteria

- Second, third and fourth degree frostbite injuries

Admission Criteria

- Greater than first degree frostbite
- Risk of refreezing exists

Non-freezing Environmental Injuries

Trench foot

- Non-freezing injury from prolonged exposure to cold, wet environment
- May cause gangrene
- Rewarm in water if needed
- Elevate to reduce edema
- Keep warm and dry
- Ibuprofen prn
- Tetanus prophylaxis (see Tetanus Protocol)

Pernio

- 12–hour to 3–day exposure to cold moist environment without freezing
- Scaling skin and edema
- Cyanotic and red skin lesions
  - Occasionally deep seated
- Use protective clothing for prevention and emollient creams for treatment
- Tetanus prophylaxis (see Tetanus Protocol)

Chilblains

- 3–6 hours of cold moist exposure without freezing
- Chronic form from recurrent Pernio
- Swelling, tender SQ vesicles with or without bluish discoloration
- Hemorrhagic bullae and skin ulcers in severe cases
- Gently rewarm, dress with dry protective bandages

- Tetanus prophylaxis (see Tetanus Protocol)

Frostnip

- Superficial and reversible ice crystal formation without tissue destruction
- Transient numbness and paresthesia that resolves after rewarming

Disposition

- Discuss with physician trench foot, Pernio and chilblains patients

Discharge instructions

- Respective cold or moisture environment aftercare instructions

Notes

References:

Cold Injuries Author: Richard F Edlich, MD, PhD, FACS, FASPS, FACEP; Chief Editor: Lars M Vistnes, MD, FRCSC, FACS emedicine.medscape.com/article/1278523

Frostbite Author: C Crawford Mechem, MD, MS, FACEP; Chief Editor: Dirk M Elston, MD emedicine.medscape.com/article/926249

ALTITUDE ILLNESS PROTOCOL

When using any protocol, always follow the Guidelines of Proper Use (page 18).

Definition

- Syndromes resulting from lack of oxygen

Differential Diagnosis

- Anxiety
- Encephalitis
- Diabetic ketoacidosis
- Meningitis
- Migraine
- Hyponatremia
- Hypoglycemia
- Hypothermia
- Cerebrovascular accident
- Transient ischemic attack
- Transient global amnesia
- Subarachnoid hemorrhage
- Subdural hemorrhage
- Carbon monoxide poisoning
- Reyes syndrome
- Nonspecific headache
- Brain tumors
- Dehydration
- Viral syndrome

Syndromes

- Acute mountain sickness (AMS)
- High-altitude cerebral edema (HAPE)
- High-altitude pulmonary edema (HACE)

Considerations

Hypoxia is primary insult

- Degree of injury dependent on rate of hypoxia onset and magnitude

- Increase minute ventilation occurs acutely with a resultant respiratory alkalosis
- Renal compensation to respiratory alkalosis occurs more slowly than compensation to respiratory acidosis
- Increased cerebral perfusion occurs
- Symptoms occur 4–10 hours after ascent
- Incidence affected by sleeping altitude
- Physical fitness not protective
- Occurs more commonly in age < 50 years

Acute Mountain Sickness (AMS)

Definition

Headache plus one of following:

- Nausea/vomiting
- Fatigue
- Dizziness
- Insomnia

Considerations

- Mild form of high altitude illness
- Generally benign
- Occurs around 6,000 feet altitude or higher with incidence of 10–40%, increasing as altitude increases
- Usually self-limited and improves over 1–3 days if no further ascent is undertaken
- Continued ascent will worsen AMS and can result in HACE
- O_2 saturation not helpful in diagnosing or managing AMS or HACE

Findings and symptoms

- Patients appear ill
- Normal neurologic examination
- Heart rate and blood pressure can vary
- May have rales, but oxygen saturation normal or near normal
- Fever is absent
- May have retinal hemorrhages
- Peripheral edema may be present

Treatment options

- Halt ascent
- Acetazolamide 250 mg PO q12hr
  - Prophylaxis — 125 mg PO q12hr starting 24 hours before ascent and continuing during ascent to at least 48 hours after arrival at highest altitude (or descent)
- Dexamethasone 4 mg PO/IM q6hr for treatment and prophylaxis (not more than 10 days)
- Ibuprofen or Tylenol for headache
- Phenergan (promethazine) prn for nausea
- Oxygen for more severe cases (4L/min to keep O_2 saturation > 92%)
- Descent for more severe symptoms

Discharge criteria

- Usually discharged

Discharge instructions

- Acute mountain sickness aftercare instructions

Consult criteria

- Discuss high altitude illness with physician

High-altitude Cerebral Edema (HACE)

Definition

- Acute Mountain Sickness with gait ataxia and altered mental status

Considerations

- Usually normal exam except for gait ataxia
- Focal neurologic deficits rare
- Continued ascent with AMS can lead to HACE
- Papilledema can occur
- Retinal hemorrhages occur
- Coma can occur

Evaluation options

- CBC
- BMP
- ABG
- CT brain

- MRI brain

Treatment

- Immediate evacuation to lower altitude
- Oxygen 4L/min to keep O_2 saturation > 92%
- Dexamethasone 8 mg PO/IM, followed by 4 mg PO/IM q6hr
- Elevate head of bed 30 degrees

Discharge criteria

- Dependent on severity

Discharge instructions

- High-altitude cerebral edema aftercare instructions if discharged

Consult criteria

- Discuss with physician

High-altitude Pulmonary Edema

Definition

- Noncardiogenic pulmonary edema from increased capillary hydrostatic pressure and pulmonary hypertension

Considerations

- Exercise at high altitude increases risk
- Fever common
- Orthopnea common
- Frothy pink sputum is a late finding
- Cyanosis can occur
- May occur with HACE

History and physical examination criteria

2 of the following:

- Weakness or decreased exercise tolerance
- Cough
- Dyspnea at rest
- Chest tightness or congestion

PLUS

2 of the following:

- Rales or wheezing

- Central cyanosis or O_2 saturation is lower than expected from elevation
- Tachycardia
- Tachypnea

Evaluation

- Chest x-ray
- Ultrasound of lungs show comet tail artifacts B–lines)
- CBC
- BMP
- BNP
- EKG
- Troponin

Treatment options

- Oxygen 6–8 liters by mask until improved then 4L/min to keep O_2 saturation > 92%
- Albuterol aerosol prn
- Immediate descent
- Bed rest
- Nifedipine 10 mg PO q6hr if oxygen not available and not hypotensive
- Cialis (tadalafil) 10 mg bid to decrease pulmonary hypertension
- Dexamethasone 8−10 mg PO/IM/IV initially then 4 mg PO/IM/IV q4hr
- Narcotic or non-narcotic cough suppressants prn
- Phenergan (promethazine) prn nausea or vomiting, and may increase respiratory stimulation

Discharge criteria

- Normal O_2 saturation (≥ 95%) breathing room air
- Significant clinical improvement
- No dyspnea at rest

Discharge instructions

- High-altitude Pulmonary Edema aftercare instructions

Admission criteria

- O_2 saturation < 95%
- Dyspnea at rest

- Inability to descend

Consult criteria

- Discuss all HAPE and high altitude illness patients with physician

Notes

References:

Altitude-Related Disorders Author: Rahul M Kale, MD, FCCP; Chief Editor: Ryland P Byrd Jr, MD
emedicine.medscape.com/article/303571

Milledge JS, Beeley JM, Broome J, Luff N, Pelling M, Smith D. Acute Mountain Sickness Susceptibility, Fitness and Hypoxic Ventilatory Response. Eur Respir J 1991;4:1000–3

NEAR DROWNING PROTOCOL

When using any protocol, always follow the Guidelines of Proper Use (page 18).

Definition

- Survival from a submersion occurring within the past 24 hours of sufficient submersion duration to warrant medical attention or survival beyond 24 hours of a submersion

Differential Diagnosis

- Child abuse
- Child neglect
- Suicide attempt
- Hypothermia
- Seizure
- Drug or toxin ingestion
- Hypoglycemia
- Head and neck trauma

Considerations

- Classified either cold water (< 20°C or 68°F) or warm water (≥ 20°C or 68°F) injury
- Very cold water injury is with water temperature ≤ 5°C (41°F)
- Most patients have an aspiration of water < 4 cc/kg
- Blood imbalances occur with aspiration > 11 cc/kg
- Electrolyte imbalances occur with aspiration > 22 cc/kg
- PO ingestion more likely to cause electrolyte imbalances
- Primary injury is hypoxemia
- Survival mainly determined by amount of brain hypoxemia and injury
- Laryngospasm can prevent aspiration
- Heimlich maneuver not effective in removing aspiration water
- Differences between freshwater and salt water submersions not clinically significant

Orlowski score — 1 point for each item

- Age 3 years or older
- Submersion time of more than 5 minutes
- No resuscitative efforts for more than 10 minutes after rescue
- Comatose on admission to the emergency department
- Arterial pH of less than 7.10
- Score of 2 or less = 90% complete recovery
- Score of 3 or more = 5% survival

History of event includes

- Submersion time
- Water temperature
- Symptoms
- Associated injuries
- Type of rescue
- Response to treatment
- Cough or shortness of breath
- Concomitant drug or alcohol use
- Past medical history (seizures, cardiac, diabetes, etc.)

Physical findings categories

- Asymptomatic
- Symptomatic
    - Abnormal vital signs
    - Dyspnea
    - Neurologic deficit
    - Altered level of consciousness
    - Anxiety
- Cardiopulmonary arrest
- Expired

Evaluation Options Depending on Severity of Presentation

- Remove wet clothing
- Chest x-ray – all patients
- O_2 saturation – all patients
- ABG

- CBC
- BMP
- LFT's
- U/A
- PT/PTT/INR
- Fibrinogen, D-dimer, fibrin split products
- Troponin useful in severe presentations for prognosis
- Toxicology as indicated
- C-spine imaging as indicated
- CT head as indicated for trauma or altered mental status
- Evaluate for associated injuries
- Core temperature
- Cardiac and O_2 saturation continuous monitoring prn

Treatment Options

- Notify physician immediately for altered mental status, neurologic abnormalities, hypoxia or hypotension
- Oxygen up to 100% FiO_2 depending on symptoms and findings
- Albuterol inhalations prn
- Correct any hypothermia (see Hypothermia Protocol)
- IV NS prn hypotension
- Vasopressors prn hypotension
- Intubation prn severe respiratory distress
- Extracorporeal cardiopulmonary resuscitation after active chest compressions may improve survival
- Steroids are of no benefit
- Hypothermia patients should be resuscitated while aggressive attempts to restore normal body temperature ensue
- Antibiotics can be given for submersion in sewage or contaminated water

Discharge Criteria

- Patients with normal examination, normal vital signs and normal chest x-ray and lab, and trivial history may be discharged after 6 hours observation
- Immersion history with mild symptoms, normal lab and chest x-ray, may be discharged after 6–12 hours of observation

Discharge instructions

- Near drowning aftercare instructions
- All discharged patients should be rechecked in 24–48 hours
- Return or see primary care provider promptly if cough, fever or shortness of breath occurs

Admission Criteria

- Hypoxia
- Acute neurologic findings
- Symptomatic patients
- Acute chest x-ray findings
- Prolonged submersion history

Consult Criteria

- Discuss all near drowning patients with physician

Notes

References:

Topjian AA, Berg RA, Nadkarni VM. Pediatric cardiopulmonary resuscitation: Advances in science, techniques, and outcomes. Pediatrics. 2008;122:1086–1098

Prognostic factors in pediatric cases of drowning and near-drowning. Orlowski JP JACEP 1979 May;8(5):176–9

Drowning Author: G Patricia Cantwell, MD, FCCM; Chief Editor: Joe Alcock, MD MS emedicine.medscape.com/article/772753

Medications

Section Contents

When using any protocol, always follow the Guidelines of Proper Use (page 18).

PAIN MANAGEMENT PROTOCOL

When using any protocol, always follow the Guidelines of Proper Use (page 18).

Considerations

- Pain is the most frequent complaint for seeking care in the emergency department or acute care settings
- Many studies have demonstrated the under-treatment of pain by Providers
- Abuse of prescription narcotics has increased in the recent past
- Under-treatment of pain can lead to pseudoaddiction — a condition where the patient actively seeks, over time, pain control
    - This is frequently perceived by Providers as drug seeking behavior
- JCAHO has standards regarding pain assessment and the right of the patient to adequate control of pain
    - This can cause the perception that the policy contributes to abuse of narcotic prescriptions
- Chronic pain is not managed well in the acute care settings
- Degree of chronic pain is not always reflected in the Provider's observation of the patient's degree of discomfort or in abnormal vital signs
    - Acute pain is reflected more so in patient's signs of discomfort and abnormal vital signs

Analgesic medication facts

- Analgesics do not alter the ability to diagnose the cause of undifferentiated abdominal pain, and they may even improve diagnostic accuracy
- Antiemetics do not enhance the analgesic effects of opioids at the commonly used doses
- There is no evidence that any NSAID provides any better analgesia than another. The analgesic effect from ketorolac is similar to other NSAIDs
- Ibuprofen 600 mg plus acetaminophen 1,000 mg has better pain relief than hydrocodone 5 mg
- Codeine has limited utility due to its low potency and frequent side effects

  - **Addiction or abuse potential significantly increases if opioids prescribed more than 3 days in opioid naïve patients**
  - It is more effective to give pain medication on a regular dosing schedule rather than waiting for the pain to be uncontrolled
  - The effective dose of Demerol can vary widely, and most patients will require at least 1.5 mg/kg
  - The increase in intrabiliary pressure is similar with meperidine and morphine. More importantly, it is of no clinical significance
  - Opioid analgesics can be an important part of pain management in patients with chronic or recurrent pain syndromes
  - When narcotics are prescribed in short courses to treat acute pain, iatrogenic addiction is rare (3 days or less is best)
  - In most studies, the analgesic effect of tramadol is equivalent or only slightly better than placebo

Evaluation

- Urine and serum drug screens are not particular routinely useful in evaluating patients
  - Drug screens may be useful if patient states they have not used controlled substances for the past 10 days to determine patient truthfulness
  - Drug screens may be useful if patient states they are taking prescription narcotics currently and the drug screen is negative, perhaps indicating that they are selling the narcotics
- If a pattern of abuse is suspected, check controlled substance prescription databases where available
- Take a history of pain treatment
- Patients who request a specific controlled substance may be more suspect for abuse behavior

Treatment Options

- Patients with chronic pain that come to the emergency department or urgent care setting should be tactfully informed that chronic pain is best managed long term by one Provider in the clinic setting
- If the Provider assesses a reasonable need to prescribe controlled pain medications, it should be of a

short course and limited number of pills (≤ 12) without refills usually
  - Exceptions are situations where a terminal cancer patient or other similar type patients with significant pain considerations that will have a delay in treatment in the outpatient office setting
- Pain amenable to local injections, such as dental pain etc., in patients with frequent repeat visits, can be treated with Marcaine (bupivacaine) local blocks depending on skill level of Provider and referred to an outpatient settings for further care
- It is appropriate to express concern for the patient's dependence on controlled substances where the Provider feels it may be productive
- There are situations where a noncontrolled substance is more effective, such as in migraine therapy, and it should be used instead
- It may be necessary to decline controlled substance treatment of pain in patients with a history of troublesome behavior of controlled substance use where appropriate
- Effective chronic pain treatment decreases visits, use of resources, improves patient care and improves patient satisfaction
- Antiemetic medication should not be used routinely with PO narcotics

Disposition

- Refer chronic pain or frequent recurrent pain patients to their primary care provider
- Referral to a Pain Clinic is appropriate in many situations
- Short courses of controlled pain medications with limited amount of pills and no refills is encouraged depending on the clinical situation
- Chronic or acute pain aftercare instructions

Notes

References:

Hooten WM, Timming R, Belgrade M, Gaul J, Goertz M, Haake B, Myers C, Noonan MP, Owens J, Saeger L, Schweim K, Shteyman G, Walker N. Assessment and management of chronic pain. Bloomington (MN): Institute for Clinical Systems Improvement (ICSI); 2013 Nov. 105

Glazier HS. Potentiation of pain relief with hydroxyzine: A therapeutic myth? Ann Pharmacother 1990;24:484–488

Pain Management In The ED: Prompt, Cost-Effective, State-Of-The-Art Strategies Michael A. Turturro, MD, FACEP

DRUG INTERACTIONS

When using any protocol, always follow the Guidelines of Proper Use (page 18).

Considerations

- Geriatric patients have a 20–30% hospitalization rate from drug effects or interactions
- Drug interactions diagnosed 25% of the time

QT Interval Prolongation

Symptoms that may occur *(not very common)*

- Syncope
- Sudden death

Drug causes

Antipsychotics	**Antiarrhythmics**	**Antibiotics**	**Antidepressants**
Pimozide	Amiodarone	Macrolides	Tricyclics
Olanzapine	Quinidine	Fluoroquinolones	Trazodone
Ziprasidone	**Antiemetics (additive)**		
Haldol	Promethazine		
Droperidol	Zofran (ondansetron)		
	Reglan (metoclopramide)		

Digoxin (digitalis) Levels

Increased by

- NSAID's
- Verapamil
- Quinidine
- Amiodarone

CYP2C9 Cytochrome Inhibition Drugs that Increase Warfarin, Sulfonylureas, Dilantin Effects or Levels

- Septra (trimethoprim/sulfamethoxazole)
- COX-II inhibitors
- Aspirin; salicylates

- ACE inhibitors
- Macrolides
- Phenobarbital
- Isoniazid
- SSRI's
- Amiodarone
- Prilosec
- Cimetidine

Serotonin Syndrome

- Caused by 2 serotonergic drug's interaction

Drugs

- Amitriptyline — Demerol (meperidine) — SSRI's
- Citalopram — Tramadol — Amphetamine
- Anafranil — Effexor — Buspar
- Robitussin — Nardil — Most antidepressants
- Fenfluramine — MAO inhibitors
- Prozac — Zoloft

Signs and symptoms

Cognitive abnormalities	Autonomic dysfunction	Neuromuscular
Confusion	Hyperthermia	Myoclonus
Agitation	Diaphoresis	Hyperreflexia
Coma	Sinus tachycardia	Rigidity
Anxiety	Hypertension	Tremor
Lethargy	Tachypnea	Hyperactivity
Seizures	Dilated pupil	Ataxia

Evaluation

- CBC
- BMP
- CPK

Treatment

- Discontinue offending drugs
- Periactin 4–8 mg PO initially prn; 4 mg PO qid prn
- Ativan or valium prn

Consult criteria

- All suspected serotonin syndromes

Notes

Reference:

Important Drug-Drug Interactions For The Emergency Physician, Gerald Maloney, DO, emedhome.com/features

Disease Management

Section Contents

When using any protocol, always follow the Guidelines of Proper Use (page 18).

Hypertension Management

When using any management guideline, always follow the Guidelines of Proper Use (page 18).

Definitions (JNC 7)

- In adults ≥ 18 years of age, hypertension classifications are the following with 2 or more averaged seated BP measurements over 2 or more office visits (initial BP may be elevated due to anxiety)
  - Normal
    - SBP < 120 mm Hg
    - DBP < 80 mm Hg
  - Prehypertension
    - SBP 120–139 mm Hg
    - DBP 80–89 mm Hg
    - Some controversy exists if this label should be given to patients without diabetic, cardiac or stroke histories
  - Stage 1 hypertension
    - SBP 140–159 mm Hg
    - DBP 90–99 mm Hg
  - Stage 2 hypertension
    - SBP ≥ 160 mm Hg
    - DBP ≥ 100 mm Hg

Considerations

- SBP > 140 mm Hg in age > 50 years is more important cardiovascular disease (CVD) risk factor than diastolic pressure
- Risk doubles for CVD for each SBP/DBP increase of 20/10 mm Hg starting at 115/75 mm Hg blood pressure (BP)
- Thiazide diuretics should be used initially or in combination with other antihypertensive medications in uncomplicated hypertension
- Most patients will require 2 or more antihypertensive medications to achieve target blood pressure of < 140/90 mm Hg in patients without diabetes or chronic kidney disease

- If blood pressure is > 20/10 mm Hg over target BP, consideration should be given to initiating 2 antihypertensive drugs, one of which should be a thiazide diuretic usually
- Clinician's judgment remains paramount in using guidelines
- Self-measured averaged blood pressures at home > 135/85 mm Hg are considered hypertensive

High risk conditions that have indications for initiation of other antihypertensive medications besides a diuretic

- Heart failure
- Postmyocardial infarction
- High coronary disease risk
- Diabetes
- Chronic kidney disease
- Recurrent stroke prevention in patients with history of stroke

Evaluation

- U/A
- CBC
- BMP and calcium level
- EKG
- Lipid profile
- Bilateral arm blood pressures
- Optic fundus examination
- Body mass index (BMI) calculation
- Auscultation for carotid, abdominal and femoral bruits
- Thyroid gland palpation
- Heart and lung examination
- Abdominal examination for masses and abdominal aortic pulsation
- Check legs for edema and arterial pulses
- Neurologic examination

JNC 8 Goals of Therapy

- Age < 60 years initiate treatment for a SBP ≥ 140 mm Hg or DBP ≥ 90 mm Hg to achieve a target SBP of <

140 mm Hg and DBP < 90 mm Hg in patients without diabetes or chronic kidney disease

- Age ≥ 60 years treat SBP ≥ 150 mm Hg or DBP ≥ 90 mm Hg to achieve SBP < 150 mm Hg and DBP < 90 mm Hg
  - If SBP < 140 mm Hg is well tolerated and without adverse effects on quality of life, then medications do not need to be adjusted
- Age ≥ 18 years with diabetes or chronic kidney disease (CKD), initiate treatment if SBP ≥ 140 mm Hg DBP ≥ 90 mm Hg to achieve SBP < 140 mm Hg and DBP < 90 mm Hg
- General nonblack population initiate treatment with either a thiazide diuretic, CCB, ACEI or ARB
- General black population
  - Initial therapy with either a thiazide diuretic or CCB
    - More effective than beta-blockers, ACEIs or ARBs
  - ACEI induced angioedema occurs 2–4 times more frequent than in other groups
    - Treat with FFP (fresh frozen plasma) if needed
- Age ≥ 18 years with CKD, initial or add-on therapy should include an ACEI or ARB
  - Improves kidney outcomes
- If blood pressure goal cannot be achieved in 1 month, increase or add a second drug from the list of thiazide diuretic, CCB, ACEI or ARB. If blood pressure control cannot be achieved with 2 drugs from the above list, add and titrate a third drug. If 3 drugs do not control blood pressure, a drug from another class can be added. Do not use an ACEI with an ARB

American Heart Association (AHA) 2017 Guidelines

- New targets for treatment: These recommend reductions in blood pressure <130/80 mm Hg in most adults (down from 140/90 mm Hg).
- Stage 1 hypertension adults with an average systolic pressure of 130 to 139/80 to 89 mm Hg (these

patients would have previously been considered as having "prehypertension").

- Atherosclerotic risk estimation to guide decisions in stage 1 hypertension: For patients at low atherosclerotic risk (10-year risk <10%), lifestyle changes alone are recommended, whereas for patients at high risk (including those with diabetes and kidney disease), lifestyle changes plus drug therapy is advised.
- Stage 2 classification: Patients with average systolic pressure >140 mm Hg or diastolic > 90 mm Hg
  - As before, drug therapy is recommended for all these patients irrespective of atherosclerotic risk
- Older adults have the same treatment target as younger patients, and drug therapy is recommended for all older adults (age >65 years) with an average systolic pressure of 130 mm Hg or greater
- Most adults with blood pressure sufficiently elevated to warrant drug therapy should be treated initially with two agents, especially patients who are black or have stage 2 hypertension.
- More accurate estimation of blood pressure: Use average of measures taken over several visits, as well as out-of-office measurements

Treatment Options without High Risk Conditions

Prehypertension

- Lifestyle modification with
  - Weight loss diet rich in potassium and calcium (DASH eating plan)
  - 2400 mg sodium diet
  - Increased physical activity
  - Moderation of alcohol consumption

Stage 1 hypertension

- Lifestyle modification
- Thiazide diuretic for most patients
- May also consider
  - Angiotensin converting enzyme inhibitor (ACEI)
  - Angiotensin receptor blocker (ARB)

  - Beta-blocker (BB)
  - Calcium channel blocker (CCB)

  OR

- Combination of above medications

Stage 2 hypertension

- Lifestyle modification
- Two drug combination of stage 1 hypertension medications usually (caution if risk of orthostatic hypotension–usually elderly)

Treatment Options with High Risk Conditions

Prehypertension

- Lifestyle modification
- Drugs as applicable in conditions below

Heart failure

- If asymptomatic give ≥ 1 medication
  - Angiotensin converting enzyme inhibitor
  - Beta-blocker
- If symptomatic give ≥ 1 medication with a loop diuretic — Lasix (furosemide) or Bumex (bumetanide)
  - Angiotensin converting enzyme inhibitor
  - Beta-blocker
  - Angiotensin receptor blocker
  - Aldosterone antagonist

Ischemic heart disease (stable angina)

- Beta-blocker

  OR

- Long acting calcium channel blocker such as Norvasc (amlodipine)

Post myocardial infarction options

- Beta-blocker
- ACEI
- Aldosterone antagonist
- Lipid management
- Low dose aspirin 160–325 mg PO qday

High risk for coronary disease options

- Thiazide diuretic
- Beta–blocker
- ACEI
- CCB
- Lipid management
- Low dose aspirin 160–325 mg PO qday

Diabetic hypertension options

Combination of ≥ 2 drugs usually needed

- Thiazide diuretic
- Beta–blocker
- ACEI or ARB (reduces diabetic nephropathy)
- CCB

Chronic kidney disease options

Definition of chronic kidney disease

- Glomerular filtration rate (GFR) < 60 cc/min
- Creatinine > 1.5 mg/dL in men and creatinine > 1.3 mg/dL in women
- Albuminuria > 300 mg/day or 200 mg of albumin/gm creatinine

Medications

- ACEI
- ARB
- Loop diuretic such as Lasix (furosemide) may be needed with creatinine > 2.5 mg/dL
- Limited rise of up to 35% of creatinine with ACEI or ARB therapy is acceptable as long as hyperkalemia does not develop

Recurrent stroke prevention options

- Thiazide diuretic
- ACEI
- Lipid management
- Low dose aspirin (160–325 mg PO qday) if hypertension reasonably controlled

Elderly patients

- Initial lower drug doses may be needed, though standard doses and multiple drugs are needed eventually in the majority to achieve BP control

- They are at risk of postural hypotension due to the frequent use of multiple medications

Follow Up and Achieving Blood Pressure Control

- Monthly follow up till blood pressure control is achieved
- Follow up every 3–6 months when blood control is achieved
- Serum creatinine and potassium should be checked 1–2 times per year
- Heart failure, diabetes and other comorbidities influence frequency of visits and tests needed
- Addition of a second drug should be in a different class if a single drug regimen was started initially and failed to achieve control
- Do not use 2 drugs in the same class at the same time (exception is Maxzide or Dyazide which are combination diuretic drugs)

Consult Criteria

- Unable to achieve target blood pressure reductions over several visits
- Blood pressure ≥ 180/110 mm Hg on 2 or more medications
- Symptomatic high risk conditions or comorbidities (CHF, progressive renal insufficiency, hyperkalemia, angina, stroke, etc.)
- More than 2 drugs needed to control blood pressure

Antihypertensive Medications (refer to PDR, drug databases or medication inserts)

Thiazide diuretics

- Chorothiazide (Diuril) 125–250 mg PO qday-bid
- Chorthalidone 12.5–25 mg PO qday
- Hydrochlorothiazide (HCTZ) 12.5–50 mg PO qday

Loop diuretics

- Lasix (furosemide) 20–40 mg PO bid
- Bumex (bumetanide) 0.5–1 mg PO bid

- Torsemide 2.5–10 mg PO qday

Potassium sparing diuretics

- Triamterene 25–50 mg PO qday-bid
- Amiloride 5 mg PO qday-bid

Aldosterone receptor blockers

- Aldactone 25–50 mg PO qday

Beta–blockers

- Atenolol 25–100 mg PO qday
- Metoprolol 50–100 mg PO qday-bid
- Corgard (Nadolol) 40–120 mg PO qday
- Toprol XL (metoprolol) 50–100 mg PO qday
- Propranolol 20–80 mg PO bid

Beta-blockers with intrinsic sympathomimetic activity

- Sectral (acebutolol) 200–400 mg PO bid
- Pindolol 5–10 mg PO bid

Combined alpha and beta-blockers

- Coreg (carvedilol) 6.25–25 mg PO bid increase every 1–2 weeks as tolerated and needed up to 25 mg bid
- Labetalol 100–400 mg PO bid

Angiotensin converting enzyme inhibitors (ACEI)

- Lisinopril 5–40 mg PO qday
- Captopril 12.5–50 mg PO bid
- Accupril (quinapril) 10–80 mg PO qday

Angiotensin receptor blockers

- Atacand (candesartan) 8–32 mg PO qday
- Cozaar (losartan) 25–50 mg PO qday-bid
- Diovan (valsartan) 80–320 mg PO qday

Calcium channel blockers—non-Dihydropyridines

- Cardizem CD (diltiazem) 180–420 mg PO qday
- Cardizem LA (diltiazem) 120–540 mg PO qday
- Calan (verapamil) SR 120–240 mg PO qday-bid

Calcium channel blockers—dihydropyridines

- Norvasc (amlodipine) 2.5–10 mg PO qday
- Procardia XL (nifedipine) 30–60 mg PO qday

Alpha-1 blockers (not first line drugs)

- Cardura (doxazosin) 1–16 mg PO qday
- Cardura (doxazosin) XL 4–8 mg PO qday
- Minipres (prazosin) 1–5 mg PO bid-tid
- Caution for orthostatic hypotension — give first dose and any increases at bedtime

Central alpha-2 agonists

- Clonidine 0.1–0.3 mg PO bid-tid
- Catapres -TTS (clonidine) patch 0.1–0.3 mg qweek

Combination drugs

- ACEI+CCB (Lotrel) amlodipine and benazepril 2.5/10–10/20 mg PO qday
- ACEI+HCTZ (Zestoretic) Lisinopril and HCTZ 10/12.5–20/25 mg PO qday
- ARBs+diuretic (Diovan-HCT) valsartan and HCTZ 80/12.5–160/50 mg PO qday
- Beta-blocker+diuretic (Tenoretic) atenolol and HCTZ 50/25 to 100/25 PO qday
- Diuretic and diuretic (Aldactazide) 25/25 to 50/50 mg PO qday-bid

Notes

References:

www.nhlbi.nih.gov/guidelines/hypertension/express.pdf

JNC 7 — The Seventh Report of the Joint National Committee on Prevention, Detection, Evaluation and Treatment of High Blood Pressure

Hypertension Treatment & Management
Author: Meena S Madhur, MD, PhD; Chief Editor: David J Maron, MD, FACC, FAHA

2014 Evidence-Based Guideline for the Management of High Blood Pressure in Adults

Report From the Panel Members Appointed to the Eighth Joint National Committee (JNC 8)

New US Hypertension Guidelines: Experts Respond
Sue Hughes December 05, 2017

CHOLESTEROL MANAGEMENT

When using any management guideline, always follow the Guidelines of Proper Use (page 18).

Considerations

- LDL (low density lipoprotein) cholesterol < 100 mg/dL is optimal
- Lowering LDL cholesterol is the primary target of therapy
- "Low HDL" (high density lipoprotein) is < 40 mg/dL
- Lowering triglycerides from levels ≥ 220 recommended
- Diabetes without ASCVD (coronary heart disease) is considered raised to ASCVD risk
- Patients with metabolic syndrome are candidates for lifestyle modification
- Complete lipoprotein profile is recommended as initial screening test
- LDL-C to levels of 40 to 60 mg/dL reduces ASCVD

4 Statin benefit groups

- Individuals with clinical ASCVD (atherosclerotic cardiovascular disease) — angina, MI, stroke, TIA or peripheral arterial disease
- Individuals with primary elevations of LDL–C ≥ 190 mg/dL
- Individuals age 40–75 years of age with diabetes and LDL–C 70–189 mg/dL without clinical ASCVD
- Individuals age 40–75 years of age without diabetes or ASCVD with LDL-C 70–189 mg/dL that have an estimated 10 year ASCVD risk ≥ 7.5%

Statin therapy

High–intensity (lowers LDL–C ≥ 50%)

- Atorvastatin 40–80 mg
- Rosuvastatin 20–40 mg

Moderate–intensity (lowers LDL–C 30 to < 50%)

- Atorvastatin 10–20 mg
- Rosuvastatin 20–40 mg

- Simvastatin 20–40 mg
- Pravastatin 40–80 mg
- Lovastatin 40 mg
- Fluvastatin 40 mg bid

Low–intensity (lowers LDL–C < 30%)

- Simvastatin 10 mg
- Pravastatin 10–20 mg
- Lovastatin 20 mg
- Fluvastatin 20–40 mg

Non-statin therapy

- Repatha (evolocumab) SQ q2weeks
    - High cost
    - May be used in statin intolerant patients
    - Lowers LDL-C > 50%
- Zetia (ezetimide) 10 mg PO qday
    - Inhibits cholesterol absorption in small intestine
- Cholestoff over the counter (plant sterols)
- Coenzyme Q–10 not proven effective in studies

Individuals with clinical ASCVD (atherosclerotic cardiovascular disease)

Age ≤ 75 years of age

- High–intensity statin
    - Moderate–intensity statin if not candidate for high–intensity statin

Age > 75 years of age

- Moderate–intensity statin

Individuals with primary elevations of LDL–C ≥ 190 mg/dL

- High–intensity statin
    - Moderate–intensity statin if not candidate for high–intensity statin

Individuals age 40–75 years of age with diabetes and LDL–C 70–189 mg/dL without clinical ASCVD

- Moderate–intensity statin
    - High–intensity statin if estimated 10 year ASCVD risk ≥ 7.5%

Individuals age 40–75 years of age without diabetes or ASCVD with LDL-C 70–189 mg/dL that have an estimated 10 year ASCVD risk ≥ 7.5%

- Moderate to high intensity statin
- clincalc.com/Cardiology/ASCVD/PooledCohort.aspx

ASCVD prevention benefit of statins may be less clear in other groups

- Primary LDL–C ≥ 160 mg/dL
- Genetic hyperlipidemias
- Family history of premature ASCVD
  - < 55 years of age of first degree male relative
  - < 65 years of age of first degree female relative
- CRP ≥ 2 mg/L
- Ankle–brachial index < 9
- Elevated lifetime risk of ASCVD

Major risk factors (excluding LDL cholesterol)

- Cigarette smoking
- Blood pressure ≥ 140–150/90 mm Hg depending on depending on JNC 8 recommendations or on hypertension medications (see hypertension management section)
- HDL cholesterol < 40 mg/dL
- Diabetes (is a risk equivalent)
- Family history of premature ASCVD
  - Male 1st degree relative age < 55 years
  - Female 1st degree relative age < 65 years
- Age
  - Men ≥ 45 years
  - Women ≥ 55 years

Testing for statin therapy initiation

- Fasting lipid profile
- ALT (evaluate unexplained increases 3X normal)
- Hemoglobin A1c (if diabetes status not known)
- CPK if indicated

- Consider evaluation for other secondary causes or conditions that influence statin safety
- Treat secondary causes of LDL
- Treat secondary of LDL-C ≥ 190 mg/dL

Secondary causes of increased LDL cholesterol

- Diabetes
- Hypothyroidism
- Obstructive liver disease
- Moderate chronic renal failure
- Drugs
    - Progestins
    - Corticosteroids
    - Anabolic steroids

ASCVD risk equivalents

- Peripheral arterial disease
- Aortic aneurysm
- Symptomatic carotid disease
- Diabetes
- Multiple risk factors that confer a 10 year risk of ASCVD or recurrent ASCVD > 20%

Metabolic syndrome

Definition

- Lipid and nonlipid risk factors of metabolic origin which enhances the risk for ASCVD

Risk factors

- Abdominal obesity
    - Men's waist size > 40 inches
    - Women's waist size > 35 inches
- Triglycerides ≥ 150 mg/dL
- HDL cholesterol
    - Men < 40 mg/dL
    - Women < 50 mg/dL
- Blood pressure ≥ 135/ ≥ 85 mm Hg
- Fasting glucose ≥ 110 mg/dL

Treatment

- Weight reduction as appropriate
- Increased physical activity

- A fibrate or nicotinic acid with a statin is no longer recommended per recent FDA determination

10 year risk estimation for ASCVD to occur (examples)

Men ≥ 20% risk	**Women ≥ 20% risk**
Age 55–59	Age 60–64
TC 200–239	TC 200–239
Smoker	Smoker
SBP ≥ 140 mm Hg	SBP ≥ 140 mm Hg

Men's and women's risk approximately ≤ 10% with above data if not a smoker

Treatment to achieve goals

- Treat any secondary causes of increased LDL cholesterol
- Weight loss and increased physical activity
- Low (saturated) fat and low cholesterol diet
- High (soluble) fiber diet of 10–25 gms/days

Time table for follow up and treatment

- Recheck in 6 weeks and if target not met
    - Add plant sterols or stanols 2 gms per day (vegetables, fruits, legumes, nuts, and seeds)
    - Increase fiber if possible
- Recheck in 4–12 weeks and if target not met
    - Start an appropriate strength statin as indicated above
- Recheck again in 4–12 weeks and if target not met
    - Intensify statin therapy
        - If a statin is not tolerated, then a nonstatin therapy such as bile acid sequestrant or nicotinic acid medication may be added in high risk patients for ASCVD
    - **ASCVD high risk patients**
        - Individuals with clinical ASCVD‡ <75 years of age

- Individuals with baseline LDL–C ≥190 mg/dL
- Individuals 40 to 75 years of age with diabetes mellitus

- Recheck in 4–12 weeks and if target still not met
    - Discuss with physician
- Recheck every 3–12 months to monitor response and adherence to therapy if targets met
- See Statin therapy section above for targets
- Monitor side effects and toxicity (myopathy, etc.)

Also treat or modify ASCVD risk factors

Notes

References:

2013 ACC/AHA Guideline on the Treatment of Blood Cholesterol to Reduce Atherosclerotic Cardiovascular Risk in Adults: A Report of the American College of Cardiology/American Heart Association Task Force on Practice Guidelines

www.nhlbi.nih.gov/guidelines/cholesterol/atp3xsum.pdf
Third Report of the National Cholesterol Education Program (NCEP) Expert Panel on Detection, Evaluation, and Treatment of High Blood Cholesterol in Adults (Adult Treatment Panel III)

[Docket No. FDA-2016-N-1127]
AbbVie Inc. et al; Withdrawal of Approval of Indications Related to the Coadministration With Statins in Applications for Niacin Extended-Release Tablets and Fenofibric Acid Delayed Release Capsules

Consultant. 2016;56(5):S2-S4. Suppl.

Glossary

ABG — arterial blood gas

ABI — ankle brachial index

AC — acromioclavicular

ACEI — angiotensin converting enzyme inhibitor

ADT — adult diphtheria tetanus

Anaphylaxis — IgE antibody release of various mediators such as histamine causing varying degrees of symptoms such as rash, pruritus, bronchospasm, GI symptoms, hypoxia, upper airway compromise, hypotension and potentially death

Angina — cardiac chest discomfort, or other discomfort or symptoms, from deficit of blood flow and oxygen delivery to the heart

Anion gap — sodium minus chloride and CO_2 (serum bicarbonate)

Anti-HBS — antibody to hepatitis B surface antigen

Aortic dissection — tearing of the wall of the aorta

ARB — Angiotensin receptor blocker

ASA — aspirin

Asthma — reversible constriction of pulmonary small airways

Asymptomatic hypertension — elevated blood pressure with no acute end-organ compromise of function

Bandemia — increased white blood cell bands from stress, infection, or inflammation

BB — beta-blocker

B-HCG — beta human chorionic gonadotropin

BID (bid) — twice a day

BMP — basic metabolic profile including sodium, potassium, chloride, carbon dioxide (CO_2), glucose, creatinine and BUN (blood urea nitrogen)

BNP — B-type natriuretic peptide, determined by stretch of cardiac muscle from CHF. Elevated in many other conditions that cause strain on the heart in addition to CHF

Bronchitis — reversible constriction of pulmonary small airways from an infection in the lungs

BSA — body surface area

Burst fracture — fracture through entire vertebral body (unstable)

CBC — complete blood count

CCB — calcium channel blocker

CHD — coronary heart disease

CHF — (Congestive heart failure) Cardiac dysfunction secondary to decreased ability of the left ventricle (LV) to eject or fill with blood

COPD — chronic obstructive pulmonary disease, usually chronic bronchitis or emphysema, or mixture of both

CPK — creatine phosphokinase (a muscle enzyme)

C-RP — C reactive protein (nonspecific marker of inflammation)

CSF — cerebral spinal fluid

C-spine — cervical spine

CXR — chest x-ray

CVA — brain neuronal death from a deficit of cerebral perfusion resulting in lack of oxygen to parts of the brain

DBP — diastolic blood pressure

D-dimer — a measurable byproduct of fibrinogen pathway indicating some level of blood clot formation

DIC — disseminated intravascular coagulation

DIP — distal interphalangeal

DJD — degenerative joint disease (osteoarthritis)

DKA — diabetic ketoacidosis (a metabolic acidotic diabetic condition resulting from insulin resistance or severe deficit of insulin, and fatty acids metabolism for energy needs, that is associated with potential mortality)

DOC — drug of choice

DUB — dysfunctional uterine bleeding

DVT — deep vein thrombosis

Dyspnea — shortness of breath

EBV — Epstein-Barr virus

Emergency hypertension — acute end-organ injury secondary to elevated blood pressure

Epley maneuver — treatment of BPV (moves otoliths out of semicircular canals). Avoid with recent neck fracture, instability or surgery, carotid disease or recent retinal detachment

ESR — erythrocyte sedimentation rate (nonspecific marker of inflammation)

ESRD — end stage renal disease

FFP — fresh frozen plasma

GC — gonococcal or gonococcus

GERD — Gastroesophageal reflux

GI — gastrointestinal

gm(s) — gram or grams

gtt — drop

HAART — highly active antiretroviral therapy with 2 NRTIs and either a protease inhibitor or NNRTI

Hallpike maneuver — patient going from sitting position to supine position rapidly with head below horizontal plane of body and head rotated quickly and carefully to the left or right. Any nystagmus and symptoms induced represent a positive test.

HBIG — hepatitis B immune globulin

HHS — hyperglycemic hyperosmolar syndrome

HIV — human immunodeficiency

HR — heart rate

HSV — herpes simplex virus

IBS — irritable bowel syndrome

IG — immune globulin

IM — intramuscular

INR — international normalized ratio (measures Coumadin therapy)

IOP — intraocular pressure

IUP — intrauterine pregnancy

IV — intravenous

Jugular venous distension — distension of the external jugular vein in the neck due to increased pressure in the right side of the heart or in the lungs (pulmonary hypertension, COPD, CHF)

KUB — kidney, ureter and bladder plain x-ray

LES — lower esophageal sphincter

LFT's — liver function tests

LP — lumbar puncture

LOC — loss of consciousness

MDI — metered dose inhaler

Metabolic acidosis — decreased serum bicarbonate

mmol/L = mEq/L on serum test levels

MP — metacarpophalangeal

MRSA — methicillin resistance staphylococcus aureus

NaHCO3 — sodium bicarbonate

NMT — no more than

Nonspecific chest pain — chest pain without evident specific cause

NNRTI — non-nucleoside reverse transcriptase inhibitor

NRTI — nucleoside reverse transcriptase inhibitor

NS — normal saline

NSAID's — nonsteroidal anti-inflammatory drugs

Nystagmus — rhythmic involuntary eye movements named for the quick component

O_2 saturation — percent of hemoglobin carrying oxygen

ORT — oral rehydration therapy

Osmolol gap — the difference between calculated and measured osmolality in the blood, usually less than 10

PAD — peripheral arterial disease

Panic disorder — state of hyperventilation causing decreased pCO_2 measurement on blood gas (respiratory alkalosis), elevated pH, resulting in feeling short of breath, acute calcium shifts into cells (can cause carpospasm), hypokalemia, paresthesias, and a sense of impending doom when more severe

PCP — primary care provider

PCR — polymerase chain reaction

PE — physical examination or pulmonary embolism (use context)

PEP — postexposure prophylaxis

PERC — pulmonary embolism rule out criteria

PID — pelvic inflammatory disease

PIP — proximal interphalangeal

PMN — polymorphonuclear neutrophil

PN — peripheral neuropathy

PO — per oral

POC — products of conception

PPI — proton pump inhibitor

PR — per rectum

PRBC — packed red blood cells

Presyncope or Near syncope — state of feeling that a fainting or syncopal episode will occur

prn — as needed

Pseudoaddiction — a condition caused by under-treatment of pain where the patient engages in an active and often repetitive search for pain medications

Pseudoseizures — seizure-like activity caused by psychiatric or functional considerations that is not a true seizure

PSVT — paroxysmal supraventricular tachycardia

Pulmonary embolism — blood clot(s) located in the lung's blood vessels that originated elsewhere, usually from veins in pelvis or proximal legs

Q or **q** — every

QID (qid) — four times a day

RCT — rotator cuff tear

Respiratory acidosis — increased pCO_2 on blood gas measurement

Respiratory alkalosis — decreased pCO_2 and elevated pH on blood gas from increased minute ventilation or hyperventilation

Respiratory failure — increasing blood gas pCO_2 and respiratory fatigue with decreasing pH, resulting in increasing somnolence, altered mental status and hypoxemia

RSV — respiratory syncytial virus

SBO — small bowel obstruction

SBP — systolic blood pressure

Sepsis — usually a bacterial infection frequently used to mean invasion of the blood stream

SLR — straight leg raise

SQ — subcutaneous

SS disease — sickle cell homozygous disease

SSRI — selective serotonin reuptake inhibitor

STD — sexual transmitted disease

SVT — supraventricular tachycardia

Syncope — loss of consciousness from decreased cerebral perfusion

TBSA — total body surface area

TC — total cholesterol

Tdap — tetanus, diphtheria and acellular pertussis vaccine

TGA — transient global amnesia

Thrombocytopenia — low platelet count

TIA — transient ischemic attack

TID (tid) — three times a day

TM — tympanic membrane

Troponin — breakdown cardiac muscle component indicating injury or death to cardiac muscle depending on level

TSH — thyroid stimulating hormone most commonly elevated in primary hypothyroidism

U/A — urine analysis

UCG — urine pregnancy test (urinary chorionic gonadotropin)

UDS — urine drug screen

UGI — upper gastrointestinal

UTI — urinary tract infection

Valsalva — straining of abdomen causing increase in intracranial and intraocular pressure

WBC — white blood count

Well's criteria — criteria developed to assess level of probability of VTE (venous thromboembolic) disease either in extremities or lungs (pulmonary embolism)

Whole bowel irrigation — giving polyethylene glycol (Miralax or Go-lytely) to flush out the intestines

Index

A

B

C

D

E

F

G

H

I

J

K

L

M

N

O

P

Q

R

S

T

U

V

W

X

Z

CPSIA information can be obtained
at www.ICGtesting.com
Printed in the USA
LVHW080809130121
676315LV00019BA/715

9 781733 157506